T0263484

Hormones and the Science of Athletic Performance

Guest Editor

PRIMUS-E. MULLIS, MD

ENDOCRINOLOGY AND METABOLISM CLINICS OF NORTH AMERICA

www.endo.theclinics.com

Consulting Editor
DEREK LEROITH, MD, PhD

March 2010 • Volume 39 • Number 1

SAUNDERS an imprint of ELSEVIER, Inc.

W.B. SAUNDERS COMPANY
A Division of Elsevier Inc.

1600 John F. Kennedy Boulevard ● Suite 1800 ● Philadelphia, Pennsylvania 19103-2899

http://www.theclinics.com

ENDOCRINOLOGY AND METABOLISM CLINICS OF NORTH AMERICA Volume 39, Number 1
March 2010 ISSN 0889-8529, ISBN-13: 978-1-4377-1816-4

Editor: Rachel Glover
Developmental Editor: Theresa Collier

Endocrinology and Metabolism Clinics of North America (ISSN 0889-8529) is published quarterly by Elsevier Inc., 360 Park Avenue South, New York, NY 10010-1710. Months of issue are March, June, September, and December. Periodicals postage paid at New York, NY and additional mailing offices. Subscription prices are USD 271.00 per year for US individuals, USD 457.00 per year for US institutions, USD 139.00 per year for US students and residents, USD 340.00 per year for Canadian individuals, USD 560.00 per year for Canadian institutions, USD 394.00 per year for international individuals, USD 560.00 per year for international institutions, and USD 206.00 per year for international and Canadian and foreign students/residents. To receive student/resident rate, orders must be accompanied by name of affiliated institution, date of term, and the signature of program/residency coordinator on institution letterhead. Orders will be billed at individual rate until proof of status is received. Foreign air speed delivery is included in all *Clinics* subscription prices. All prices are subject to change without notice. **POSTMASTER:** Send address changes to *Endocrinology and Metabolism Clinics of North America*, Elsevier Health Sciences Division, Subscription Customer Service, 3251 Riverport Lane, Maryland Heights, MO 63043. **Customer Service: Telephone: 1-800-654-2452** (U.S. and Canada); **1-314-447-8871** (outside U.S. and Canada). **Fax: 1-314-447-8029. E-mail: journalscustomerservice-usa@elsevier.com** (for print support); **journalsonlinesupport-usa@elsevier.com** (for online support).

Reprints. For copies of 100 or more, of articles in this publication, please contact the Commercial Rights Department, Elsevier Inc., 360 Park Avenue South, New York, NY 10010-1710; phone: (+1) 212-633-3813; fax: (+1) 212-462-1935; e-mail: reprints@elsevier.com.

Endocrinology and Metabolism Clinics of North America is covered in *MEDLINE/PubMed (Index Medicus)*, *EMBASE/Excerpta Medica*, *Current Contents/Clinical Medicine*, *Current Contents/Life Sciences*, *Science Citation Index*, *ISI/BIOMED*, *BIOSIS*, and *Chemical Abstracts*.

Printed and bound in the United Kingdom
Transferred to Digital Print 2011

Contributors

CONSULTING EDITOR

DEREK LeROITH, MD, PhD
Chief, Division of Endocrinology, Metabolism, and Bone Diseases, Mount Sinai School of Medicine, New York, New York

GUEST EDITOR

PRIMUS-E. MULLIS, MD
Professor, Division of Paediatric Endocrinology, Diabetology & Metabolism, University Children's Hospital Inselspital, University of Bern, Bern, Switzerland

AUTHORS

BRUNO ALLOLIO, MD
Professor of Medicine, Endocrinology and Diabetes Unit, Department of Medicine I, University of Würzburg, Würzburg, Germany

NORBERT BACHL, MD
Department of Sports and Exercise Physiology, Centre for Sports Sciences and University Sports, University of Vienna, Vienna, Austria

MARTIN BIDLINGMAIER, MD
Head, Endocrine Research Laboratories, Medizinische Klinik – Innenstadt, Ludwig-Maximilians University, Munich, Germany

VITA BIRZNIECE, MD, PhD
Pituitary Research Unit, Garvan Institute of Medical Research, Darlinghurst, New South Wales, Australia

MARTINE DUCLOS, MD, PhD
Professor of Medicine; Head of the Department of Sport Medicine and Functional Explorations, University-Hospital (CHU), Hopital G. Montpied; INRA; University Clermont, UFR Médecine; Centre de Recherche en Nutrition Humaine d'Auvergne, Clermont-Ferrand, France

WOUTER EILERS, MSc
Institute for Biomedical Research into Human Movement and Health, Manchester Metropolitan University, Manchester, United Kingdom

IOULIETTA EROTOKRITOU-MULLIGAN, PhD
Statistician, Endocrinology & Metabolism Unit, Developmental Origins of Health and Disease Division, University of Southampton School of Medicine, Southampton, Hampshire, United Kingdom

ULRICH FLENKER, Dipl-Sportwiss
Research Scientist, Manfred Donike Institute, DSHS, Cologne, Germany

MARTIN FLUECK, PhD
Professor in Muscle Cell Physiology, Institute for Biomedical Research into Human Movement and Health, Manchester Metropolitan University, Manchester, United Kingdom

HANS GEYER, PhD
Deputy Director, Institute of Biochemistry, Center for Preventive Doping Research, German Sport University Cologne, Cologne, Germany

GEOFFREY GOLDSPINK, PhD, ScD, FRCS
Department of Surgery; Department of Anatomy and Developmental Biology, University College Medical School, University of London, England, United Kingdom

STEFANIE HAHNER, MD
Endocrinology and Diabetes Unit, Department of Medicine I, University of Würzburg, Würzburg, Germany

KEN K.Y. HO, FRACP, MD
Professor, Pituitary Research Unit, Garvan Institute of Medical Research, Darlinghurst, New South Wales, Australia

RICHARD I.G. HOLT, PhD, FRCP
Professor in Diabetes and Endocrinology, Endocrinology & Metabolism Unit, Developmental Origins of Health and Disease Division, University of Southampton School of Medicine, Southampton, Hampshire, United Kingdom

MATTHIAS KAMBER, PhD
Director, Antidoping Switzerland, Bern, Switzerland

WILFRIED KINDERMANN, MD, PhD
Institute of Sports and Preventive Medicine, University of Saarland, Saarbruecken, Germany

SÉVERINE LAMON, MSc
Swiss Laboratory for Doping Analyses, University Center of Legal Medicine, West Switzerland, Epalinges, Switzerland

JENNY MANOLOPOULOU, PhD
Research fellow, Endocrine Research Laboratories, Medizinische Klinik – Innenstadt, Ludwig-Maximilians University, Munich, Germany

FELICIA A. MENDELSOHN, MD
Women's Health Scholar; Associate Research Scientist; Assistant Professor of Clinical Medicine, Department of Obstetrics and Gynecology, Columbia College of Physicians and Surgeons, Greenwich, Connecticut

PRIMUS-E. MULLIS, MD
Professor, Division of Paediatric Endocrinology, Diabetology & Metabolism, University Children's Hospital Inselspital, University of Bern, Bern, Switzerland

ANNE E. NELSON, PhD
Pituitary Research Unit, Garvan Institute of Medical Research, Darlinghurst, New South Wales, Australia

MARIA K. PARR, PhD
Research Scientist, Institute of Biochemistry, German Sport University Cologne (DSHS), Cologne, Germany

NEIL ROBINSON, PhD
Swiss Laboratory for Doping Analyses, University Center of Legal Medicine, West Switzerland, Epalinges, Switzerland

CHRISTOPHE SAUDAN, PhD
Swiss Laboratory for Doping Analyses, University Center of Legal Medicine, West Switzerland, Epalinges, Switzerland

MARTIAL SAUGY, PhD, PD
Swiss Laboratory for Doping Analyses, University Center of Legal Medicine, West Switzerland, Epalinges, Switzerland

WILHELM SCHÄNZER, PhD
Professor for Biochemistry; Chief, Institute of Biochemistry, German Sport University Cologne (DSHS), Cologne, Germany

N.C. CRAIG SHARP, BVMS, PhD, DSc, FIBiol, FBASES, MRCVS
Emeritus Professor of Sports Medicine, Centre for Sports Medicine and Human Performance, Brunel University, Uxbridge, West London, United Kingdom

GERD SIGMUND, MSc
Chemist, Institute of Biochemistry, Center for Preventive Doping Research, German Sport University Cologne, Cologne, Germany

PIERRE-EDOUARD SOTTAS, PhD
Swiss Laboratory for Doping Analyses, University Center of Legal Medicine, West Switzerland, Epalinges, Switzerland

MARIO THEVIS, PhD
Professor, Institute of Biochemistry, Center for Preventive Doping Research, German Sport University Cologne, Cologne, Germany

HARALD TSCHAN, PhD
Department of Sports and Exercise Physiology, Centre for Sports Sciences and University Sports, University of Vienna, Vienna, Austria

MICHELLE P. WARREN, MD
Wyeth-Ayerst Professor of Women's Health, Department of Obstetrics and Gynecology and Medicine, Columbia College of Physicians and Surgeons, New York, New York

BARBARA WESSNER, PhD
Department of Sports and Exercise Physiology, Centre for Sports Sciences and University Sports, University of Vienna, Vienna, Austria

BERND WOLFARTH, MD
Department of Preventive and Rehabilitative Sports Medicine, Technical University Munich, Munich, Germany

JAN C. WUESTENFELD, MD
Department of Sports Medicine, Institute for Applied Training Science (IAT), Leipzig, Germany

Contents

This article describes the worldwide endeavor to combat doping in sports. It describes the historical reasons the movement began and outlines the current status of this effort by international sports groups, governments, and the World Anti-Doping Agency. The purposes, strengths, and limitations of the various entities are illustrated; and recommendations for improvements are made.

Human growth hormone (GH) is widely abused by athletes; however, there is little evidence that GH improves physical performance. Replacement of GH in GH deficiency improves some aspects of exercise capacity. There is evidence for a protein anabolic effect of GH in healthy adults and for increased lean body mass following GH, although fluid retention likely contributes to this increase. The evidence suggests that muscle strength, power, and aerobic exercise capacity are not enhanced by GH administration, however GH may improve anaerobic exercise capacity. There are risks of adverse effects of long-term abuse of GH. Sustained abuse of GH may lead to a state mimicking acromegaly, a condition with increased morbidity and mortality.

Catching athletes abusing human growth hormone (GH) by official anti-doping tests is challenging because of specific properties of the hormone. Furthermore, the chemical structure of recombinant GH (rGH) is identical to that of the main GH isoform secreted by the pituitary, making it difficult to discriminate between endogenous and injected GH molecules by biochemical tests. The approaches developed to solve the problem include the "marker approach," which measures changes in concentration of GH-dependent proteins that are inappropriately elevated after rGH injection, and the "isoform approach," which detects changes in the spectrum of circulating GH isoforms after administration of rGH. A more widespread use of these tests in out-of-competition controls will enhance the likelihood to detect GH doping.

It is believed that insulin and insulin-like growth factor I (IGF-I) are abused by professional athletes, either alone or in combination with growth hormone (GH) and anabolic steroids. The recent introduction of IGF-I to clinical practice is likely to increase its availability and abuse. Insulin and IGF-I work together with GH to control the supply of nutrients to tissues in the fasted and fed state. The actions of insulin and IGF-I that may enhance performance include increased protein anabolism and glucose uptake and storage. The detection of IGF-I and insulin abuse is challenging. There are established mass spectrometry methods for insulin analogs. The feasibility of using GH-dependent markers to detect IGF-I use is being assessed.

Testosterone is the principal male sex hormone. As with all natural steroids, it is biosynthesized from cholesterol. Phase I metabolism employs some very specific enzymes and pathways. Phase II metabolism and excretion follow more general patterns. The effects of testosterone are twofold: anabolic and androgenic. Because of its anabolic effects, testosterone is frequently abused in sports. Because of its endogenous nature, testosterone doping is difficult to detect. The standard procedure is based on the evaluation of the urinary steroid profile. Conspicuous samples then are submitted to compound-specific $^{13}C/^{12}C$ analysis. Synthetic and endogenous steroids differ in this measure. Numerous xenobiotic compounds have been derived from testosterone. The modifications typically aim at a reduction of the androgenic properties while maintaining the anabolic potential. Most of these compounds have been withdrawn from the legal market. However, they are found to be illicitly added to otherwise inefficient nutritional supplements. These products represent a major problem to doping control. Recently, clinical trials with selective androgen receptor modulators have been started.

The Athlete Biological Passport (ABP) is an individual electronic document that collects data regarding a specific athlete that is useful in differentiating between natural physiologic variations of selected biomarkers and deviations caused by artificial manipulations. A subsidiary of the endocrine module of the ABP, that which here is called Athlete Steroidal Passport (ASP), collects data on markers of an altered metabolism of endogenous steroidal hormones measured in urine samples. The ASP aims to identify not only doping with anabolic–androgenic steroids, but also most indirect steroid doping strategies such as doping with estrogen receptor antagonists and aromatase inhibitors. Development of specific markers of steroid doping, use of the athlete's previous measurements to define individual limits, with the athlete becoming his or her own reference, the inclusion of heterogeneous factors such as the UDPglucuronosyltransferase B17 genotype of the athlete, the knowledge of potentially confounding effects such as heavy alcohol consumption, the development of an external quality control system to control analytical uncertainty, and finally the use of Bayesian inferential methods to evaluate the value of indirect evidence have made the ASP a valuable alternative to deter steroid doping in elite sports. The ASP can be used to target athletes for gas chromatography/ combustion/ isotope ratio mass spectrometry (GC/C/IRMS) testing, to withdraw temporarily the athlete from competing when an abnormality has been detected, and ultimately to lead to an antidoping infraction if that abnormality cannot be explained by a medical condition. Although the ASP has been developed primarily to ensure fairness in elite sports, its application in endocrinology for clinical purposes is straightforward in an evidence-based medicine paradigm.

The potential ergogenic effects of asthma medication in athletes have been controversially discussed for decades. The prevalence of asthma is higher in elite athletes than in the general population. The highest risk for developing asthmatic symptoms is found in endurance athletes and swimmers. In addition, asthma seems to be more common in winter-sport athletes. Asthmatic athletes commonly use inhaled β2-agonists to prevent and treat asthmatic symptoms. However, β2-agonists are prohibited according to the "Prohibited List of the World Anti-Doping Agency" (WADA). Until the end of 2009 an exception was only allowed for the substances formoterol, salbutamol, salmeterol, and terbutaline by inhalation, as long as a so-called therapeutic use exemption has been applied for and was granted by the relevant anti-doping authorities. From 2010 salbutamol and salmeterol are allowed by inhalation requiring a so called declaration of use.

Stimulants have been frequently detected in doping control samples and represent a structurally diverse class of compounds. Comprehensive sports drug-testing procedures have been developed using gas or liquid chromatography combined with mass spectrometric detection, and they have revealed various adverse analytical findings, as demonstrated with 2 examples, 4-methylhexan-2-amine and methoxyphenamine. Moreover, the necessity of controlling the use or misuse of stimulating agents is outlined by means of pseudoephedrine, a compound that was prohibited in sports until the end of 2003. Since the ban was lifted, monitoring programs proved a significant increase in pseudoephedrine applications as determined from urine samples collected in competition. As a consequence, a reimplementation of this drug in future doping controls was decided.

Certain international sports federations are requesting that glucocorticoids (GCs) be removed from the World Antidoping Agency's list of banned products. Their arguments are based on the fact that GCs are in wide-spread use in sports medicine and have no demonstrated ergogenic activity. This article shows that there is scientific evidence that GCs mediate ergogenic effects in animals and humans. Moreover, the health risks of using GCs are well characterized. GCs are doping agents and should remain on the World Antidoping Agency's list of banned products.

Dehydroepiandrosterone (DHEA) is secreted by the zona reticularis of the adrenal cortex and is converted into potent sex steroids in peripheral target cells. As oral DHEA administration can lead to dose-dependent increases in circulating androgens, which may reach high supraphysiologic levels in women, it has been included in the list of prohibited substances by the World Anti-Doping Agency (WADA). However, evidence for an ergogenic activity of DHEA is still largely nonexistent. Randomized trials in elderly subjects with an age-dependent decrease in DHEA have provided little or no evidence for enhanced physical performance after long-term administration of DHEA, 50 mg/d, and smaller short-term studies in healthy male athletes using higher doses were completely negative. Thus the widely perceived performance-enhancing activity of DHEA is still more myth than reality. However, because studies in female athletes are still lacking, an ergogenic activity of high-dose DHEA in this population cannot be excluded but is expected to be associated with adverse events like hirsutism, acne, and alopecia.

Hemoglobin concentration is one of the principal factors of aerobic power and, consequently, of performance in many types of physical activities. The use of recombinant human erythropoietin is, therefore, particularly powerful for improving the physical performances of patients, and, more generally, improving their quality of life. This article discusses procedures for monitoring recombinant erythropoietin and its analogues in doping for athletic performance.

The female athlete triad is an increasingly prevalent condition involving disordered eating, amenorrhea, and osteoporosis. An athlete can suffer from all 3 components of the triad, or just 1 or 2 of the individual conditions. The main element underlying all the aspects of the triad is an adaptation to a negative caloric balance. Screening for these disorders should be an important component of an athlete's care. Prevention and treatment should involve a team approach, including a physician, a nutritionist, and a mental health provider.

This article discusses the inevitable use of growth factors for enhancing muscle strength and athletic performance. Much effort has been expended on developing a treatment of muscle wasting associated with a range of diseases and aging. Frailty in the aging population is a major socioeconomic and medical problem. Emerging molecular techniques have made it possible to gain a better understanding of the growth factor genes and how they are activated by physical activity. The ways that misuse of growth factors may be detected and verified in athletes and future challenges for detecting manipulation of signaling pathways are discussed.

Endurance athletes demonstrate an exceptional resistance to fatigue when exercising at high intensity. Much research has been devoted to the contribution of aerobic capacity for the economy of endurance performance. Important aspects of the fine-tuning of metabolic processes and power output in the endurance athlete have been overlooked. This review addresses how training paradigms exploit bioenergetic pathways in recruited muscle groups to promote the endurance phenotype. A special focus is laid on the genome-mediated mechanisms that underlie the conditioning of fatigue resistance and aerobic performance by training macrocycles and complements. The available data on work-induced muscle plasticity implies that different biologic strategies are exploited in athletic and untrained populations to boost endurance capacity. Olympic champions are probably endowed with a unique constitution that renders the conditioning of endurance capacity for competition particularly efficient.

Hugh Montgomery's discovery of the first of more than 239 fitness genes together with rapid advances in human gene therapy have created a prospect of using genes, genetic elements, and cells that have the capacity to enhance athletic performance (to paraphrase the World Anti-Doping Agency's definition of gene doping). This brief overview covers the main areas of interface between genetics and sport, attempts to provide a context against which gene doping may be viewed, and predicts a futuristic legitimate use of genomic (and possibly epigenetic) information in sport.

FORTHCOMING ISSUES

RECENT ISSUES

THE CLINICS ARE NOW AVAILABLE ONLINE!

Access your subscription at:
www.theclinics.com

Foreword

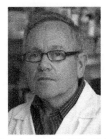

Derek LeRoith MD, PhD
Consulting Editor

Doping in sports has a long history, and Drs. Kamber and Mullis describe the history of the abuse and the establishment of world bodies that arose as anti-doping regulators. The World Anti-doping Agency (WADA) was created following years of scandals and controversy. Its job is to test and regulate doping in sport—a very challenging task! This historical perspective is a great introduction to the topic of this issue.

Birzniece, Nelson, and Ho develop the theme as to whether administration of growth hormone (GH) is safe and effective for athletic performance. They remind the readers that GH administration to GH-deficient individuals is very helpful in improving lean body mass, protein synthesis, and strength, but has little real effects on healthy individuals and many potential side-effects, including peripheral edema, carpal tunnel syndrome, arthralgias, myalgias, insulin resistance, diabetes, cardiomyopathy, and possibly malignancy.

Detecting GH abuse in athletes poses many problems, as outlined in the article by Drs. Bidlingmaier and Manolopoulou, because recombinant human GH (rhGH) is identical to endogenous GH. One approach has been the isoform measurement; rhGH is the 22 kDa form, and exogenous injection suppresses endogenous GH release and reduction of the other circulating isoforms. The second approach used by the WADA involves measuring markers of GH's biologic effects that would be altered by exogenous rhGH administration to a level inappropriate for the normal situation. Both of these techniques are used and are problematic.

Like GH, insulin and insulin-like growth factor-1 (IGF-1) are indeed anabolic, enhancing protein synthesis and nutrient storage and availability. As Drs. Erotokritou-Mulligan and Holt discuss, they are considered and have been used by sports people for physique enhancement and improved performance. Detecting abuse in sports people is challenging unless analogs that can be detected by sophisticated separation techniques are used.

Measurement of steroids, particularly testosterone and related products, are described in a technical article by Drs. Parr, Flenker, and Schänzer. In addition to the classic mass spectrometry they describe isotope ratio mass spectrometry, a very sensitive technique. These and other techniques are critical for evaluation of

Endocrinol Metab Clin N Am 39 (2010) xiii–xv
doi:10.1016/j.ecl.2009.11.006
0889-8529/10/$ – see front matter © 2010 Elsevier Inc. All rights reserved.

endo.theclinics.com

steroid abuse, because many athletes take xenobiotics that are derived from testosterone and are purported to be without androgenic effects but maintaining anabolic effects.

Drs. Sottas, Saugy, and Saudan describe another concept, the Athlete Biological Passport, which collects data electronically. The passport records data from gas chromatography/mass spectrometry; selective biomarkers that are affected by steroid abuse, especially androgenic compounds but also estrogens, are recorded.

Surprisingly, athletes and swimmers may have an increased incidence of asthma. Most asthmatics use β-2 adrenergic agonists as therapy, however they are banned substances by WADA even though they have not been shown to be effective in improving ergogenics in healthy individuals. As Drs. Wolfarth, Wuestenfeld, and Kinderman mention, the anti-doping agency does allow their use in competitive athletes under the "therapeutic use exemption" clause.

In addition to the classic hormones that are abused by sports people, other stimulants including pseudoephedrine, and some herbal supplements containing stimulants have been used. Drs. Thevis, Sigmund, Geyer, and Schänzer strongly propose that in addition to using techniques to determine the abuse, pseudoephedrine should be banned.

Can glucocorticoids be considered doping agents?, asks Dr. Duclos. Animal and human studies indicate that they can have positive effects on athletic performance, and they are therefore included in testing by the WADA. Unfortunately, the side-effects of glucocorticoids are numerous and severe. It is to be hoped that athletes are educated enough to not even consider their use.

Dehydroepiandrosterone (DHEA) is a banned substance by the WADA, as discussed by Drs. Hahner and Allolio. DHEA is readily converted to androgen and women taking sufficient quantities develop hirsutism, alopecia, and acne. On the other hand, there is absolutely no evidence that it affects exercise performance in men, and very little evidence in women.

Erythropoietin (EPO) has the ability to raise hemoglobin levels significantly, and human recombinant EPO (rhEPO) is currently used in the treatment of anemia in several serious medical conditions. Not surprisingly, this profound effect on hemoglobin levels has found its way to use in athletes. As discussed by Drs. Lamon, Robinson, and Saugy in their article, identifying doping with rhEPO is a challenge, because the amount in urine is small and plasma levels of rhEPO are difficult to distinguish between the identical endogenous form.

The American College of Sports Medicine has defined a triad of disorders in adolescent and young female athletes that includes eating disorders, amenorrhea, and osteoporosis. As pointed out by Drs. Mendelsohn and Warren, this triad resembles anorexia nervosa and bulimia and is associated with low energy availability. These elements should be screened for by the physician in conjunction with a nutritionist, and even in collaboration with a mental health specialist.

Drs. Goldspink, Wessner, Tschan, and Bachl discuss their recent findings of a so-called muscle mechano growth factor (MGF) that was found to be capable of stimulating muscle progenitor cells. The proposed protein is a splice variant of the normal IGF-1 molecule that has similar properties in muscle growth. The value of these protein(s) is in enhancing muscle strength or preventing the aging process. Whether MGF will ever be used by athletes will depend on its availability.

The bioenergetics of exercise performance is discussed in an informative article by Dr. Flueck and Eilers. Athletes improve endurance by increasing cardiac and skeletal muscle oxidative metabolism. These changes in mitochondrial function include changes in gene expression that could be studied further and theoretically for the specific requirements of those individuals, to ensure maximum effectiveness.

As researchers develop an interest in the value of genomics and epigenetics in understanding and possibly treating diseases, so may athletes turn to gene therapy for performance enhancement. Although this possibility is futuristic, as Dr. Sharp points out, the International Olympic Council and WADA are aware of the possibility.

This issue on doping in sports brings together physiologists, endocrinologists, experts on measurements, those with expertise on the topic of abuse, and organizations involved in controlling abuse. Dr. Mullis has compiled an informative issue with much insight and is to be complimented together with the authors.

Derek LeRoith, MD, PhD
Division of Endocrinology, Metabolism, and Bone Diseases
Mount Sinai School of Medicine
One Gustave L. Levy Place
Box 1055, Altran 4-36
New York, NY 10029, USA

E-mail address:
derek.leroith@mssm.edu (D. LeRoith)

Preface

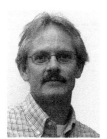

Primus-E. Mullis, MD
Guest Editor

The extensive use of drugs in society, and specifically in sport, is by no means a new phenomenon. What has changed, however, are the methods applied, and the drugs used are now more sophisticated. Throughout history there are plenty of indications that athletes have used "magic" potions to give them an extra punch to gain an unfair advantage and hopefully win.

The development of new test methods and substances come and go very quickly, and we all have to accept that the battle against doping is far from being won. Although sport is hopefully or perhaps fairer than at any time, we must be conscious of the ever-present possibility that the winner, and clearer not only the winner, in any athletic event may not be the best. If this issue, focusing on drugs used and methods to detect them, helps to advance our understanding and our quest for honest competition, then it will have served its purpose.

Primus-E. Mullis, MD
Division of Paediatric Endocrinology, Diabetology & Metabolism
University Children's Hospital Inselspital
University of Bern
CH-3010 Bern, Switzerland

E-mail address:
primus.mullis@insel.ch (P-E. Mullis)

Endocrinol Metab Clin N Am 39 (2010) xvii
doi:10.1016/j.ecl.2009.11.005
0889-8529/10/$ – see front matter

The Worldwide Fight Against Doping: From the Beginning to the World Anti-Doping Agency

Matthias Kamber, PhD[a],*, Primus-E. Mullis, MD[b]

KEYWORDS

- World Anti-Doping Agency • World Anti-Doping Program
- Sports doping • Banned substances

It is nothing remarkable to observe that doping (like other forms of cheating) in sports is neither new nor rare. As soon as the opportunity to gain publicity, status, money, and prestige through athletic competition arises, the temptation to achieve this through doping is present. This began in antiquity and continues today. The substances and methods—and the measures to combat doping—have changed over time.

THE FIGHT AGAINST DOPING: THE BEGINNING

The current fight against doping began in the 1970s. Following various fatalities due to doping abuse (eg, the Danish racing cyclist Knut Jensen in 1960 and the British racing cyclist Tom Simpson in 1967), individual organizations began to take up the fight against doping. Countries such as France, Greece, and Belgium (1965), and Turkey and Italy (1971), passed laws against doping.[1] The Council of Europe adopted a resolution against doping in sports on June 20, 1967.[2] The increased pressure on organized sports affected by the resolution led the International Olympic Committee (IOC) to restructure its medical commission in 1967. From then on, the commission advised the IOC on the fight against doping and observed its progress. Other individual international associations, such as the International Cycling Union and the International Association of Athletics Federations introduced doping regulations and tests.

The first lists of banned substances were compiled by the international soccer association Fédération Internationale de Football Association (FIFA) (1966), the International Cycling Union (1967), and the International Union of the Modern Pentathlon (1967).[3]

[a] Antidoping Switzerland, P.O. Box 606, CH-3000 Bern 22, Switzerland
[b] Division of Paediatric Endocrinology, Diabetology & Metabolism, University Children's Hospital Inselspital, University of Bern, CH-3010 Bern, Switzerland
* Corresponding author.
E-mail address: matthias.kamber@antidoping.ch (M. Kamber).

Endocrinol Metab Clin N Am 39 (2010) 1–9
doi:10.1016/j.ecl.2009.10.009
0889-8529/10/$ – see front matter © 2010 Elsevier Inc. All rights reserved.

They were primarily comprised of narcotics and stimulants such as amphetamines, ephedrine, or cocaine, and varied from sport to sport.

THE MEDICAL COMMISSION OF THE IOC

The medical commission of the IOC issued a list of banned substances for the first time in 1968 for the Olympic Games of Grenoble and Mexico City. A definition of doping was not given; simply, tests were performed at competitions. The list contained substances such as sympathomimetic amines (such as amphetamines or ephedrine), centrally stimulating substances (such as strychnine and analeptics), narcotics (such as morphine), antidepressants (such as monoamine oxidase [MAO] inhibitors), and tranquilizers (such as phenothiazine). The number of initial tests was moderate (Grenoble: 86; Mexico City: 667, 1 positive test). The first comprehensive tests (2,079; 7 positive tests) took place in 1972 in Munich. A wider scope of testing was made possible through the introduction of instrumental analysis (gas chromatography with nitrogen selective detector). Despite this, the first tests were not numerous worldwide. The reasons were high costs and ambiguity about who should lead the fight against doping. Regardless of such tentative first steps, the IOC developed, little by little, a leading position in the worldwide fight against doping—mainly because it was the only way that the integrity of the Olympic spirit could be protected. In September 1988, the International Olympic Charter against Doping in Sport was adopted. During the following years, it would serve as a reference for sport in the fight against doping. With it, a set of rules and regulations for doping tests was determined. Because the quality of the laboratories that had emerged around the world differed greatly, a system for the accreditation of doping analysis laboratories was also created. These rules were, in turn, adopted by various international sport associations. The medical commission of the IOC also revised the doping list yearly; new substances and methods were included (eg, anabolic steroids in 1975, beta blockers and blood doping in 1985, diuretics in 1987, erythropoietin in 1990, and gender doping in 1995).

THE TURNING POINT

In the late 1980s, various doping scandals in several countries led to fundamental changes in antidoping policies. On one hand, scientific researchers were given access to the doping policies in the countries of the former Eastern Bloc after its collapse.[4,5] On the other hand, doping scandals and allegations of covered-up doping activity in countries including Australia, the United Kingdom, and Canada led to fundamental public discussion and to rethinking the fight against doping. In Australia, publications on alleged systematic doping in the most prestigious athletics school, the Australian Institute of Sport, led to a public scandal and an investigation by the Australian parliament in 1987. The fact-finding committee under Senator Black (The Black Report) disclosed that the testing system at that time could be systematically undermined and that athletes and their networks were acting in collusion. The main effect of the report was the foundation of the Australian Sports Drug Agency (now, the Australian Sports Anti-Doping Authority—ASADA) in 1990. The foundation of the agency was based on a legal decree, marking governmental encroachment into the hitherto autonomous field of sport. Today, ASADA is the largest antidoping agency in the world and can even work closely with customs and police institutions when a doping offense is suspected.

Development of antidoping measures took a similar course in Canada. After the positive doping case of the 100 m runner Ben Johnson at the 1988 Olympic Games in Seoul, an independent fact-finding commission (the Dublin Inquiry) was created to clear up the background of the doping scandal and to make recommendations for improving the fight against doping. The final report[6] revealed a gloomy snapshot of the existing measures in Canada and a sports association that was reluctant to fight doping and that was incapable of fighting it effectively. One of the 70 recommendations in the final report was the creation of an independent organization, the Canadian Center for Drug-Free Sport (today Canadian Center for Ethics in Sport), which, since 1991, has been responsible for the Canadian testing system, for preventative measures, and for recommendations and guidelines for the sports associations on how to implement their anti-doping policies.

However, the same degree of harmonization was not achieved in the area of standardization of penalties for identical doping offenses. This was particularly attributable to the fact that independent jurisdictions existed for each sports association at the national and international level, hindering the standardization of sanctions.

THE ANTIDOPING CONVENTION OF THE COUNCIL OF EUROPE

Various countries recognized early on that the rules of the IOC alone could not eliminate the problem of doping in sports, but rather that coordinated and harmonized rules and support on the governmental level was needed. The Nordic Anti-Doping Convention — ratified by Sweden, Norway, Denmark, Finland, and Iceland in 1985 — envisions a harmonization of testing procedures at and outside of competitions. This constitutes the basis of reciprocal acknowledgment of test results. Other countries including Russia, the United States, Australia, Canada, and England followed suit with similar conventions.

The development of antidoping regulations through the Council of Europe mirrors the growing realization that governments have an important role to play in the fight against doping. The resolution on doping[2] was already written in 1967 and was further developed into a charter against doping in 1984 because of growing public discussion of the topic at the time. Growing political will to fight doping was expressed with this move, while, even more important from a practical standpoint, a series of recommendations on the buildup of national and international rules and policies was created to fight doping effectively at all levels. Furthermore, these recommendations contained a call to governments to limit the availability of drugs, to support financially the national organizations responsible for fighting doping, and to facilitate the endeavors of international sports organizations to harmonize doping rules and proceedings. The charter had the status of a recommendation and was not legally binding. Although it has always been a sensitive matter when the state intervenes in the otherwise autonomous field of sport, the charter found great response among nations and nongovernmental organizations. Within a year of its publication, the IOC and the General Association of International Sports Federations passed resolutions supporting the charter. Recognition also came from United Nations Educational, Scientific and Cultural Organization (UNESCO), the European Union, and the World Health Organization. Furthermore, countries outside of Europe (such as Canada) showed interest in the charter in that they aligned their national antidoping policies to the guidelines of the document.[1] Because of the charter's success and the intensification of doping worldwide, it was agreed to develop it into a legally binding convention against doping.[7]

The Convention of the Council of Europe has so far been signed by 46 European and 4 non-European states. Most European countries have thereby reached remarkable political consensus and have committed themselves to fighting drug abuse in sport as and to enhancing prevention. The Convention of the Council of Europe is the first international agreement with the force of law in the area of doping in sport. It embraces the goal of reducing and, when possible, eliminating doping completely from sports, bringing about domestic coordination of measures, and fostering cross-national harmonization of proceedings. The implementation of the Convention is reviewed by a sophisticated system. One element is the Monitoring Group, to which all signatory states are members and which meets twice a year to exchange ideas and monitor progress. In addition, other Advisory Groups exist (currently in Legal, Education, Science, and Database Development) that handle tasks and questions addressed to the Monitoring Group and make proposals accordingly.

In April 2004, an additional protocol to the Convention[8] came into effect that aimed for reciprocal acknowledgment of doping tests between states and improved application of the Convention. Acknowledgment should follow if a certified (eg, ISO) testing system exists within a country. Thus, the bilateral and multilateral agreements between states or national antidoping agencies, which would otherwise be essential, are no longer necessary.

With regard to the reinforcement of the application of the Convention, the Protocol sets up a binding monitoring mechanism (Compliance with Commitments). This monitoring is performed by an evaluation team, which makes a visit to the country concerned, followed by an evaluation report. The Protocol means that the Anti-Doping Convention becomes one of the few international conventions to have a real binding control mechanism.

This Compliance with Commitment Project was originally prepared to allow the examination of all conventions of the Council of Europe. However, to the authors' knowledge, it is less successfully applied to other conventions than to the Anti-Doping Convention. It consists of a multilevel process.[9] States that develop an antidoping system can make a request through the Council of Europe for a consultation visit by experts from other countries and thus benefit from their experience and suggestions. On the other hand, states that already have a well-developed system to fight doping can have it reviewed through the Council of Europe, which, in turn, assembles experts from other countries.[10] The evaluation team prepares a final report for the Council of Europe and the reviewed state that provides recommendations for improving the existing system. As a rule, the reviewed state then submits a progress report within 2 years of evaluation. The program is very successful. By the end of 2008, 18 consultation visits and 17 evaluation visits had already taken place.[11] In various countries, the program has led to improvements in legal, structural, and financial aspects, in the fight against doping.

Although accession to the Convention of the Council of Europe is also open to non-European countries, those countries that do not yet have a fully developed system to fight doping have hesitated to join, since compliance with the Convention of the Council of Europe presents a high hurdle to overcome. Despite this, the Convention is a success and marks a milestone in the development of governmental antidoping measures. Until 2005, no other region in the world had an organ similar to the Monitoring Group of the Council of Europe, in which governments had a platform for direct exchange about measures to fight doping. It is thus not surprising that the Monitoring Group played a formative role in the development of the World Anti-Doping Program (WADP) of 2003 and 2009 as well as the UNESCO Convention of 2005.

THE WORLD ANTI-DOPING AGENCY

The events of the 1998 Tour de France led to significant changes in the fight against doping, nationally and internationally. Through the intervention of the French justice system, doping schemes surfaced that had particularly strained athletes' networks. The impertinence with which athletes, team doctors and other team workers had built up a system of cheating was appalling.[12] The intensive intervention of the French police and public prosecutor's office represented the first instance of intervention by a state authority in the otherwise autonomous field of sport. Because of these revelations and with pressure from various mostly European states, a World Conference on Doping was held in February 1999 through the IOC. As a result of the Conference, it was possible to pass a declaration which served as the basis for the foundation of an independent World Anti-Doping Agency (WADA).

The WADA was established as a foundation according to Swiss law on November 10, 1999, on the initiative of the IOC and with the support of intergovernmental organizations, governments, public authorities, and other public and private bodies. Its mission is the advancement and harmonization of antidoping measures in international sport. The agency consists of equal representatives from the Olympic Movement and public authorities. Funding is likewise provided equally by the Olympic Movement and by governments. The current yearly budget is around 25 million United States' dollars.

WADA is composed of a Foundation Board, an Executive Committee, and several committees. The 38-member Foundation Board is WADA's supreme decision-making body. It is composed equally of representatives from the Olympic Movement and governments. WADA Foundation Board delegates the actual management and running of the Agency, including the performance of activities and the administration of assets, to the Executive Committee, WADA's ultimate policy-making body. The 12-member Executive Committee is also composed equally of representatives from the Olympic Movement and governments.

Several expert committees also exist, which WADA advises and supports in specific tasks. There are committees for Finance and Administration, Education and Health, and Medical and Research. The latter committee is also responsible for the compilation of the yearly doping list.

WADA's main activities and responsibilities can be summarized as follows[13]:

Code compliance monitoring. Facilitate sport and government acceptance of the World Anti-Doping Code (Code) and its principles to ensure a harmonized approach to antidoping in all sports and all countries, and monitoring implementation of and compliance with the Code

Cooperation with law enforcement. Develop protocols to ensure evidence gathering and information sharing between the sports movement and governments; cooperate with Interpol, in collaboration with UNESCO, with the aim to develop laws to restrict the availability of prohibited substances or methods to athletes

Science and medicine. Promote global research to identify and detect doping substances and methods; exploring new models for enhanced detection; develop and maintain the annual List of Prohibited Substances and Methods. Develop and maintain a system for accrediting antidoping laboratories worldwide

Antidoping coordination. Develop and maintain a web-based database management system to help stakeholders coordinate anti-doping activities

Antidoping development: facilitate the coordination of regional antidoping organizations in regions with no or limited antidoping activities to pool resources to implement antidoping activities

Education and outreach. Lead and coordinate effective doping prevention strategies and education, assist stakeholders, and be present at major sport events

WADP

A milestone in the short history of the WADA is the WADP. It was passed by the WADA Foundation Board on March 5, 2003, at the Second World Conference on Doping in Sport in Copenhagen, after international sports organizations and the approximately 80 government representatives present agreed to it. It consists of the Code, 4 technical standards, and several nonbinding best-practice models.

The introduction and implementation of the WADP has facilitated worldwide progress in the harmonization and standardization of the fight against doping in recent years. In turn, this has shown that the foundation of the WADA in 1999 was a correct and important step. Never had such great progress in the worldwide fight against doping been possible as after the foundation of the WADA. The model of the independent agency supported cooperatively by sports organizations and governments was subsequently implemented in many countries—in Switzerland, in 2008, with the establishment of the Antidoping Switzerland Foundation.

The application of the WADP has shown in recent years that there is room for improvement in various provisions such as sanctions, roles and responsibilities, and education or implementation. The WADP was revised and passed at the November 2007 Third World Conference on Doping in Madrid in extensive and transparent proceedings that included all partners. It came into effect on January 1, 2009.

The aims of the revised WADP can be described as follows:

To protect the athletes' fundamental right to participate in doping-free sport and thus promote health, fairness, and equality for athletes worldwide.

To ensure harmonized, coordinated, and effective antidoping programs at the international and national levels with regard to detection, deterrence, and prevention of doping

The WADP encompasses all of the elements needed to ensure optimal harmonization and best practice in international and national antidoping programs, and specifies the responsibilities of its stakeholders.

The WADP is based on a three-tier model. The first tier is made up of the Code, the second tier consists of a series of international standards, and the third provides models of best practice in implementation and guidelines. Implementing the Code and the international standards is mandatory. Models of best implementation practice place state-of-the-art solutions in different areas at the disposal of all the partners; they are recommended but not binding.

Signatories of the WADP are the IOC, the International Paralympic Committee, international sports federations, national Olympic and Paralympic committees, major event organizations, national antidoping organizations, and the WADA. They are obligated to transfer and implement the rules of the WADP into their own rules and statutes. The WADA is obligated, pursuant to Article 23.4 of the Code,[14] to monitor the correct application and implementation of the WADP by the signatories. Toward this end, the signatories must submit their sets of rules and regulations and compose a compliance report for the WADA every 2 years. Signatories that do not fulfill WADP requirements can be penalized, for example, by not being allowed to host or take part in major international events.

After the Olympic Movement, governments are the second, equally powerful body responsible for the WADA, but cannot sign the WADP. Sovereign states cannot be bound by the rules of an organization operating under private law. To accommodate this situation, governments were bound by the so-called Copenhagen Declaration, agreed to at the Second World Conference against Doping, in March 2003, in

Copenhagen, during which the first WADP was adopted. The purpose of the Declaration is to articulate a political and moral understanding among participants to recognize the role of and support for WADA, support for the World Anti-Doping Code, to sustain international intergovernmental cooperation in advancing harmonization in antidoping policies and practices in sport, and to support a timely process leading to an international convention against doping in sport.[15]

UNESCO subsequently showed its readiness to create an international agreement against doping within its legal framework. The Convention was developed within a record time of just under 2 years. It is based on the Convention of the Council of Europe of 1989, but does not go as far in some fundamental points (eg, measuring compliance). Within comparison to the Convention of the Council of Europe, it refers to the WADP and the role of the WADA in the international fight against doping. With its accession to the UNESCO Convention and the application of the Convention on national level, a state fulfills its responsibility to fight doping.

THE UNESCO CONVENTION AGAINST DOPING IN SPORT

UNESCO developed the International Convention against Doping in Sport, which came into force on February 1, 2007, so that all countries around the world could apply the force of international law against doping. The Convention provides a framework for harmonizing antidoping rules and policies worldwide, and ensures the effectiveness of the World Anti-Doping Code. It calls upon governments to join efforts to strengthen ethics, personal responsibility, and integrity in sport.

The Convention consists of 43 articles, 2 integral appendices, and 3 attachments. The Convention and 2 appendices (lists of banned substances and methods and a section of the standards on the granting of therapeutic-use exemptions) are intergovernmentally binding and are not self-executing. The World Anti-Doping Code and the two international standards for laboratories and for doping tests are attachments for informational purposes and are not integral elements of the Convention.

The Convention should contribute to anchoring the regulations and principles of the World Anti-Doping Code in the laws of the contracting parties. In this regard, the governments have broad flexibility in the chosen approach. The Convention can be applied through legislation, regulations, political means, or administrative provisions. Contracting parties must take measures to:

Reduce the availability of banned substances and methods (other than those used for legitimate medical purposes), including taking measures against their distribution

Facilitate doping tests in their own country and financial support of national doping test programs

Discontinue financial contributions to athletes and their networks when they violate doping regulations, and to sports organizations that do not fulfill the stipulations of the Code

Encourage producers and distributors of dietary supplements to introduce best practice guidelines for the labeling, marketing, and sale of products that may contain banned substances

Support doping prevention for athletes and, overall, promote a sportsmanlike environment

Around 120 states have already adhered to the Convention, which makes it one of the most successful UNESCO conventions and again demonstrates the will of the community of states to fight doping together in cooperation with private law.

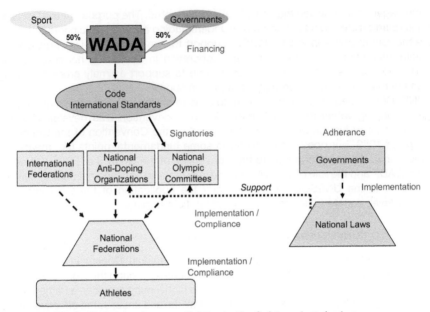

Fig. 1. Simplified relations and responsibilities in the fight against doping.

Compliance checks take place through reporting by the states themselves and through the conference for signatory states that takes place every 2 years. These measures do not come close to those of the Compliance with Commitments Project of the Council of Europe, but the guidelines can still be improved.

SUMMARY

Following the first isolated and tentative attempts to combat doping in the 1970s, the fight against doping has gathered momentum in recent years. The current system, with all stakeholders and partners integrated into the WADP and UNESCO, is comprehensive and well thought out. However, it is complex and often far from transparent for outsiders. In particular, athletes often do not understand who is now responsible for them and which procedures they have to follow. In the flow of today's body of rules and regulations, they are placed at the end (**Fig. 1**).

There is room for improvement—above all among jurisdictions (eg, between national organizations and international sport federations)—during proceedings such as that for therapeutic-use exemptions or during testing procedures (obligation to report) and regarding the contents of the doping list (concentration on significant substances and methods). Furthermore, the WADA should further develop in the direction of taking on the role of quality assurance and auditing during examinations of compliance with the WADP. A reliable but complex model is already available in the Compliance with Commitment Project of the Council of Europe and could be adapted to the needs of the WADP.

Despite the current minor weaknesses of the WADP and the UNESCO Convention, stakeholders and partners should now be given enough time to implement provisions before a new, larger revision of the regulations begins. The introduction of the WADP in 2003, and then in 2009, greatly strained and challenged international sports federations and national antidoping organizations, both during participation and contribution to the WADP and in introduction and implementation the WADP. It is one thing to introduce a series of rules and regulations, but an entirely different thing to implement them so that they are understood and accepted by those most affected: the athletes and their entourage.

REFERENCES

1. Houlihan B. Dying to win, doping in sport and the development of anti-doping policy. Strasbourg, France: Council of Europe Publishing; 1999.
2. Council of Europe Resolution (67) 12 on the doping of athletes, Strasbourg, France, 1967.
3. Clasing D. Doping und seine Wirkstoffe. Balingen, Germany: Spitta Verlag; 2004. p. 30.
4. Berendonk B. Doping—von der Forschung zum Betrug. Aktualisierte und erweiterte Neuauflage. Hamburg, Germany: Rowohlt; 1992.
5. Singler A, Treutlein G. Doping im Spitzensport—Sportwissenschaftliche Analysen zur nationalen und internationalen Leistungsentwicklung. Aachen, Germany: Meyer & Meyer; 2000.
6. Commission of inquiry into the use of drugs and banned practices intended to increase athletic performance. Ottawa, Canada: Canadian Government Publishing Centre; 1990.
7. Council of Europe, Anti-Doping Convention (ETS 135), Strasbourg, France, 1989.
8. Council of Europe, Additional Protocol to the Anti-Doping Convention (ETS 188), Strasbourg, France, 2002.
9. Council of Europe, Committee for the Development of Sport (CDDS), Standing Committee of the European Convention on Spectator Violence (T-RV), Monitoring Group of the Anti-Doping Convention (T-DO), Compliance with Commitments project. Procedural Guidelines "HANDBOOK" 2nd edition (2004), Document prepared by the Secretariat in consultation with the Group on Compliance with Commitments. CDDS (2003) 59 rev, Strasbourg, 21 June 2004.
10. Council of Europe. Operating procedures for the evaluations. Rules adopted by the Monitoring Group in accordance with article 2.4 of the Additional Protocol. T-DO (2003) 6 rev 5, Strasbourg, France, 10 February 2004.
11. Council of Europe, Monitoring Group of the Anti-Doping Convention (T-DO) Compliance with Commitments. An overview of the project and timetable. T-DO (2008) 1, Strasbourg, France, 30 January 2008.
12. Voet W. Massacre à la chaîne...Révélations sur 30 ans de tricheries. Paris: Calman-Lévy; 1999.
13. Available at: http://www.wada-ama.org/en/dynamic.ch2?pageCategory.id=255.
14. World Anti-Doping Code. World Anti-Doping Agency. Montreal: Canada; 2009. Available at: http://www.wada-ama.org/rtecontent/document/code_v2009_En.pdf.
15. Council of Europe, Anti-Doping Convention, Copenhagen Declaration on Anti-Doping in Sport. T-DO (2003) Inf 4 Final, Strasbourg, France, 13 March 2003.

Growth Hormone Administration: Is It Safe and Effective for Athletic Performance

Vita Birzniece, MD, PhD, Anne E. Nelson, PhD,
Ken K.Y. Ho, FRACP, MD*

KEYWORDS

- Growth hormone • Physical performance • Athletes
- Muscle strength • Anaerobic exercise capacity • Side effects

Growth hormone (GH) is listed in the 2008 Prohibited List (http://www.wada-ama.org/rtecontent/document/2008_List_En.pdf) because of its theoretical potential to enhance sports performance, its violation of the spirit of sports, and the health risks that it poses to athletes. Doping with GH is a well-known problem in the world of sports and its abuse has increased since the availability of recombinant GH in the late 1980s. Its increasing popularity stems from its anabolic and lipolytic properties, and the difficulty of detection.[1] There is anecdotal evidence that GH is abused in doses of between 5 to 15 times that of the daily production rate.[2,3] Despite large doses being administered, the evidence of a beneficial effect on performance is weak.

Fitness correlates positively with GH status[4,5] and physical training increases levels of GH and insulin-like growth factor I (IGF-I) in healthy subjects.[6-9] The maximum peak of GH is detected at the end of prolonged exercise[9] with a minor gender difference in the timing of the peak GH response, which occurs earlier in female athletes.[6] The link between GH and exercise suggests a physiologic role of GH in the regulation of physical health.

This article examines effects of GH on physical performance in the state of GH deficiency and in healthy adults, and also examines the health risks posed by long-term abuse.

GROWTH HORMONE DEFICIENCY
Consequences of Growth Hormone Deficiency on Body Composition

The effects of GH replacement in GH-deficient adults provide a useful model to understand its role in adult life. GH deficiency (GHD) results in a reduction of lean body

Pituitary Research Unit, Garvan Institute of Medical Research, 384 Victoria Street, Darlinghurst, New South Wales 2010, Australia
* Corresponding author.
E-mail address: k.ho@garvan.org.au (K.K.Y. Ho).

Endocrinol Metab Clin N Am 39 (2010) 11–23
doi:10.1016/j.ecl.2009.10.007
endo.theclinics.com

mass, muscle atrophy, and an increase in fat mass and central abdominal obesity.[10] GH has a regulatory role in optimizing body composition through its anabolic and lipolytic actions.[11] These effects are demonstrated when patients with GHD are replaced with GH. GH reverses muscle atrophy and reduces central and total body fat mass.[12,13] In adults with GHD, long-term GH replacement reduces fat mass by up to 20% and increases lean body mass (LBM) by about 3% to 7%, depending on the GH dose and the duration of treatment.[13–17]

Consequences of Growth Hormone Deficiency on Muscle Strength

Muscle strength is also reduced in patients with GHD.[18] The reduced muscle mass and strength could be an effect of reduced muscle cross-sectional area in GHD patients.[19] It could also be caused by a reduction in the power generated per muscle area,[20] suggesting that contractile properties and neural activation might be additional factors determining the reduction in muscle strength in adult GHD patients. Most open studies report that GH replacement increases muscle strength in GHD subjects but the effect is not uniform.[18] Some double-blind placebo-controlled studies show that GH replacement increases certain aspects of muscle strength,[21] whereas other studies report no beneficial effect.[22] A recent meta-analysis of nine randomized placebo-controlled studies of mean duration 6.7 months showed that short-term GH replacement does not significantly improve muscle strength in GHD patients.[23] However, Jorgensen and colleagues[24] reported an improvement in isometric knee flexion by 10% and extension by 7% after 12 months of GH treatment. After 3 years of GH replacement, the improvement in muscle strength was maintained but remained only 66% that of healthy subjects.[25] Other studies also show a small although persistent increase in muscle strength.[26] Therefore, with long-term GH replacement a certain degree of improvement in muscle strength can be expected.

Consequences of Growth Hormone Deficiency on Exercise Capacity

In addition to reduced muscle strength, aerobic exercise capacity is impaired in GH-deficient adults. Aerobic exercise capacity is typically measured by assessing maximal oxygen consumption while exercising at maximum capacity (VO_2max). VO_2max is reduced in GHD patients by about 20% compared with predicted VO_2max for age, gender, and height.[18] Cuneo and colleagues[27] in 1991 reported a 17% increase in VO_2max after 6 months of GH replacement compared with only 6% increase in the placebo group. After 5 years of GH replacement, VO_2max was maintained at the level close to that of expected VO_2max for age and gender.[28] Nass and colleagues[29] have shown in a double-blind placebo-controlled 6-month study that GH replacement in GHD adults increased VO_2max, maximal power output, and exercise time compared with placebo-treated patients. However, when VO_2max was expressed per kilogram lean body mass, there were no effects of GH compared with placebo, suggesting that increase in VO_2max may depend on changes in muscle mass from the GH supplementation.[29] A meta-analysis by Widdowson and Gibney[30] of 11 placebo-controlled studies shows that GH replacement improves VO_2max and maximal power output in GH-deficient subjects independent of GH dose.

Several factors may contribute to the reduced exercise capacity in GHD. Respiratory muscle weakness[31] and a reduction in cardiac function, such as left ventricular ejection fraction and diastolic filling at rest, have been reported in patients with GH deficiency.[32] In addition, GHD is associated with an increase in plasma viscosity and a reduction in plasma volume that may affect oxygen delivery and availability to the tissues, rendering reduction in aerobic exercise capacity.[33,34] Central effects, such as reduction in general well-being, may also contribute to the reduced exercise capacity in GH-deficient patients.[18] Thus, following GH replacement, upon improvement of cardiorespiratory function and quality of life, exercise capacity may improve as well.

In summary, replacement of GH in GH deficiency improves some aspects of exercise capacity but causes no further increase in muscle mass or strength, beyond that expected for healthy adults of the same age and gender.

HEALTHY ADULTS
Protein Metabolism

There is unequivocal evidence that GH induces a protein anabolic effect in healthy adults. This is supported by tracer studies at the tissue and the whole body levels. An increase in whole body protein synthesis upon treatment with GH is clearly demonstrated in untrained men.[35] In a placebo-controlled study, Healy and colleagues[36] reported that GH treatment significantly reduced whole body protein oxidation, thus reducing irreversible protein loss, and increased protein synthesis rate in trained men. A program of resistance exercise also increased protein synthesis in muscle[35] and, in a further study, the effect of resistance training was shown to be maintained for up to 24 hours after exercise.[37] On a whole body level, protein oxidation is also stimulated during exercise.[36] When GH was administered for 4 weeks, it resulted in a smaller increase in protein oxidation compared with that induced by 30 minutes of exercise alone, with concurrent stimulation of protein synthesis.[36] Thus, GH may conserve protein during exercise. However, administration of GH for 12 weeks in combination with training did not have an additional effect on muscle protein metabolism when compared with placebo treatment.[35] Thus, there is little evidence that supra-physiologic doses of GH administration confer an additional protein anabolic effect over and above that induced by exercise in healthy adults.

Although GH induces whole body protein synthesis in untrained men, this effect appears to be lost in highly trained athletes. When Yarasheski and colleagues[38] administered high-dose GH (40 μg/kg/d for 14 days) to experienced athletes during weight-training routines, they found no change in whole body protein synthesis. This finding suggests that GH administration modifies protein metabolism in untrained individuals but is unlikely to induce a major anabolic stimulus to skeletal muscle in highly trained athletes despite substantial increase in IGF-I levels.

Body Composition

There is good evidence that GH supplementation increases LBM in athletes. The LBM is heterogeneous, comprising an inert compartment of extracellular water (ECW) and a functional cellular compartment of mostly muscle, the body cell mass. Most methods for evaluation of LBM, such as dual-energy x-ray absorptiometry (DXA), do not distinguish lean solid tissue from fluid. Therefore, change in LBM measured by DXA alone does not distinguish between changes in muscle mass and ECW. ECW can be quantified separately using techniques such as bromide dilution[39] and when subtracted from the LBM, can be used to provide an estimate of body cell mass.

In a systematic review on the effects of GH recently undertaken by Liu and colleagues,[40] GH increased LBM by an average of 2.1 kg by meta-analysis of nine studies involving an average treatment duration of 4 weeks. What is not clear is whether increase in LBM reflects an increase in muscle mass or increase in fluid retention. Moller and colleagues[41] have reported that 2 weeks of GH treatment in healthy men increased ECW, but not intracellular water, a measure of body cell mass. Another study showed that GH treatment for 1 month reduced body fat by 7% and increased ECW by 10%.[42] As no significant increase in intracellular water was found, the increase in lean body mass by 5% is likely accounted for by an increase in ECW volume. In a double-blind placebo-controlled study from our group, growth hormone for 8 weeks significantly increased LBM as estimated by DXA by about 2.5 kg.[43] However, there was a concomitant expansion of the ECW volume by 2 L as estimated by concurrent bromide dilution. The data provide strong evidence that fluid retention accounts for most of the increase of LBM induced by GH.

EFFECTS OF GROWTH HORMONE ON PHYSICAL PERFORMANCE IN HEALTHY ADULTS

The effect of GH on physical performance in healthy adults has not been studied rigorously. Most of the studies available have evaluated GH effects in small groups of subjects and almost exclusively in men (**Table 1**). Liu and colleagues[40] have also undertaken a systematic review of the effects of GH on various measures of athletic performance, such as muscle strength and endurance. Twenty-seven studies comprising a total number of 303 physically fit participants with mean age of 27 years and mean body mass index (BMI) of 24 kg/m^2 were considered suitable for analyses. Participants from 7 studies received GH as only one injection but 20 of the studies used GH treatment for an average of 20 days with average daily dose of 36 µg/kg. Change in strength was evaluated in two studies and exercise capacity outcomes were measured in six studies. The authors concluded that claims that GH enhances physical performance are not supported by the scientific literature.[40] However, they stressed that more research is required to conclusively determine the effect of GH on athletic performance. Recently, there has been evidence for improved physical performance following short-term GH administration in a single-blind study; however, this study was undertaken using the specific model of abstinent anabolic androgenic steroid dependents.[48]

Here we review double-blind placebo-controlled studies evaluating the effect of GH on physical performance in healthy subjects including that of a large double-blind placebo-controlled study from our center. The information is summarized in **Table 1**. Effects of GH in this section are discussed according to different measures of physical performance, namely muscle strength and power, and aerobic and anaerobic exercise capacity.

Effects on Muscle Strength

There is little information on the effects of GH on muscle strength in healthy adults. Only three studies have appropriately evaluated muscle strength and none showed any improvement after GH treatment (see **Table 1**).[35,43,44] In one study involving eight athletes, 6 weeks of GH treatment revealed no positive effect on maximal voluntary strength of biceps and quadriceps muscles.[44] Similarly, in a large group of recreational athletes, our group has recently reported that both muscle strength, assessed by dead lift dynamometer, and muscle power, assessed by jump height, were not affected by GH treatment.[43] Athletes often administer a cocktail of performance-enhancing drugs, which contains androgens and GH. However, we showed in healthy trained men, that co-administration of testosterone with GH in pharmacologic doses for 8 weeks also failed to improve muscle strength or power.[43]

Exercise is the most potent stimulant for improving muscle strength. Exercise has been shown to increase GH secretion; however, it is not known whether GH may add to the beneficial effect of exercise on muscle strength. It can be postulated that when GH administration is combined with exercise, it may increase muscle strength more than exercise alone. However, this is not supported by a study in healthy untrained men, which showed that addition of GH to resistance exercise training for

Table 1
GH effect on physical performance in healthy subjects

Study	Study Type	Subjects	GH Dose	Treatment Duration	Outcome Measures
Yarasheski et al, 1992[35]	Double-blind placebo-controlled parallel study	18 untrained men	40 μg/kg/d for 5 d/wk + resistance exercise	12 weeks	Muscle strength improved with exercise, but similar in placebo and GH groups
Deyssig et al, 1993[44]	Double-blind placebo-controlled parallel study	22 lean men (power athletes)	30 μg/kg/d	6 weeks	No effect on biceps and quadriceps strength
Lange et al, 2002[45]	Double-blind placebo-controlled cross-over study	7 highly trained men	2.5 mg	4 hours pre-exercise	Bicycling speed did not change, but GH prevented 2 subjects from completing the exercise protocol; VO_2max did not change
Irving et al, 2004[46]	Randomized within-subject design of 5 GH and 1 placebo studies	9 fit lean men	10 μg/kg	0.75 to 3.75 hours pre-exercise	VO_2max reduced without a drop-off in power output
Berggren et al, 2005[47]	Double-blind placebo-controlled parallel study	30 active volunteers (15 men, 15 women)	33 μg/kg/d 67 μg/kg/d	4 weeks	VO_2max, power output, muscle mass did not change
Meinhardt et al, in press[43]	Double-blind placebo-controlled parallel study	96 recreational athletes (63 men, 33 women)	2 mg/d	8 weeks	VO_2max, muscle strength, power did not change; anaerobic sprint capacity increased

12 weeks did not further improve muscle strength compared with that achieved by training alone.[35] Taken together, these studies show that in healthy subjects, muscle strength and power do not improve after administration of GH in supraphysiological doses.

Effects on Aerobic Exercise Capacity

Aerobic exercise capacity is assessed by measuring VO_2max, which depends not only on muscle function, but also on cardiorespiratory function and on motivation. Several studies have found no significant effect of GH on VO_2max in healthy adults, as reviewed by Liu and colleagues.[40]

In a study involving 30 healthy young men and women, Berggren and colleagues[47] found no significant effect on VO_2max or on maximum achieved power output during exercise after 4 weeks of GH treatment at two different doses, approximately 5 to 10 times daily production rate. There was no relationship between changes in IGF-I and changes in oxygen uptake or maximum achieved power output.[47] This negative finding has been confirmed by our recent large study in 96 recreationally trained athletes (see **Table 1**). GH administration for 8 weeks did not significantly change VO_2max in either men or women, and co-administration of testosterone also failed to increase VO_2max in men.[43]

It has been shown that acute GH administration may be detrimental. Irving and colleagues[46] reported that acute administration of GH reduced oxygen uptake during exercise but did not affect total work and ratings of perceived exertion. In addition, administration of GH 4 hours before exercise reduced performance in well-trained young adults.[45] Two subjects were unable to complete the 90-minute moderate- to high-intensity exercise after receiving the GH treatment.[45]

These findings differ from the beneficial effects of GH replacement in enhancing exercise capacity in GHD subjects. The duration of GH administration in studies in athletes may have been too short, and treatment for months or years may be required to show beneficial effect on physical performance, however observations in acromegaly suggest this is unlikely. Prolonged excess of GH in acromegaly causes myopathy with hypertrophic, but functionally weaker muscles,[49,50] and significantly lower VO_2max is observed in acromegaly patients, to that predicted for healthy sedentary adults of the same age, gender, and height.[51] Importantly, reduction in IGF-I following treatment of acromegaly correlates with improvement in exercise capacity.[51]

Thus, GH administration in healthy adults does not induce a stimulation of aerobic exercise capacity.

Effects on Anaerobic Exercise Capacity

There is little published evidence on assessment of GH effects on anaerobic capacity. Anaerobic capacity assesses the ability to generate a relatively high power output of brief duration and represents capacity to exercise using predominately anaerobic sources of energy, derived from phosphocreatinine degradation and glycogenolysis. It is usually measured by the Wingate test, which is a 30-second all-out sprint capacity test.

We have recently shown a novel enhancing effect of GH on muscle performance that is dependent on the anaerobic metabolism.[43] This is the first study assessing the effect of GH on anaerobic capacity in healthy men and women. Eight weeks of GH improved sprint capacity by about 6%. The effect was slightly greater in men when co-administered with testosterone, with the increase approaching 9%. This study provides the first evidence that growth hormone enhances anaerobic exercise capacity.[43]

In summary, there is no evidence from double-blind placebo-controlled studies that GH enhances muscle strength or aerobic capacity in trained adult athletes despite evidence for an anabolic effect of GH in GH-deficient patients (see **Table 1**). However, there is evidence from a recent study that GH improves anaerobic exercise capacity.

POTENTIAL BENEFITS OF GROWTH HORMONE ADMINISTRATION IN ELITE ATHLETES

There are no published studies on the effects of GH treatment in elite athletes and it is unlikely that these studies will ever be conducted for ethical reasons. Even if these studies were undertaken, it is unlikely they could be sufficiently powered to detect differences of 0.5% to 1.0% in physical performance, the small differences that separate Olympic champions from other finishing positions (http://en.beijing2008.cn/). Another factor that may influence performance relates to the potential psychological effect of any substance administration, namely the placebo effect. A positive effect of placebo treatment has been found in many conditions, such as pain and movement disorders, and depression.[52] Placebo treatment may modulate pain pathways, increase endogenous opioids and neurotransmitters, and influence the neuroendocrine and immune systems.[52,53] In addition, placebo has been shown to increase physical performance and pain endurance, and reduce muscle fatigue perception.[53–55]

Finally, there is the possibility that GH may be beneficial in accelerating recovery from soft tissue injury. This is based on the known effects of GH on connective tissue formation, as indicated by an increase in collagen turnover markers.[56,57] Animal studies show that tendons heal faster after treatment with IGF-I.[58] Thus, the increase in IGF-I, which parallels GH treatment, may have potential beneficial effects on recovery from injury in athletes, although evidence from human studies are lacking.

GROWTH HORMONE SIDE EFFECTS

Saugy and colleagues[3] have reported that athletes may be using GH in dosages ranging from approximately 10 to 25 IU per day three to four times a week. These doses are approximately 5 to 10 times the daily production rate, and are higher than dosages used in most studies of GH administration. There are side effects from GH that arise from its antinatriuretic, metabolic, and growth-promoting properties. Most of the acute side effects reported in trials in healthy adults arise from fluid retention (**Fig. 1**). These include edema, "pins and needles," carpal tunnel syndrome, and arthralgias.[40,42,57] Other side effects, including sweating, fatigue, and dizziness, have been reported after GH administration in healthy subjects.[40,60] However, serious side effects, including diabetes, may arise from its anti-insulin properties, especially with high doses.[61] The severity of these adverse effects may be worsened by concurrent abuse of anabolic steroids, which could have synergistic effects with GH, such as effects on fluid retention[62] and on the myocardium.[63,64]

Excess levels of GH negatively affect cardiac function. The effects of two doses (0.03 or 0.06 mg/kg/d) of GH on cardiac output and morphology were examined in a group of 30 young healthy men and 30 women treated for 4 weeks.[59] Although the lower dose of GH did not significantly affect echocardiographic parameters, the higher dose increased cardiac output and left ventricular mass index. The accompanying increase in left ventricular wall thickness indicates that GH induces concentric left ventricular remodeling.[59] The effect of massive doses of anabolic androgenic steroids without or with GH on left ventricular mass was studied by Karila and colleagues[63] in 20 male power athletes. They found a significant association between androgenic steroids dose and left ventricular mass increase. Concomitant treatment

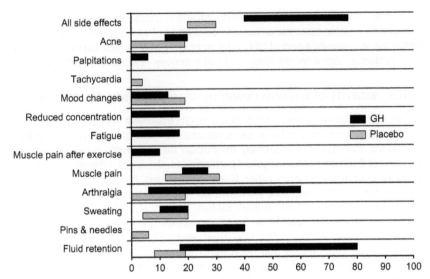

Fig. 1. Summary of side effects reported in seven double-blind placebo-controlled trials in healthy subjects of GH administration for 4 to 12 weeks with median GH dose of 40 μg/kg/day.[35,36,42,43,47,56,59] Data are presented as a range of percent of the subjects reporting side effects after treatment with GH (*black bars*) and placebo (*gray bars*).

with GH further increased left ventricular mass and was associated with concentric remodeling.[63]

The potential health risks of chronic abuse of GH can be gleaned from acromegaly, which presents with cardiac, metabolic, and articular complications with increased risk of malignant neoplasms and shortened life expectancy. Systolic and diastolic functions are impaired in acromegaly.[65] Morphologic studies of the heart in acromegaly report ventricular hypertrophy with increased fibrosis and extracellular collagen, which coexists with myofibrillar derangement, myocyte necrosis, and lymphomononuclear infiltration, resembling a pattern of myocarditis.[5,65] The incidence of hypertension,[66] as well as cardiovascular and cerebrovascular mortality is increased in acromegaly.[67]

GH impairs insulin action and hepatic and peripheral insulin sensitivity.[68–70] Therefore, prolonged and sustained use of GH conveys a state of insulin resistance, predisposing to the development of diabetes. Indeed, diabetes is found in up to 40% of patients with untreated acromegaly.[4,66] There is also some evidence that prolonged use of GH may be associated with increased risk of neoplasms.[67,71] The incidence of colon polyps, thyroid nodules, and prostate hypertrophy is increased in acromegaly. Whether this translates into increase in cancer risk is not clear.[72] However, the mortality rate of colon cancer is significantly increased in patients with acromegaly compared with the control population,[72] suggesting that a milieu of GH excess accelerates the growth of malignancy.

GH excess induces dysregulated growth of cartilage, causing arthralgia.[73] These changes in articular cartilage are irreversible. This is exemplified by a study in a group of patients cured of acromegaly, in whom the authors reported radiological evidence of osteoarthritis in 99% and clinical osteoarthritis in 63%.[74]

Life expectancy is reduced in acromegaly, which is normalized by achieving disease control. Overall standardized mortality rates are approximately two times higher than in the general population, relating to an average reduction in life expectancy of approximately 10 years.[67]

In summary, many of the acute side effects of GH arise from fluid retention. The features of the acromegaly indicate the potential health risks of chronic abuse of GH, which include cardiac complications, arthralgia, insulin resistance, and increased risk of diabetes and malignancy. Finally, a potential risk is that of abusers acquiring fatal Creutzfelt-Jakob disease from the use of cadaveric pituitary-derived GH that is still available on the black market because of the high cost of recombinant human GH (rhGH).[75]

SUMMARY

Contrary to improvements in exercise capacity by GH replacement in GH-deficient adults, the evidence suggests that in healthy adults, muscle strength, power, and aerobic exercise capacity are not enhanced by GH administration. Recent data indicate that GH may improve a selective aspect of performance, that of anaerobic exercise capacity. There are, however, serious adverse effects of long-term abuse of GH, including fluid retention, carpal tunnel syndrome, arthralgias, myalgias, insulin resistance, and increased risk of diabetes, cardiomyopathy, and malignancy. Thus, there are serious health risks and potential increase in mortality rate from prolonged use of GH in healthy adults.

ACKNOWLEDGMENTS

Dr Vita Birzniece was supported by the National Health and Medical Research Council of Australia. Dr Anne E. Nelson was supported by the World Anti-Doping Agency and by the Australian Government through the Anti-Doping Research Program and the Department of Communications, Information Technology, and the Arts.

REFERENCES

1. Holt RI, Sonksen PH. Growth hormone, IGF-I and insulin and their abuse in sport. Br J Pharmacol 2008;154:542.
2. Holt RI, Erotokritou-Mulligan I, Sonksen PH. The history of doping and growth hormone abuse in sport. Growth Horm IGF Res 2009;19(4):320–6.
3. Saugy M, Robinson N, Saudan C, et al. Human growth hormone doping in sport. Br J Sports Med 2006;40(Suppl 1):i35.
4. Ezzat S, Forster MJ, Berchtold P, et al. Acromegaly. Clinical and biochemical features in 500 patients. Medicine (Baltimore) 1994;73:233.
5. Fazio S, Cittadini A, Biondi B, et al. Cardiovascular effects of short-term growth hormone hypersecretion. J Clin Endocrinol Metab 2000;85:179.
6. Ehrnborg C, Lange KH, Dall R, et al. The growth hormone/insulin-like growth factor-I axis hormones and bone markers in elite athletes in response to a maximum exercise test. J Clin Endocrinol Metab 2003;88:394.
7. Giannoulis MG, Boroujerdi MA, Powrie J, et al. Gender differences in growth hormone response to exercise before and after rhGH administration and the effect of rhGH on the hormone profile of fit normal adults. Clin Endocrinol (Oxf) 2005;62:315.
8. Wallace JD, Cuneo RC, Baxter R, et al. Responses of the growth hormone (GH) and insulin-like growth factor axis to exercise, GH administration, and GH withdrawal in trained adult males: a potential test for GH abuse in sport. J Clin Endocrinol Metab 1999;84:3591.

9. Wallace JD, Cuneo RC, Bidlingmaier M, et al. The response of molecular isoforms of growth hormone to acute exercise in trained adult males. J Clin Endocrinol Metab 2001;86:200.

10. Carroll PV, Christ ER, Bengtsson BA, et al. Growth hormone deficiency in adulthood and the effects of growth hormone replacement: a review. Growth Hormone Research Society Scientific Committee. J Clin Endocrinol Metab 1998;83:382.

11. Gibney J, Healy ML, Sonksen PH. The growth hormone/insulin-like growth factor-I axis in exercise and sport. Endocr Rev 2007;28:603.

12. Gibney J, Wallace JD, Spinks T, et al. The effects of 10 years of recombinant human growth hormone (GH) in adult GH-deficient patients. J Clin Endocrinol Metab 1999;84:2596.

13. Rodriguez-Arnao J, Jabbar A, Fulcher K, et al. Effects of growth hormone replacement on physical performance and body composition in GH deficient adults. Clin Endocrinol (Oxf) 1999;51:53.

14. Attanasio AF, Bates PC, Ho KK, et al. Human growth hormone replacement in adult hypopituitary patients: long-term effects on body composition and lipid status—3-year results from the HypoCCS Database. J Clin Endocrinol Metab 2002;87:1600.

15. Burt MG, Gibney J, Hoffman DM, et al. Relationship between GH-induced metabolic changes and changes in body composition: a dose and time course study in GH-deficient adults. Growth Horm IGF Res 2008;18:55.

16. Gotherstrom G, Svensson J, Koranyi J, et al. A prospective study of 5 years of GH replacement therapy in GH-deficient adults: sustained effects on body composition, bone mass, and metabolic indices. J Clin Endocrinol Metab 2001;86:4657.

17. Wolthers T, Hoffman DM, Nugent AG, et al. Oral estrogen antagonizes the metabolic actions of growth hormone in growth hormone-deficient women. Am J Physiol Endocrinol Metab 2001;281:E1191.

18. Woodhouse LJ, Mukherjee A, Shalet SM, et al. The influence of growth hormone status on physical impairments, functional limitations, and health-related quality of life in adults. Endocr Rev 2006;27:287.

19. Sartorio A, Narici MV. Growth hormone (GH) treatment in GH-deficient adults: effects on muscle size, strength and neural activation. Clin Physiol 1994;14:527.

20. Cuneo RC, Salomon F, Wiles CM, et al. Skeletal muscle performance in adults with growth hormone deficiency. Horm Res 1990;33(Suppl 4):55.

21. Cuneo RC, Salomon F, Wiles CM, et al. Growth hormone treatment in growth hormone-deficient adults. I. Effects on muscle mass and strength. J Appl Physiol 1991;70:688.

22. Woodhouse LJ, Asa SL, Thomas SG, et al. Measures of submaximal aerobic performance evaluate and predict functional response to growth hormone (GH) treatment in GH-deficient adults. J Clin Endocrinol Metab 1999;84:4570.

23. Widdowson MW, Gibney J. The effect of growth hormone (GH) replacement on muscle strength in patients with GH-deficiency: a meta-analysis. Clin Endocrinol (Oxf) 2009, in press.

24. Jorgensen JO, Pedersen SA, Thuesen L, et al. Long-term growth hormone treatment in growth hormone deficient adults. Acta Endocrinol (Copenh) 1991;125:449.

25. Jorgensen JO, Thuesen L, Muller J, et al. Three years of growth hormone treatment in growth hormone-deficient adults: near normalization of body composition and physical performance. Eur J Endocrinol 1994;130:224.

26. Svensson J, Sunnerhagen KS, Johannsson G. Five years of growth hormone replacement therapy in adults: age- and gender-related changes in isometric and isokinetic muscle strength. J Clin Endocrinol Metab 2003;88:2061.

27. Cuneo RC, Salomon F, Wiles CM, et al. Growth hormone treatment in growth hormone-deficient adults. II. Effects on exercise performance. J Appl Physiol 1991;70:695.

28. Cenci MC, Soares DV, Spina LD, et al. Effects of 5 years of growth hormone (GH) replacement therapy on cardiac parameters and physical performance in adults with GH deficiency. Pituitary 2009;12(4):322–9.

29. Nass R, Huber RM, Klauss V, et al. Effect of growth hormone (hGH) replacement therapy on physical work capacity and cardiac and pulmonary function in patients with hGH deficiency acquired in adulthood. J Clin Endocrinol Metab 1995;80:552.

30. Widdowson WM, Gibney J. The effect of growth hormone replacement on exercise capacity in patients with GH deficiency: a metaanalysis. J Clin Endocrinol Metab 2008;93:4413.

31. Merola B, Longobardi S, Sofia M, et al. Lung volumes and respiratory muscle strength in adult patients with childhood- or adult-onset growth hormone deficiency: effect of 12 months' growth hormone replacement therapy. Eur J Endocrinol 1996;135:553.

32. Colao A, Di Somma C, Cuocolo A, et al. The severity of growth hormone deficiency correlates with the severity of cardiac impairment in 100 adult patients with hypopituitarism: an observational, case-control study. J Clin Endocrinol Metab 2004;89:5998.

33. El-Sayed MS, Ali N, El-Sayed Ali Z. Haemorheology in exercise and training. Sports Med 2005;35:649.

34. Moller J, Frandsen E, Fisker S, et al. Decreased plasma and extracellular volume in growth hormone deficient adults and the acute and prolonged effects of GH administration: a controlled experimental study. Clin Endocrinol (Oxf) 1996;44:533.

35. Yarasheski KE, Campbell JA, Smith K, et al. Effect of growth hormone and resistance exercise on muscle growth in young men. Am J Physiol 1992;262:E261.

36. Healy ML, Gibney J, Russell-Jones DL, et al. High dose growth hormone exerts an anabolic effect at rest and during exercise in endurance-trained athletes. J Clin Endocrinol Metab 2003;88:5221.

37. Chesley A, MacDougall JD, Tarnopolsky MA, et al. Changes in human muscle protein synthesis after resistance exercise. J Appl Physiol 1992;73:1383.

38. Yarasheski KE, Zachweija JJ, Angelopoulos TJ, et al. Short-term growth hormone treatment does not increase muscle protein synthesis in experienced weight lifters. J Appl Physiol 1993;74:3073.

39. Miller ME, Cosgriff JM, Forbes GB. Bromide space determination using anion-exchange chromatography for measurement of bromide. Am J Clin Nutr 1989;50:168.

40. Liu H, Bravata DM, Olkin I, et al. Systematic review: the effects of growth hormone on athletic performance. Ann Intern Med 2008;148:747.

41. Moller J, Jorgensen JO, Moller N, et al. Expansion of extracellular volume and suppression of atrial natriuretic peptide after growth hormone administration in normal man. J Clin Endocrinol Metab 1991;72:768.

42. Ehrnborg C, Ellegard L, Bosaeus I, et al. Supraphysiological growth hormone: less fat, more extracellular fluid but uncertain effects on muscles in healthy, active young adults. Clin Endocrinol (Oxf) 2005;62:449.

43. Meinhardt U, Nelson AE, Hansen JL, et al. The effects of growth hormone on body composition and physical performance in recreational athletes: a randomized placebo-controlled trial. Ann Intern Med, in press.

44. Deyssig R, Frisch H, Blum WF, et al. Effect of growth hormone treatment on hormonal parameters, body composition and strength in athletes. Acta Endocrinol (Copenh) 1993;128:313.
45. Lange KH, Larsson B, Flyvbjerg A, et al. Acute growth hormone administration causes exaggerated increases in plasma lactate and glycerol during moderate to high intensity bicycling in trained young men. J Clin Endocrinol Metab 2002; 87:4966.
46. Irving BA, Patrie JT, Anderson SM, et al. The effects of time following acute growth hormone administration on metabolic and power output measures during acute exercise. J Clin Endocrinol Metab 2004;89:4298.
47. Berggren A, Ehrnborg C, Rosen T, et al. Short-term administration of supraphysiological recombinant human growth hormone (GH) does not increase maximum endurance exercise capacity in healthy, active young men and women with normal GH-insulin-like growth factor I axes. J Clin Endocrinol Metab 2005;90:3268.
48. Graham MR, Baker JS, Evans P, et al. Physical effects of short-term recombinant human growth hormone administration in abstinent steroid dependency. Horm Res 2008;69:343.
49. Brumback RA, Barr CE. Myopathy in acromegaly. A case study. Pathol Res Pract 1983;177:41.
50. Nagulesparen M, Trickey R, Davies MJ, et al. Muscle changes in acromegaly. Br Med J 1976;2:914.
51. Thomas SG, Woodhouse LJ, Pagura SM, et al. Ventilation threshold as a measure of impaired physical performance in adults with growth hormone excess. Clin Endocrinol (Oxf) 2002;56:351.
52. Price DD, Finniss DG, Benedetti F. A comprehensive review of the placebo effect: recent advances and current thought. Annu Rev Psychol 2008;59:565.
53. Pollo A, Carlino E, Benedetti F. The top-down influence of ergogenic placebos on muscle work and fatigue. Eur J Neurosci 2008;28:379.
54. Beedie CJ, Foad AJ. The placebo effect in sports performance: a brief review. Sports Med 2009;39:313.
55. Benedetti F, Pollo A, Colloca L. Opioid-mediated placebo responses boost pain endurance and physical performance: is it doping in sport competitions? J Neurosci 2007;27:11934.
56. Longobardi S, Keay N, Ehrnborg C, et al. Growth hormone (GH) effects on bone and collagen turnover in healthy adults and its potential as a marker of GH abuse in sports: a double blind, placebo-controlled study. The GH-2000 Study Group. J Clin Endocrinol Metab 2000;85:1505.
57. Nelson AE, Meinhardt U, Hansen JL, et al. Pharmacodynamics of growth hormone abuse biomarkers and the influence of gender and testosterone: a randomized double-blind placebo-controlled study in young recreational athletes. J Clin Endocrinol Metab 2008;93:2213.
58. Kurtz CA, Loebig TG, Anderson DD, et al. Insulin-like growth factor I accelerates functional recovery from Achilles tendon injury in a rat model. Am J Sports Med 1999;27:363.
59. Cittadini A, Berggren A, Longobardi S, et al. Supraphysiological doses of GH induce rapid changes in cardiac morphology and function. J Clin Endocrinol Metab 2002;87:1654.
60. Keller A, Wu Z, Kratzsch J, et al. Pharmacokinetics and pharmacodynamics of GH: dependence on route and dosage of administration. Eur J Endocrinol 2007;156:647.
61. Young J, Anwar A. Strong diabetes. Br J Sports Med 2007;41:335.

62. Johannsson G, Gibney J, Wolthers T, et al. Independent and combined effects of testosterone and growth hormone on extracellular water in hypopituitary men. J Clin Endocrinol Metab 2005;90:3989.
63. Karila TA, Karjalainen JE, Mantysaari MJ, et al. Anabolic androgenic steroids produce dose-dependant increase in left ventricular mass in power athletes, and this effect is potentiated by concomitant use of growth hormone. Int J Sports Med 2003;24:337.
64. Mark PB, Watkins S, Dargie HJ. Cardiomyopathy induced by performance enhancing drugs in a competitive bodybuilder. Heart 2005;91:888.
65. Meyers DE, Cuneo RC. Controversies regarding the effects of growth hormone on the heart. Mayo Clin Proc 2003;78:1521.
66. Colao A, Baldelli R, Marzullo P, et al. Systemic hypertension and impaired glucose tolerance are independently correlated to the severity of the acromegalic cardiomyopathy. J Clin Endocrinol Metab 2000;85:193.
67. Ayuk J, Sheppard MC. Does acromegaly enhance mortality? Rev Endocr Metab Disord 2008;9:33.
68. Bratusch-Marrain PR, Smith D, DeFronzo RA. The effect of growth hormone on glucose metabolism and insulin secretion in man. J Clin Endocrinol Metab 1982;55:973.
69. Fowelin J, Attvall S, von Schenck H, et al. Characterization of the insulin-antagonistic effect of growth hormone in man. Diabetologia 1991;34:500.
70. Rizza RA, Mandarino LJ, Gerich JE. Effects of growth hormone on insulin action in man. Mechanisms of insulin resistance, impaired suppression of glucose production, and impaired stimulation of glucose utilization. Diabetes 1982;31:663.
71. Perry JK, Emerald BS, Mertani HC, et al. The oncogenic potential of growth hormone. Growth Horm IGF Res 2006;16:277.
72. Orme SM, McNally RJ, Cartwright RA, et al. Mortality and cancer incidence in acromegaly: a retrospective cohort study. United Kingdom Acromegaly Study Group. J Clin Endocrinol Metab 1998;83:2730.
73. Colao A, Pivonello R, Scarpa R, et al. The acromegalic arthropathy. J Endocrinol Invest 2005;28:24.
74. Wassenaar MJ, Biermasz NR, van Duinen N, et al. High prevalence of arthropathy, according to the definitions of radiological and clinical osteoarthritis, in patients with long-term cure of acromegaly: a case-control study. Eur J Endocrinol 2009;160:357.
75. Brown P, Preece M, Brandel JP, et al. Iatrogenic Creutzfeldt-Jakob disease at the millennium. Neurology 2000;55:1075.

Detecting Growth Hormone Abuse in Athletes

Martin Bidlingmaier, MD*, Jenny Manolopoulou, PhD

KEYWORDS

• Growth hormone • Immunoassay • Antibodies
• Isoforms • Binding protein • Standardization

The availability of recombinant growth hormone (rGH) for treatment of GH deficiency in 1983 was a major step forward for patients, making treatment more safe and effective. However, the drug immediately also made its way into the arena of sport. Data demonstrating the efficacy of GH in healthy subjects are scarce, and experts continue to discuss if GH has any performance-enhancing effects in trained healthy athletes.[1] But there is no doubt that GH is used by athletes. Several former athletes have confessed abuse of rGH, and ampoules containing GH have been found in the possession of athletes and trainers. Although scientific studies supporting the performance-enhancing effects of GH in trained healthy individuals might be missing, the rumors about its tremendous efficacy appear to be seducing.[2] Consequently, the International Olympic Committee (IOC) banned GH in 1989, and GH is still listed as a banned substance on the World Anti-Doping Agency's (WADA) 2008 prohibited list. Since the mid 1990s, the IOC and national doping control authorities have funded research projects to develop a test method to detect doping with GH. Later, WADA took over leadership in coordinating the research projects.[3] Since the beginning, researchers mainly followed two different approaches, namely the "marker approach" and the "isoform approach."[4] It took until the summer of 2004, during the Olympic Games in Athens, when a test to detect GH doping was officially introduced. The development did not stop, and both strategies are subjects of ongoing research projects to validate and improve the methods. This article describes the difficulties associated with developing a test to detect GH doping, and shows the progress made until today.

PHYSIOLOGICAL, BIOCHEMICAL, AND ANALYTICAL DIFFICULTIES

The difficulties of developing a test to detect the illicit use of performance-enhancing drugs can occur at different levels. If an athlete is using a substance not naturally

Endocrine Research Laboratories, Medizinische Klinik – Innenstadt, Ludwig-Maximilians University, Ziemssenstr. 1, 80336, Munich, Germany
* Corresponding author.
E-mail address: martin.bidlingmaier@med.uni-muenchen.de (M. Bidlingmaier).

Endocrinol Metab Clin N Am 39 (2010) 25–32
doi:10.1016/j.ecl.2009.10.006   endo.theclinics.com
0889-8529/10/$ – see front matter © 2010 Elsevier Inc. All rights reserved.

occurring in the human body, the situation is comparably simple because the demonstration of the presence of such a substance might be evidence enough to convince a jury. The development of methods in these cases usually is focused on improvements in sensitivity of the measurement or on the development of measurement techniques for new substances. The situation is more complex when cheating athletes are using substances that also are produced by the human body. Obviously, the presence of the substance alone in these cases cannot be used as an indication for abuse. Typical examples for this situation are the peptide hormones, which are available in a recombinant form for treatment of diseases. Usually, the molecular structure of the recombinant hormones is very similar if not identical to the form naturally occurring in the human body. Depending on the degree of homology between the recombinant and the endogenous peptide hormones, discrimination by biochemical methods is difficult or impossible. In the case of recombinant erythropoietin (EPO), researchers were able to develop a test to discern the close similarity between endogenous EPO and its recombinant form.[5,6] Although identical in amino acid sequence, the EPO molecules as produced by recombinant expression systems differ slightly in their glycosylation pattern from the EPO molecules produced by the human body. Unfortunately, such differences in the glycosylation pattern do not occur between endogenous and rGH, making it impossible to use the test principle of the EPO test for a GH test.

One might think that eventually the absolute concentration of the hormone could help to identify the cheaters. If the concentration is inappropriately elevated, the exogenous origin of the circulating molecules could be suspected. However, unfortunately several hormones that are abused to enhance performance physiologically are secreted in a pulsatile rather than a continuous fashion, leading to highly variable concentrations in the bloodstream. This is especially true in the case of GH, which is secreted by the pituitary gland in a pulsatile fashion and also has a very short half-life in circulation.[7] The release is enhanced in response to various stimuli including sleep, stress, and exercise. Therefore, even if very high, the absolute concentration of GH in a blood sample cannot prove administration of rGH.[8]

Another problem that might have delayed the development, acceptance, and implementation of test methods to detect GH doping is related to the laboratory methods used. Over decades, the measurement of peptide hormones in biological fluids has been done using immunological methods, namely immunoassays. These methods can be very sensitive and can be applied to complex biological matrices like blood. However, immunoassays inherently are "relative measurements"—what is translated into a signal is the interaction between an antibody and a respective analyte, not the absolute amount of a substance present in the sample. In contrast, classical doping tests were based on laboratory methods frequently referred to as "higher-order measurements," allowing absolute quantification of the analytes. Such methods are used as "reference methods" in laboratory medicine, and usually comprise a combination of gas chromatography or liquid chromatography and mass spectrometry (MS). The WADA-accredited antidoping laboratories have longstanding experience with such MS-based methods,[9] but immunoassays were not frequently used. The application of these MS-based techniques to the analysis of peptide hormones, including GH, was not possible for a long time. Today, application of MS to the analysis of peptide hormones is a rapidly developing field, and also for GH promising data have recently been reported.[10,11] However, the extremely low concentrations together with the complex biological matrix represent problems for these methods, and immunoassays are still the most frequently used methods for measuring peptide hormones in clinical medicine. The approaches to detect GH doping described later in this article are based on immunoassay measurement of GH or GH-dependent peptide markers. Therefore, the antidoping laboratories, and also the institutions involved in the jurisdiction in doping cases, would have to implement and accept immunoassays as proof for the illicit use of substances. This addition to the methodological spectrum used in doping tests has already been reflected by the inclusion of immunoassays into the current WADA International Standard for Laboratories.

Finally, it is important to keep in mind that in the past most doping tests were based on collection and analysis of urine samples. However, the measurement of peptide hormones in urine, although possible, is associated with several problems. In the case of GH, it has been clearly demonstrated that urinary GH is highly variable in concentration, and not sufficiently associated with differences in the GH secretory status to allow its use in a clinical context.[12] Therefore, blood-based methods to detect rGH application are considered more promising.[13] This requires the implementation of blood sampling into routine doping controls, which is expensive and requires sophisticated logistics, especially when out-of-competition controls are needed.

DETECTING GROWTH HORMONE DOPING BASED ON PHARMACODYNAMIC END POINTS OF GROWTH HORMONE ACTION

As a consequence of the molecular identity of rGH and the main isoform of GH as naturally secreted by the pituitary gland and of the short half-life of GH in circulation, an international team of researchers (GH2000) decided to follow a strategy to detect rGH doping that is based not on measurements of GH itself but on a panel of proteins that physiologically are induced by GH.[14] If it would be possible to show that concentrations of these proteins usually do not exceed certain thresholds unless exogenous GH was applied, measurement of those proteins could be used as an indirect proof of illicit use of GH. The rationale behind this strategy, often referred to as the "marker approach," is that indeed GH in the human body exerts many of its effects not directly, but through the stimulation of the secretion of other proteins.[15] These proteins, namely those belonging to the insulin-like growth-factor I (IGF-I)/IGF binding protein (IGFBP) system, exhibit a much longer half-life than GH itself, therefore potentially allowing a longer window of opportunity for detection of rGH administration. One problem of such an approach is that under physiological conditions, the concentrations of IGFs and IGFBPs are also determined by a variety of factors other than GH, such as age, sex, exercise, nutritional status, and others. Therefore, it was crucial to show that changes in the markers induced by GH doping clearly exceed those fluctuations occurring under physiological conditions. In their initial proof-of-principle studies, the GH2000 consortium demonstrated that indeed several components of the GH/IGF system were much more sensitive to the application of moderate doses of rGH than to the short-term increases in endogenous GH levels seen after acute exercise.[16] The consortium also investigated changes in several markers of bone and collagen turnover after administration of rGH. It is known that many factors involved in the regulation of bone and collagen can be influenced by GH, and the consortium focused on bone-specific alkaline phosphatase, carboxy-terminal propeptide of type I procollagen, amino-terminal extension peptide of type III procollagen (PIIIP), and carboxy-terminal cross-linked telopeptide of type I collagen (ICTP). Especially for PIIIP and ICTP it could be shown that changes after administration of rGH by far exceeded changes seen after acute exercise.[17,18] To further increase the reliability and sensitivity of a potential doping test based on measurement of GH-dependent markers, it was proposed to analyze a combination of more than one factor. Most promising is a combination of the markers IGF-I and PIIIP, which in a blinded study allowed identifying subjects who had taken rGH for several days after cessation of treatment. To achieve this, specific formulae have been developed, which take into account the influence of gender on the index calculated from both markers.[19] During the past years, several studies have been performed to validate the marker approach in different cohorts of subjects and with respect to different potentially confounding factors. With respect to gender, it is known that GH-deficient males are more sensitive to GH administration than GH-deficient females.[20] In agreement with this, it seems that a higher percentage of males than females exhibit a pronounced increase in the index calculated from the concentrations of the markers, and that the window of opportunity to detect administration of rGH is longer in males than in females.[21] It is well known that, in addition to gender, age also has major influences on GH secretory capacity, and as a consequence on the concentrations of the markers. Consequently, a correct interpretation of the concentrations of the markers found in samples taken from athletes would require age-adjusted normative data. A large cross-sectional study was performed in athletes from several disciplines.[22] The study confirmed that age was the major determinant for the variability of the markers. To make the reference data even more reliable, the effect of ethnic background was also studied. Older studies had indicated ethnic differences in endogenous GH secretion,[23] but the previously mentioned cross-sectional study had included mainly White athletes. Several studies meanwhile have shown that ethnic differences in circulating concentrations are mainly seen for IGFBPs, but not for IGF-I.[24,25] Overall, the impact of ethnic background on the index used to detect previous administration of GH by the marker approach seems to be limited.[24] Furthermore, in another study the authors were able to demonstrate that the between-individual variability in the index is much greater than the within-individual changes observed when no GH was administered. They conclude that the variability is mainly determined genetically, and that an "athlete's passport" documenting the individual marker levels over time could be a possibility to enhance the sensitivity of the test.[26] In an independent study on the within-individual variability and the analytical imprecision,[27] it was confirmed that the variability is comparably small and that use of a Bayesian approach allows prediction of future IGF-I values from a single measurement in an untreated individual with sufficient reliability. Another aspect investigated by GH2000 was the impact of injury on the test outcome in an athlete. Injury of course could affect markers of bone and connective tissue turnover. In an observational longitudinal study investigating the serum levels of the markers after musculoskeletal or soft tissue injury, it was found that levels of IGF-I did not change, but levels of PIIIP increased by about 40% in the weeks after injury. However, when the discriminate functions for the "marker approach" were applied, no subject would have been erroneously declared positive for GH doping. The authors conclude that the order of magnitude of the changes in PIIIP seen after injury was unable to invalidate the marker approach.[28]

Similar to the "isoform approach" described later in this article, the "marker approach" is based on quantification of serum proteins in blood samples by immunoassays. It has been repeatedly demonstrated that protein concentrations as revealed by immunoassay measurement are highly dependent on the specific method used. This is mainly a consequence of the different antibodies used in different immunoassays. Therefore, it would be highly desirable that doping test authorities such as WADA were in a position where they have control over the antibodies used in such assays to guarantee consistency of the assay results obtained. For the same reason of consistency over time, the use of monoclonal antibodies for assays used in the context of doping controls must be preferred. Otherwise, it might be necessary to re-establish normative data for each new assay or assay lot used. However, in view of the promising and extensive studies conducted during the past decade to validate the marker approach, it seems to be very appropriate to also investigate the development of standardized assay methods that then should be available for long-term use in WADA-accredited laboratories.

DETECTING GROWTH HORMONE DOPING BASED ON ANALYSIS OF GROWTH HORMONE ISOFORMS

The second major strategic approach to detect GH doping was first described in 1999[29] and is based on the direct analysis of GH, or more precisely, analysis of various molecular isoforms of GH in circulation. The rationale behind this approach is that rGH is identical only to the monomer of the most abundant GH isoform in circulation, the 22-kD GH isoform. However, GH as occurring in the human body normally consists of a large spectrum of different isoforms.[30–32] To further increase complexity, those isoforms exist as homo- and heterodimers or multimers. Pituitary secretion of endogenous GH isoforms is suppressed when rGH is injected,[33,34] and therefore the 22-kD isoform becomes the only or at least the predominant GH isoform in circulation. Given that sensitive and specific assays to asses the isoform composition in an athlete's sample are available, a doping test could be designed where an inappropriately high percentage of 22-kD GH in a sample would indicate illicit use of rGH. The isoform approach in its classical form[29] consists of two assays: One assay preferentially recognizes the monomeric 22-kD isoform (also named "rec assay"), whereas the other recognizes a broad spectrum of GH isoforms (also called "pit assay"). Each sample is tested by both assays. In a sample taken after administration of rGH, the relative abundance of 22-kD GH is increased, and therefore the result in assay one (the "rec assay") tends to be higher, whereas because of the suppression of the other isoforms the result in assay two (the "pit assay") tends to be lower. The ratio between both results ("rec/pit ratio") is used as an index to detect previous rGH application, and this ratio is increased if the sample is taken after rGH application.[4,35] It could be shown that based on analysis of the rec/pit ratios it is possible to clearly discriminate between subjects with and without rGH administration.[29,36] Further validation was done by analysis of the impact of acute exercise on GH isoforms in circulation. It could be demonstrated that, although during exercise 22-kD GH increases slightly more than the other isoforms, whereas after exercise the other isoforms tend to become somewhat more predominant, the corresponding changes in the rec/pit ratio are only marginal.[37,38] Of course, because the half-life of GH in circulation is very short, the window of opportunity for detection is limited. It had been shown that in some individuals suppression of GH isoforms other than 22-kD lasts for more than 30 hours,[33,36] but detecting a cheating athlete is most likely during the first 24 hours. This has raised concerns about the usefulness of this test during competitions,[14] as athletes easily can avoid a positive test result by stopping medication a few days in advance of the competition. Clearly, the potential of this isoform approach lies in the implementation for routine out-of-competition testing, and it is also mandatory to dramatically increase the number of blood samples taken during such tests. As mentioned previously for the marker method, the isoform approach also relies on immunoassays. To fulfill the requirements for test methods used in an antidoping laboratory as specified by WADA guidelines, it is necessary to have a second, independent assay to confirm the results of any measurement obtained by immunoassays. This independent assay must be based on independent antibodies, recognizing an epitope that is different from the epitope used in the first test. In the case of the isoform approach this made it necessary to develop two pairs of rec- and pit-assays.[35] Meanwhile, the assays are available to WADA-accredited laboratories in a certified and standardized format, and the epitopes of the antibodies used in the assays have been published.[36] Based on research reagents, the assays had already been used in a test period in WADA-accredited laboratories during the Athens Olympic Games in the summer of 2004 and during the Torino Olympic Games in the winter of 2006.[39] However, the first use of the official certified format of the tests was made during the Beijing Olympic Games in the summer of 2008, where about 500 samples were tested. Not really to the surprise of the experts, no positive test result was reported; again it became clear that most likely the test is most successfully used in an out-of-competition setting because of the limited window of opportunity. A substantial increase in the number of blood samples taken in out-of-competition tests is required to increase the chance of catching the cheaters.

Meanwhile, the principle of the isoform approach has also been applied using other assays. For example, it is also possible to use specific immunoassays for 20-kD GH to detect the suppression of 20-kD GH after injection of 22 kD and to obtain the ratio of 20-kD GH over 22-kD GH as an indicator of rGH use. In addition, it has been proposed to use immunoassays based on surface plasmon resonance to investigate isoform composition in an athlete's samples.[40] Other new developments include the use of 2-dimensional gel electrophoresis to visualize the isoforms present in a sample,[10] and also to identify the isoforms from the spots in the gel via mass spectrometry.[11] Overall, the field of methods based on the isoform approach is developing, and it might be expected that in the future more than one method will be used to increase the possibility to detect doping with GH.[41]

SUMMARY

In summary, the work of several groups during the past decade has allowed the development and validation of two independent strategies to detect abuse of GH. The marker approach is in the final stages of validation, whereas the isoform approach is already implemented in many WADA-accredited laboratories. Each of the methods has its difficulties, but both clearly demonstrate that detection of GH doping is possible "beyond reasonable doubt."[42] Full implementation of the isoform assays in WADA-accredited laboratories, organization of sufficient supplies with assays of consistent quality for the markers, and subsequent implementation in the laboratories as well as significant increases in the number of blood samples taken during doping controls worldwide remain the challenges for the next years.

REFERENCES

1. Rennie MJ. Claims for the anabolic effects of growth hormone: a case of the emperor's new clothes? Br J Sports Med 2003;37:100.
2. Holt RI, Erotokritou-Mulligan I, Sonksen PH. The history of doping and growth hormone abuse in sport. Growth Horm IGF Res 2009;19:320.
3. Barroso O, Schamasch P, Rabin O. Detection of GH abuse in sport: past, present and future. Growth Horm IGF Res 2009;19:369.
4. Bidlingmaier M, Strasburger CJ. Technology insight: detecting growth hormone abuse in athletes. Nat Clin Pract Endocrinol Metab 2007;3:769.
5. Lasne F. Double-blotting: a solution to the problem of non-specific binding of secondary antibodies in immunoblotting procedures. J Immunol Methods 2001; 253:125.
6. Lasne F, de Ceaurriz J. Recombinant erythropoietin in urine. Nature 2000;405: 635.

7. Veldhuis JD, Bidlingmaier M, Anderson SM, et al. Impact of experimental blockade of peripheral growth hormone (GH) receptors on the kinetics of endogenous and exogenous GH removal in healthy women and men. J Clin Endocrinol Metab 2002;87:5737.
8. Armanini D, Faggian D, Scaroni C, et al. Growth hormone and insulin-like growth factor I in a Sydney Olympic gold medallist. Br J Sports Med 2002;36:148.
9. Bowers LD. Analytical advances in detection of performance-enhancing compounds. Clin Chem 1997;43:1299.
10. Kohler M, Puschel K, Sakharov D, et al. Detection of recombinant growth hormone in human plasma by a 2-D PAGE method. Electrophoresis 2008;29:4495.
11. Kohler M, Thomas A, Puschel K, et al. Identification of human pituitary growth hormone variants by mass spectrometry. J Proteome Res 2009;8:1071.
12. Leger J, Reverchon C, Porquet D, et al. The wide variation in urinary excretion of human growth hormone in normal growing and growth hormone-deficient children limits its clinical usefulness. Horm Res 1995;44:57.
13. Saugy M, Cardis C, Schweizer C, et al. Detection of human growth hormone doping in urine: out of competition tests are necessary. J Chromatogr B Biomed Appl 1996;687:201.
14. Sonksen P. The International Olympic Committee (IOC) and GH-2000. Growth Horm IGF Res 2009;19:341.
15. Le Roith D, Bondy C, Yakar S, et al. The somatomedin hypothesis: 2001. Endocr Rev 2001;22:53.
16. Wallace JD, Cuneo RC, Baxter R, et al. Responses of the growth hormone (GH) and insulin-like growth factor axis to exercise, GH administration, and GH withdrawal in trained adult males: a potential test for GH abuse in sport. J Clin Endocrinol Metab 1999;84:3591.
17. Longobardi S, Keay N, Ehrnborg C, et al. Growth hormone (GH) effects on bone and collagen turnover in healthy adults and its potential as a marker of GH abuse in sports: a double blind, placebo-controlled study. The GH-2000 Study Group. J Clin Endocrinol Metab 2000;85:1505.
18. Wallace JD, Cuneo RC, Lundberg PA, et al. Responses of markers of bone and collagen turnover to exercise, growth hormone (GH) administration, and GH withdrawal in trained adult males. J Clin Endocrinol Metab 2000;85:124.
19. Erotokritou-Mulligan I, Bassett EE, Kniess A, et al. Validation of the growth hormone (GH)-dependent marker method of detecting GH abuse in sport through the use of independent data sets. Growth Horm IGF Res 2007;17:416.
20. Burman P, Johansson AG, Siegbahn A, et al. Growth hormone (GH)-deficient men are more responsive to GH replacement therapy than women. J Clin Endocrinol Metab 1997;82:550.
21. Powrie JK, Bassett EE, Rosen T, et al. Detection of growth hormone abuse in sport. Growth Horm IGF Res 2007;17:220.
22. Healy ML, Dall R, Gibney J, et al. Toward the development of a test for growth hormone (GH) abuse: a study of extreme physiological ranges of GH-dependent markers in 813 elite athletes in the postcompetition setting. J Clin Endocrinol Metab 2005;90:641.
23. Wright NM, Renault J, Willi S, et al. Greater secretion of growth hormone in black than in white men: possible factor in greater bone mineral density—a clinical research center study. J Clin Endocrinol Metab 1995;80:2291.
24. Erotokritou-Mulligan I, Bassett EE, Cowan DA, et al. Influence of ethnicity on IGF-I and procollagen III peptide (P-III-P) in elite athletes and its effect on the ability to detect GH abuse. Clin Endocrinol (Oxf) 2009;70:161.

25. Nelson AE, Howe CJ, Nguyen TV, et al. Influence of demographic factors and sport type on growth hormone-responsive markers in elite athletes. J Clin Endocrinol Metab 2006;91:4424.
26. Erotokritou-Mulligan I, Eryl Bassett E, Cowan D, et al. The use of growth hormone (GH)-dependent markers in the detection of GH abuse in sport: physiological intra-individual variation of IGF-I, type 3 pro-collagen (P-III-P) and the GH-2000 detection score. Clin Endocrinol (Oxf), 2009 [Epub ahead of print].
27. Nguyen TV, Nelson AE, Howe CJ, et al. Within-subject variability and analytic imprecision of insulinlike growth factor axis and collagen markers: implications for clinical diagnosis and doping tests. Clin Chem 2008;54:1268.
28. Erotokritou-Mulligan I, Bassett EE, Bartlett C, et al. The effect of sports injury on insulin-like growth factor-I and type 3 procollagen: implications for detection of growth hormone abuse in athletes. J Clin Endocrinol Metab 2008;93:2760.
29. Wu Z, Bidlingmaier M, Dall R, et al. Detection of doping with human growth hormone. Lancet 1999;353:895.
30. Baumann G. Growth hormone heterogeneity in human pituitary and plasma. Horm Res 1999;51:2.
31. Baumann G. Growth hormone heterogeneity: genes, isohormones, variants, and binding proteins. Endocr Rev 1991;12:424.
32. Baumann GP. Growth hormone isoforms. Growth Horm IGF Res 2009;19:333.
33. Keller A, Wu Z, Kratzsch J, et al. Pharmacokinetics and pharmacodynamics of GH: dependence on route and dosage of administration. Eur J Endocrinol 2007;156:647.
34. Leung KC, Howe C, Gui LY, et al. Physiological and pharmacological regulation of 20-kDa growth hormone. Am J Physiol Endocrinol Metab 2002;283:E836.
35. Bidlingmaier M, Wu Z, Strasburger CJ. Test method: GH. Baillieres Best Pract Res Clin Endocrinol Metab 2000;14:99.
36. Bidlingmaier M, Suhr J, Ernst A, et al. High-sensitivity chemiluminescence immunoassays for detection of growth hormone doping in sports. Clin Chem 2009;55: 445.
37. Wallace JD, Cuneo RC, Bidlingmaier M, et al. Changes in non-22-kilodalton (kDa) isoforms of growth hormone (GH) after administration of 22-kDa recombinant human GH in trained adult males. J Clin Endocrinol Metab 2001;86:1731.
38. Wallace JD, Cuneo RC, Bidlingmaier M, et al. The response of molecular isoforms of growth hormone to acute exercise in trained adult males. J Clin Endocrinol Metab 2001;86:200.
39. Saugy M, Robinson N, Saudan C, et al. Human growth hormone doping in sport. Br J Sports Med 2006;40(Suppl 1):i35.
40. Gutierrez-Gallego R, Bosch J, Such-Sanmartin G, et al. Surface plasmon resonance immuno assays—a perspective. Growth Horm IGF Res 2009;19:388.
41. Segura J, Gutierrez-Gallego R, Ventura R, et al. Growth hormone in sport: beyond Beijing 2008. Ther Drug Monit 2009;31:3.
42. Holt RI. Beyond reasonable doubt: catching the growth hormone cheats. Pediatr Endocrinol Rev 2007;4:228.

Insulin-like Growth Factor I and Insulin and Their Abuse in Sport

Ioulietta Erotokritou-Mulligan, PhD*,
Richard I.G. Holt, PhD, FRCP

KEYWORDS

• Insulin-like growth factor I • Insulin • Doping in sport

It is widely accepted that growth hormone (GH) is abused by athletes for its lipolytic and anabolic properties, and over the last decade several high profile athletes have admitted to using GH as part of their training regimens despite its inclusion in the World Anti-Doping Agency (WADA) Prohibited Substances List.[1,2]

The anabolic effects of GH are mediated at least in part by the generation of the mitogenic polypeptide, insulin-like growth factor-I (IGF-I). Together with insulin, GH and IGF-I form part of a complex mechanism that regulates the supply of nutrients to tissues during fasting and feeding.[3] It is therefore perhaps unsurprising that there are now reports that insulin and IGF-I increasingly are being abused by athletes with GH to form a powerful cocktail to enhance performance.[1]

Insulin and recombinant human (rh)GH have been widely available for clinical use for many years but only recently have commercial preparations for rhIGF-I been developed.[4,5] Together with less pure compounds that are produced for scientific research but are not intended for human use, the wide accessibility to these hormones is likely to lead to an increase in their misuse.

The aim of this article is to discuss what is known about the misuse of IGF-I and insulin, the reasons why athletes choose these hormones, and the methodologies that are being developed to detect their use. The use of GH is discussed in a separate article in this publication.

The GH-2004 project is supported by the World Anti-Doping Agency and US Anti-Doping Agency.

Endocrinology & Metabolism Unit, Developmental Origins of Health and Disease Division, University of Southampton, School of Medicine, Southampton, Hampshire, UK
* Corresponding author. The Institute of Developmental Sciences (IDS Building), MP887, Southampton General Hospital, Tremona Road, Southampton S016 6YD, Hampshire, UK.
E-mail address: I.E.Mulligan@soton.ac.uk (I. Erotokritou-Mulligan).

DOPING WITH IGF-I

Until recently, IGF-I was only available in limited supply, partly because there is no natural source for this hormone and partly because there were no pharmaceutical preparations. The only available form of recombinant IGF-I was produced by biotechnology companies for use in research into cellular growth and into the treatment of conditions such as myotonic dystrophy. Its complex molecular structure precluded amateur synthesis, and as such, doping with IGF-I has not been as extensive as GH or insulin.

This situation has changed recently with the development of two compounds, Mecasermin Tercica (Increlex) by Tercica (Brisbane, CA) and Mecasermin Rinfabate (iPLEX) by Insmed (Richmond, VA).[4,5] The former is rhIGF-I alone, while the latter is a compound containing rhIGF-I bound to rhIGFBP-3, its major binding protein, in equimolar proportions. Both preparations have received US Food and Drug Administration (FDA) approval for clinical use in the treatment of growth failure in children with severe primary IGF-I deficiency or with GH gene deletion who have developed neutralizing GH antibodies. Future possible clinical indications for rhIGF-I include other growth disorders, severe insulin resistance syndromes such as Rabson-Mendenhall syndrome, osteopenia, and burns. Clinical trials also have suggested that rhIGF-I may be beneficial for treating patients with type 1 diabetes, although further development in this area has been halted because of concerns over the potential development of diabetic retinopathy.

Despite the limited production and availability, it would appear that IGF-I already is being abused by athletes and bodybuilders. There are over 100,000 hits on the Internet describing IGF-I in the context of bodybuilding. IGF-I is reported to be much more powerful than rhGH, and its purported benefits include improvements in energy and endurance, tissue repair, muscle growth, sexual enhancement and endurance, immune balance, bone density, anti-aging, fat loss, rebuilding of cartilage (through high concentrations of glucosamine sulfate), ligament repair, skin rejuvenation, blood glucose level improvement, stress reduction, and improved mood and mental acuity, as well as acting as an anti-inflammatory and nerve regeneration agent.

There are many sites advertising the sale of IGF-I on the black market, although the veracity of these claims has not been established. The genie appears to be out of the bottle, and as its supply increases, it seems likely that the misuse of IGF-I will increase.

DOPING WITH INSULIN

Unlike IGF-I, insulin and insulin analogs are widely available in clinical practice. Although a prescription-only medication in the UK, a pharmacist may dispense insulin as an emergency medicine if he or she believes the patient has diabetes. Although there is a charge for this, this is considerably lower than the black market price.[6]

Similar to the situation regarding rhGH, there is only vague information about the use of insulin by professional athletes, and most of this is anecdotal. The first suggestions of insulin as an anabolic agent were published in two bodybuilding magazines in 1996, which were commented upon in the British Journal of Sports Medicine in 1997.[6] Dawson also raised concerns about the increase in the use of insulin following a regular increase in the number of inquiries about insulin as an anabolic agent. In the same letter, Dawson stated that 6 out of 200 clients attending a drugs in sport clinic admitted to using insulin.

At the Winter Olympic Games in Nagano in 1998, a Russian medical officer enquired whether the use of insulin was restricted to type 1 diabetes.[7] This drew attention to its role as a potential performance-enhancing drug and immediately led to its ban by the

International Olympic Committee. Athletes with insulin requiring diabetes, however, may use insulin with a therapeutic use exemption certificate.

As part of his attempt to be included in the 2008 British Olympic team, the sprinter Dwain Chambers provided the British Authorities with a description of what he was taking when he failed his drug test in 2003, including how much he was taking of each substance and when exactly he was taking them. The account was written by Victor Conte, the founder and owner of the Bay Area Laboratory Co-operative. The report describes how insulin was used after strenuous weight training sessions during the off-season. Three units of the fast-acting insulin lispro were injected immediately after the workout sessions together with a glucose and protein drink with the purpose of replenishing glycogen and adenosine triphosphate (ATP) quickly and promoting protein synthesis and muscle growth.

Further anecdotal evidence comes from Conte, who alleged that he personally provided Marion Jones and other athletes with a number of performance enhancing concoctions that included a number of peptide hormones including insulin, erythropoietin, and human GH.

The biggest case involving IGF-I and insulin abuse was also Spain's biggest doping scandal, which was coded by the Spanish police as Operación Puerto. This case focused on Dr. Eufemiano Fuentes and his accomplices. Following several police raids, evidence was gathered suggesting that nearly 200 high-profile athletes including Tyler Hamilton and Alberto Contador were provided with a large variety of performance-enhancing substances in carefully designed doping regimens by Fuentes and his colleagues. The trial has been ongoing since May 2006, and as doping is not a criminal offense in Spain, it is unlikely that the case will result in a prosecution.

WHY DO ATHLETES ABUSE IGF-I AND INSULIN?

To understand why athletes abuse IGF-I and insulin, it is important to review the physiology of the GH-IGF axis and the actions of IGF-I and insulin. It is also important to understand how these three hormones act in a coordinate manner regulating nutrient supply during the fed and fasting states.

IGF-I Physiology

GH is secreted from the anterior pituitary gland in a pulsatile fashion and exerts its anabolic actions at least in part by the generation of IGF-I. IGF-I is a small peptide of 7.5 kDa, comprising 70 amino acids with structural homology to insulin.[8] Most circulating IGF-I is derived from the liver, but it is believed that IGF-I is produced almost ubiquitously. IGF-I exerts its effects through endocrine, paracrine, and autocrine actions.

The importance of GH in regulating the production of IGF-I is shown in people with acromegaly who have elevated IGF-I concentrations. In contrast, people with GH deficiency have low IGF-I concentrations. Furthermore, as GH secretion falls with aging, there is a concomitant decline in serum IGF-I.[9]

In addition to GH, there are several other important regulators of IGF-I production including insulin and nutritional status. Although overnight fasting and feeding have little effect on IGF-I, with more prolonged fasting, IGF-I concentrations fall. In contrast, insulin increases IGF-I production by the liver in response to GH. Thyroid status and estrogen and cortisol levels all affect IGF-I production.

Less than 1% to 5% of circulating IGF-I is free IGF-I, with most of the rest (75% to 90%) existing in a ternary protein complex bound to IGF binding protein-3 (IGFBP-3) and an acid labile subunit (ALS). The effect of this association is to prolong the circulating half-life of IGF-I from a few minutes to approximately 12 to 15 hours.[10] Consequently, serum IGF-I is much more stable than GH, and many factors that influence GH concentrations such as circadian rhythm or the pulsatile nature of pituitary hGH release have minimal or no effect on IGF-I. This has important consequences for the therapeutic use of IGF-I. When IGF-I is administered by subcutaneous injection to healthy volunteers, the peak IGF-I concentration is reached after about 7 hours, and IGF-I is cleared with a half-life of approximately 20 hours.[11]

Actions of IGF-I

Anabolic actions

The metabolic and anabolic actions of GH first were identified in the 1930s.[12] GH alters body composition by increasing muscle mass and decreasing fat mass through its actions on protein synthesis and lipolysis.[13] IGF-I is an important mediator of the growth promoting effects of GH. This was first shown in the classic experiments of Salmon and Daughaday in 1957.[14] Normal rat serum stimulates sulfate uptake into cartilage, whereas serum from hypophysectomized animals does not, even if GH is added to the serum. The somatomedin subsequently was identified as IGF-I. The endocrine function of IGF-I recently has been called into question by experiments involving transgenic animals in which the gene for IGF-I is selectively deleted in the liver. These animals grow normally despite having only 10% to 25% of serum IGF-I concentrations compared with controls, indicating the importance of local paracrine and autocrine effects.[15,16]

When administered exogenously, IGF-I has potent anabolic effects that are similar to the effects to GH. IGF-I promotes protein synthesis directly,[17] in part by enhancing the uptake of amino acids for muscle synthesis, provided there is an adequate supply of amino acids (**Fig. 1**). Using radiolabeled amino acids, human studies have shown that infusions of rhIGF-I reduced proteolysis[18] and increased protein synthesis.[17] The increased protein synthesis may have functional benefits as has been demonstrated in mice where IGF-I is selectively overexpressed in skeletal muscle. These mice develop functional myocyte hypertrophy that is resistant to age-related muscle atrophy and other disease-related cachexia.[19]

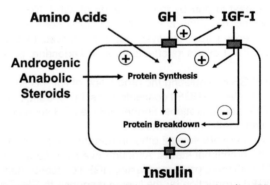

Fig. 1. This diagram illustrates the synergistic actions between insulin, IGF-I, and GH in regulating protein synthesis. GH and IGF-I stimulate protein synthesis directly, while insulin is mainly anabolic through the inhibition of protein breakdown. The anabolic action of both GH and IGF-I appears to be mediated through induction of amino acid transporters in the cell membrane.

IGF-I administration reverses the catabolic effects of a calorie-restricted diet in normal volunteers, and this reversal is enhanced substantially when IGF-I is given concomitantly with GH.[20]

Children with GH insensitivity syndrome provide the best evidence of the effect of IGF-I on linear growth. These individuals who lack the GH receptor have profound growth retardation that is reversed by treatment with IGF-I.[21]

Glucose metabolism

IGF-I has important actions on glucose metabolism.[22] The IGF-I hepatic knock-out mice are hyperinsulinemic and develop insulin resistance, despite being leaner than wild-type mice.[23] Similarly, in patients with GH insensitivity syndrome, there is a decrease in carbohydrate oxidation and an increase in hepatic glucose production.[21]

When IGF-I is given to rats as an intravenous infusion, it causes hypoglycemia by stimulating peripheral glucose uptake, glycolysis, and glycogen synthesis, but it only has a minimal effect on hepatic glucose production.[24] The effect in people is similar: a single intravenous dose of 100 µg/kg results in the rapid onset of symptomatic hypoglycemia and is equipotent to 0.15 IU/kg of insulin.[25] Insulin sensitivity is increased with respect to glucose by IGF-I through increased peripheral glucose uptake and decreased hepatic glucose production.[26]

There was interest in treating patients with type 1 diabetes with IGF-I at a replacement dose to correct the derangements of the GH-IGF axis and exploit its hypoglycemic actions.[22] Although IGF-I improved glycemic control and reduced insulin requirements, these studies were halted because of concerns about the development of diabetic retinopathy. Nevertheless, the effects on glucose metabolism may be exploited by an athlete to allow rapid replenishment of muscle glycogen following a bout of exercise.

Lipid metabolism

IGF-I administration increases the rates of lipolysis and lipid oxidation, although the mechanism remains unclear. The action may be indirect through a suppression of circulating insulin by rhIGF-I, but the presence of IGF-I receptors in mature human adipocytes raises the possibility that rhIGF-I has direct lipolytic effects on adipose tissue.[27] By contrast, it appears that GH induces lipolysis directly by acting on adipose tissue, acting through GH receptors that are abundantly expressed on adipocytes. Increased lipolysis may have several benefits for performance. First, it would provide an abundant fuel source for endurance events while preserving glycogen stores and protein. Furthermore, in the longer term, fat mass may reduce.

INSULIN PHYSIOLOGY

Insulin is a 51 amino acid peptide hormone comprising two polypeptide chains, which are linked by disulphide bridges. Insulin is synthesized and secreted in a coordinated pulsatile fashion from the β-cells of the islets of Langerhans in the pancreas into the portal vein in a characteristic biphasic pattern. Pancreatic β-cells secrete 0.25 to 1.5 units of insulin per hour during the fasting state, accounting for over 50% of total daily insulin secretion, with the remainder being meal-related insulin secretion. Glucose is the principal stimulus for insulin secretion, although other macronutrients and hormonal and neuronal factors also may alter this response.

Actions of Insulin

Insulin exerts its biologic actions by binding to the heterotetrameric insulin receptor on the target cell surface, initiating a cascade of intracellular signaling. Insulin is considered as a hormone that signals the fed state and as the pivotal hormone regulating cellular energy supply and macronutrient balance and directing anabolic processes during the fed state. It has major anabolic actions on intermediate metabolism, affecting glucose, lipid, and protein metabolism. The major insulin-sensitive tissues are the liver, skeletal muscle, and adipose tissue. Approximately 60% of insulin is cleared during the first pass through the liver, so portal vein insulin concentrations reaching the liver are almost threefold higher than in the peripheral circulation.

Glucose Metabolism

Normally plasma glucose concentration is maintained within a narrow range despite wide fluctuations in nutrient supply and demand, with insulin being the prime regulator. Insulin regulates hepatic glucose output by inhibiting gluconeogenesis and promoting glycogen storage. Similarly, in muscle cells, insulin-mediated glucose uptake enables glycogen to be synthesized and stored, and for carbohydrates, rather than fatty acids or amino acids, to be utilized as the immediately available energy source for muscle contraction. The many actions of insulin on carbohydrate metabolism are shown in **Table 1**. The use of insulin following a bout of exercise may replenish glycogen and ATP stores more quickly than rest or feeding alone.

Table 1
Insulin actions on carbohydrate and fat metabolism

Action	Mechanism
Glucose metabolism	
Increases glucose uptake into cells	Translocation of GLUT-4 glucose transporter to cell surface
Increases glycogen synthesis	Activates glycogen synthase by dephosphorylation
Inhibits glycogen breakdown	Inactivates glycogen phosphorylase kinase by dephosphorylation
Inhibits gluconeogenesis	Dephosphorylation of pyruvate kinase and 2,6 biphosphate kinase
Increases glycolysis	Dephosphorylation of pyruvate kinase and 2,6 biphosphate kinase
Converts pyruvate to acetyl-CoA	Activates the intra-mitochondrial enzyme complex pyruvate dehydrogenase
Fat metabolism	
Increases fatty acid synthesis	Activation and increased phosphorylation of acetyl-CoA carboxylase
Suppression of fatty acid oxidation	Inhibition of carnitine acyltransferase
Increases triglyceride synthesis	Stimulates esterification of glycerol phosphate
Inhibits triglyceride breakdown	Dephosphorylation of hormone sensitive lipase
Increases cholesterol synthesis	Activation and dephosphorylation of 3-hydroxy-3-methyl-glutary-CoA (IHMG CoA) reductase
Inhibition of cholesterol ester breakdown	Dephosphorylation of cholesterol esterase

Lipid Metabolism

Insulin promotes the storage of lipids and suppresses adipose tissue fat breakdown. It increases the rate of lipogenesis in several ways in adipose tissue and the liver and controls the formation and storage of triglyceride (see **Table 1**). The critical step in lipogenesis is the activation of the insulin-sensitive lipoprotein lipase in the capillaries, allowing the uptake of fatty acids into adipose tissue. Triglyceride synthesis is stimulated by esterification of glycerol phosphate, while triglyceride breakdown is suppressed by dephosphorylation of hormone-sensitive lipase.

Protein Metabolism

While insulin stimulates the uptake of amino acid into cells and promotes protein synthesis in a range of tissues at high insulin concentrations, the major action of insulin is to inhibit the breakdown of proteins, which occurs at lower insulin concentrations (see **Fig. 1**).

INTEGRATED ACTIONS OF GH, IGF-I, AND INSULIN DURING FEEDING AND FASTING

Although IGF-I and insulin have distinct important roles in protein and carbohydrate metabolism, their actions are interlinked, regulating fluctuations in energy supply and demand.[3] During the fed state, insulin concentrations rise while GH is low. As the individual moves toward the postabsorptive period, insulin concentrations begin to decline while GH increases. In the fed state, IGFBP-1 falls, which may increase the bioavailability of free IGF-I.[22] In contrast to this acute regulation, the effect of GH on IGF-I is more chronic.

There is considerable evidence that under normal physiologic conditions these three hormones act in a coordinated way to regulate nutrient supply during fasting and feeding. During feeding, insulin is the major anabolic hormone storing all fuels, while GH is the major anabolic hormone during feeding and stress, including exercise, sparing glucose and protein at the expense of lipids. When there are conditions of energy surplus, nitrogen retention is promoted, but when food is sparse, GH alters fuel consumption from the use of carbohydrates and protein to the use of lipids, thereby allowing conservation of vital protein stores.

There is anecdotal evidence that athletes are using a combination of GH, IGF-I, and insulin to exploit this effect.

THE EFFECT OF IGF-I AND INSULIN ON EXERCISE PERFORMANCE

At present there are no clinical or scientific trials that have shown a performance benefit for either IGF-I or insulin, either alone or in combination with other drugs.[1] This is not to say, however, that there is no performance benefit. Most scientists regard randomized controlled trials (RCTs) as the gold standard for determining cause and effect; however, the format of these trials may not be the best way of determining whether IGF-I or insulin has a performance benefit. Most RCTs do not have the power to detect the small differences that might mean the difference between a gold medal and not even making the final. Furthermore, most trials are designed to test one or at most two interventions, while as illustrated previously, athletes frequently combine performance-enhancing drugs. It seems likely that the athletes using the "n=1" design are in a better position to address the question whether these hormones are performance-enhancing, and one may need to accept that trials may never establish whether IGF-I or insulin enhances performance.

POTENTIAL ADVERSE EFFECTS OF IGF-I AND INSULIN ADMINISTRATION

There is only limited clinical experience with the use of rhIGF-I; therefore, most of the known adverse effects relate to short-term usage only from the clinical trials involving people with diabetes or GH insensitivity syndrome. The adverse effects that have been reported with Increlex, the pure rhIGF-I preparation, include hypoglycemia, jaw pain, headache, myalgias, and fluid retention.[28] Mecasermin Rinfabate (rhIGF-I bound to rhIGFBP-3 in equimolar proportions) appears to be associated with fewer adverse effects, because the drug forms a ternary complex with ALS more readily than rhIGF-I alone.[5] This prolongs its half-life and clinical efficacy while buffering the acute effects of rhIGF-I. The most common adverse effects observed so far with the use of Mecasermin Rinfabate include local injection site erythema and lipohypertrophy, although headaches, increased liver and kidney size, and altered liver function tests also have been reported.

Current knowledge of the long-term effects of IGF-I comes from an IGF-I administration study of up to 12 years involving children with GH insensitivity syndrome. In this study, a significant number of children showed increased tonsillar and adenoidal tissue growth during treatment, but this reverted back to the original condition following discontinuation of treatment.[29]

It also seems reasonable to hypothesize that IGF-I could result in adverse effects that are similar to acromegaly, as the anabolic effects of GH are closely related to the production of IGF-I in different tissues. There is, therefore, a potential risk of an acromegalic-like cardiomyopathy that is characterized by concentric biventricular hypertrophy, valve dysfunction, and diastolic dysfunction initially, which can progress to systolic dysfunction at rest if left untreated.[30] There is also concern about the risk of cancer, as in vitro studies show that IGF-I stimulates proliferation of transformed neoplastic cell clones and the growth of pre-existing tumor tissues.[31] Furthermore, a positive correlation has been observed between circulating IGF-I concentrations and the incidence of prostate and colorectal cancers.[32,33] Although there is a continued debate about the risk of cancer in acromegaly, vigilance will be required.

The adverse effects of insulin are well documented from experience in treating people with diabetes. The most commonly experienced adverse effect is hypoglycemia. Weight gain is also a problem in people with diabetes, but this is probably less of an issue for athletes whose diet and training regimen are closely monitored.

DETECTION OF IGF-I ABUSE IN SPORT

At present there is no specific test to detect IGF-I abuse. The main challenge lies in distinguishing exogenous IGF-I from endogenously produced IGF-I, as rhIGF-I is structurally identical to endogenous IGF-I. As a result, techniques such as electrophoresis, which rely on electrical charge differences to distinguish endogenous and exogenous forms of prohibited hormones such as erythropoietin,[34] cannot be used to detect IGF-I administration.

The GH-2000 team and subsequently the GH-2004 team have developed a methodology for the detecting GH abuse. This methodology involves the measurement of serum IGF-I and type 3 procollagen in combination with discriminant function analysis. It may be possible to use a similar approach to detect IGF-I abuse, not least because IGF-I is one of the markers proposed by the GH-2000 project.[1] IGF-I is also known to have a major role in the regulation of bone turnover.[35]

This approach is attractive, because it would allow the doping authorities to use a single test to detect doping with either GH or IGF-I, and WADA recently funded a further study by the GH-2004 team to assess whether a marker approach can be used to detect the administration of exogenous IGF-I.[36]

At present, the marker approach used by the GH-2004 team relies on the use of immunoassays, but a mass spectrometry method is under development.[37] This method has provided lower limits of detection (LLODs) between 20 and 50 ng/mL, and precision less than 15% at the LLOD and at higher concentration levels. There was a reasonable correlation with values obtained from a commercially available immunoradiometric assay, but the absolute concentrations were lower for the mass spectrometry procedure.

DETECTION OF INSULIN ABUSE IN SPORT

Many of the challenges in the detection of IGF-I are equally applicable to insulin. Although there are commercially available insulin assays, these do not differentiate between endogenous and exogenous insulin. Insulin may degrade after collection, and the results also may be adversely affected by hemolysis or the presence of circulating antiinsulin antibodies.

Although no test is available to detect human insulin, there are both urine and blood mass spectrometry methods that can detect insulin analogs.[38] Insulin analogs have been designed to alter their pharmacokinetics by genetic substitutions of one or two amino acids from human insulin. These small differences can be utilized to differentiate between native and exogenous insulin.

SUMMARY

There is anecdotal evidence that insulin and IGF-I are abused by professional athletes, often in combination with GH and anabolic steroids. Although insulin is widely available, IGF-I only recently was approved by the FDA for use in people. This is likely to increase its availability and consequently its abuse. Insulin and IGF-I work together with GH to control the supply of nutrients to tissues in the fasted and fed state. Actions that may enhance performance include the promotion of protein anabolism, glucose uptake, and storage as lipolysis. The detection of IGF-I and insulin abuse is challenging. There are established mass spectrometry methods for insulin analogs and an on-going study examining the feasibility of using GH-dependent markers to detect IGF-I use.

ACKNOWLEDGMENTS

The authors thank the rest of the GH-2004 team: Peter Sönksen, Eryl Bassett, David Cowan, Nishan Guha, and Christiaan Bartlett. They acknowledge the support of UK Sport (Michael Stow and Andy Parkinson), the Wellcome Trust Clinical Research Facility (WT-CRF) at Southampton General Hospital and its nurses, and the numerous Southampton medical students who have assisted in the authors' research.

REFERENCES

1. Holt RI, Sonksen PH. Growth hormone, IGF-I and insulin and their abuse in sport. Br J Pharmacol 2008;154(3):542–56.
2. World Anti-Doping Agency. The World Anti-Doping Code—the 2009 prohibited list International Standard. Available at: http://www.wada-ama.org/rtecontent/document/2009_Prohibited_List_ENG_Final_20_Sept_08.pdf. Accessed July 29, 2009.

3. Moller N, Jorgensen JO. Effects of growth hormone on glucose, lipid, and protein metabolism in human subjects. Endocr Rev 2009;30(2):152–77.
4. Norman P. Mecasermin tercica. Curr Opin Investig Drugs 2006;7(4):371–80.
5. Kemp SF. Mecasermin rinfabate. Drugs Today (Barc) 2007;43(3):149–55.
6. Dawson RT, Harrison MW. Use of insulin as an anabolic agent. Br J Sports Med 1997;31(3):259.
7. Sonksen PH. Insulin, growth hormone and sport. J Endocrinol 2001;170(1):13–25.
8. Rinderknecht E, Humbel RE. The amino acid sequence of human insulin-like growth factor I and its structural homology with proinsulin. J Biol Chem 1978; 253(8):2769–76.
9. Toogood AA. Growth hormone (GH) status and body composition in normal ageing and in elderly adults with GH deficiency. Horm Res 2003;60(Suppl 1): 105–11.
10. Guler HP, Zapf J, Schmid C, et al. Insulin-like growth factors I and II in healthy man. Estimations of half-lives and production rates. Acta Endocrinol 1989; 121(6):753–8.
11. Grahnen A, Kastrup K, Heinrich U, et al. Pharmacokinetics of recombinant human insulin-like growth factor I given subcutaneously to healthy volunteers and to patients with growth hormone receptor deficiency. Acta Paediatr Suppl 1993; 82(Suppl 391):9–13.
12. Houssay BA, Biasotti A. La diabetes pancreatica de los perros hipofiseoprivos. Rev Soc Argent Biol 1930;6:251–96.
13. Salomon F, Cuneo RC, Hesp R, et al. The effects of treatment with recombinant human growth hormone on body composition and metabolism in adults with growth hormone deficiency. N Engl J Med 1989;321(26):1797–803.
14. Salmon WD Jr, Daughaday WH. A hormonally controlled serum factor which stimulates sulfate incorporation by cartilage in vitro. J Lab Clin Med 1957;49(6): 825–36.
15. Sjogren K, Liu JL, Blad K, et al. Liver-derived insulin-like growth factor I (IGF-I) is the principal source of IGF-I in blood but is not required for postnatal body growth in mice. Proc Natl Acad Sci U S A 1999;96(12):7088–92.
16. Yakar S, Liu JL, Stannard B, et al. Normal growth and development in the absence of hepatic insulin-like growth factor I. Proc Natl Acad Sci U S A 1999; 96(13):7324–9.
17. Russell Jones DL, Umpleby AM, Hennessy TR, et al. Use of a leucine clamp to demonstrate that IGF-I actively stimulates protein synthesis in normal humans. Am J Phys 1994;267:591–8.
18. Fryburg DA. Insulin-like growth factor I exerts growth hormone- and insulin-like actions on human muscle protein metabolism. Am J Phys 1994;267: 331–6.
19. Musaro A, McCullagh K, Paul A, et al. Localized Igf-1 transgene expression sustains hypertrophy and regeneration in senescent skeletal muscle. Nat Genet 2001;27(2):195–200.
20. Clemmons DR, Smith-Banks A, Underwood LE. Reversal of diet-induced catabolism by infusion of recombinant insulin-like growth factor-I in humans. J Clin Endocrinol Metab 1992;75(1):234–8.
21. Laron Z. The essential role of IGF-I: lessons from the long-term study and treatment of children and adults with Laron syndrome. J Clin Endocrinol Metab 1999;84(12):4397–404.
22. Holt RI, Simpson HL, Sonksen PH. The role of the growth hormone–insulin-like growth factor axis in glucose homeostasis. Diabet Med 2003;20(1):3–15.

23. Sjogren K, Wallenius K, Liu JL, et al. Liver-derived IGF-I is of importance for normal carbohydrate and lipid metabolism. Diabetes 2001;50(7):1539–45.
24. Jacob R, Barrett E, Plewe G, et al. Acute effects of insulin-like growth factor I on glucose and amino acid metabolism in the awake fasted rat. Comparison with insulin. J Clin Invest 1989;83(5):1717–23.
25. Zenobi PD, Graf S, Ursprung H, et al. Effects of insulin-like growth factor-I on glucose tolerance, insulin levels, and insulin secretion. J Clin Invest 1992;89(6):1908–13.
26. Russell Jones DL, Bates AT, Umpleby AM, et al. A comparison of the effects of IGF-I and insulin on glucose metabolism, fat metabolism, and the cardiovascular system in normal human volunteers. Eur J Clin Invest 1995;25(6):403–11.
27. Mauras N, O'Brien KO, Welch S, et al. Insulin-like growth factor I and growth hormone (GH) treatment in GH-deficient humans: differential effects on protein, glucose, lipid, and calcium metabolism. J Clin Endocrinol Metab 2000;85(4):1686–94.
28. Williams RM, McDonald A, O'Savage M, et al. Mecasermin rinfabate: rhIGF-I/rhIGFBP-3 complex: iPLEX. Expert Opin Drug Metab Toxicol 2008;4(3):311–24.
29. Chernausek SD, Backeljauw PF, Frane J, et al. Long-term treatment with recombinant insulin-like growth factor (IGF)-I in children with severe IGF-I deficiency due to growth hormone insensitivity. J Clin Endocrinol Metab 2007;92(3):902–10.
30. Colao A, Marzullo P, Di Somma C, et al. Growth hormone and the heart. Clin Endocrinol 2001;54(2):137–54.
31. Wu Y, Yakar S, Zhao L, et al. Circulating insulin-like growth factor-I levels regulate colon cancer growth and metastasis. Cancer Res 2002;62(4):1030–5.
32. Nam RK, Trachtenberg J, Jewett MA, et al. Serum insulin-like growth factor-I levels and prostatic intraepithelial neoplasia: a clue to the relationship between IGF-I physiology and prostate cancer risk. Cancer Epidemiol Biomarkers Prev 2005;14(5):1270–3.
33. Giovannucci E, Pollak MN, Platz EA, et al. A prospective study of plasma insulin-like growth factor-1 and binding protein-3 and risk of colorectal neoplasia in women. Cancer Epidemiol Biomarkers Prev 2000;9(4):345–9.
34. Catlin DH, Breidbach A, Elliott S, et al. Comparison of the isoelectric focusing patterns of darbepoetin alfa, recombinant human erythropoietin, and endogenous erythropoietin from human urine. Clin Chem 2002;48(11):2057–9.
35. Kasukawa Y, Miyakoshi N, Mohan S. The anabolic effects of GH/IGF system on bone. Curr Pharm Des 2004;10(21):2577–92.
36. Guha N, Sonksen PH, Holt RI. IGF-I abuse in sport: Current knowledge and future prospects for detection. Growth Horm IGF Res 2009;19(4):408–11.
37. Bredehoft M, Schanzer W, Thevis M. Quantification of human insulin-like growth factor-1 and qualitative detection of its analogues in plasma using liquid chromatography/electrospray ionisation tandem mass spectrometry. Rapid Commun Mass Spectrom 2008;22(4):477–85.
38. Thevis M, Lohmann W, Schrader Y, et al. Use of an electrochemically synthesised metabolite of a selective androgen receptor modulator for mass spectrometry-based sports drug testing. Eur J Mass Spectrom 2008;14(3):163–70.

Sports-Related Issues and Biochemistry of Natural and Synthetic Anabolic Substances

Maria K. Parr, PhD[a], Ulrich Flenker, Dipl-Sportwiss[b], Wilhelm Schänzer, PhD[a],*

KEYWORDS

• Doping • Testosterone • Anabolic-androgenic steroids
• Selective androgen receptor modulators

Testosterone represents the principal male sex hormone. It is responsible for the growth of muscles, for the development of sexual organs, and for the maintenance of sexual functions. At the same time, it features psychotropic effects, where mostly aggressiveness appears to be promoted. These characteristics evidently render the substance an attractive compound to athletes. Testosterone remains one of the most frequently abused doping agents. Certainly the trend is supported by the fact that it is an endogenous substance, which—in contrast to xenobiotics—is relatively difficult to detect. Moreover, it may well be speculated that among dopers there is a perception that endogenous compounds are "natural." Hence, some might think such compounds have no harmful properties.

Of course, some reasons for exploiting the beneficial effects of this hormone can be perfectly ethical. For example, researchers have tried to use the testosterone molecule as a template for anabolic pharmaceuticals to treat excessive loss of muscle mass, which is a dramatic symptom of various diseases. As the androgenic effects typically are detrimental during treatment of weight loss, researchers have tried to chemically modify the molecule to enhance anabolic and diminish androgenic properties. Researchers have also sought pharmacologic improvements to enhance bioavailability and extend effectiveness.

Because of unacceptable side effects, most of these compounds have disappeared from the (legal) pharmaceutical market. However, the substitution of testosterone for treatment of sexual disorders still has some relevance. Pharmaceuticals have been designed to enhance female libido and to treat climacterium virile. For this,

[a] Institute of Biochemistry, German Sport University Cologne (DSHS), Am Sportpark Müngersdorf 6, 50933 Cologne, Germany
[b] Manfred Donike Institute, DSHS, Am Sportpark Müngersdorf 6, 50933 Cologne, Germany
* Corresponding author.
E-mail address: w.schaenzer@biochem.dshs-koeln.de (W. Schänzer).

Endocrinol Metab Clin N Am 39 (2010) 45–57
doi:10.1016/j.ecl.2009.11.004
0889-8529/10/$ – see front matter © 2010 Elsevier Inc. All rights reserved.

endo.theclinics.com

testosterone itself is the compound of choice. Typically it is applied transdermally in small doses that are continuously and frequently repeated.

In short, these effects render testosterone and related molecules promising products for the still expanding market of "anti-aging" products. Near mythical effects have been attributed to dehydroepiandrosterone (DHEA), which is a physiologic precursor of testosterone but also appears to have some endocrine potential itself. In several countries, the commercial promotion of DHEA certainly is related to its legal status rather than to its physiologic effects. For example, in the United States, DHEA is available over-the-counter while testosterone is classified as a controlled substance.

Demand is strong from both athletes and nonathletes to enhance fitness and appearance beyond what can be achieved by physical training alone. Inevitably, products appear on the market that promise corresponding effects. If consumers enjoy any beneficial effects at all, they are not in a position to fully understand the immediate cause. Evidence has shown that some unscrupulous manufacturers have blended otherwise inefficient products with anabolic steroids.

This article introduces the reader to the issues related to testosterone use and abuse, provides a brief introduction to the biochemistry and physiology of this important hormone and related substances, and describes elements of related analytical work.

TESTOSTERONE

Testosterone represents the principle human androgen. It is mainly secreted from the testes in males and from the ovaries and the placenta in females. The adrenal glands also release testosterone in small amounts. The effects of testosterone, mediated by the cytosolic androgen receptor (NR3C4), can be classified as anabolic and androgenic. The term *anabolic* refers to hypertrophic processes, such as nitrogen retention and net protein synthesis (ie, protein anabolism), as well as to use of energy for synthetic metabolism, rather than for storage in adipose tissue. This results in increased lean body mass and decreased fat mass. The effects also encompass growth and maintenance of muscle mass and strength, increased bone density and stability, and stimulation of linear growth and bone maturation. The androgenic effects are characterized by development and maintenance of male sex characteristics (ie, maturation of the sex organs; deepening of the voice; and growth of the beard, axillary, and pubic hair). Testosterone is reported to mainly induce development of the primary male sex organs, while its metabolite 5α-dihydrotestosterone (DHT) is mainly responsible for the secondary male characteristics.[1] DHT also exerts androgenic effects in the skin and prostate. Many countries have approved the use of testosterone preparations for hormonal replacement therapy, especially for the treatment of erectile dysfunction or osteoporosis.

In sports, testosterone is abused because of its performance-enhancing anabolic effects. It is the drug most often detected in human sports doping control in recent years. The World Anti-Doping Agency's (WADA's) list of prohibited substances explicitly mentions testosterone under the class "S1.1.b Endogenous Anabolic Androgenic Steroids" as a subclass of "S1. Anabolic Agents." Its use by athletes is therefore prohibited both in and out of competition.

Testosterone is derived from cholesterol in the leydig cells, thecal cells, and zona reticularis via pregnenolone and DHEA or androstenedione. It structurally is closely related to cholesterol. The backbone is known as androstane and lacks the cholesterol side chain at C-17 (C-20–C-27). The biosynthesis of steroid hormones, including testosterone, always employs cholesterol as an intermediate.[2] Remarkably, we still do not know whether production of testosterone in humans preferably starts from dietary cholesterol, whether de novo synthesis predominates, and to what degree cholesterol yielded by organs other than the sexual glands is processed. Textbooks differ largely concerning the proportions of testosterone derived from different possible cholesterol sources. However, just like most animal cells, testicular cells feature all enzymes required for the acetate/mevalonate pathway. The latter yields all isoprenoid lipids, including sterols and corresponding derivates.[3] Therefore steroid hormones may be produced from scratch.

Complete de novo synthesis from acetate thus is possible. Whether this pathway is actually employed very probably depends on substrate availability. But even a diet completely free from cholesterol leaves the possibility of predominant or even exclusive use of low-density lipoprotein.

PROHORMONES

Once the cholesterol sidechain has been cleaved, the pathway to testosterone may proceed via two parallel and related pathways. Pregnenolone is generated from cholesterol by a single but multifunctional enzyme called P450scc. It still features the 5-6 double bond of cholesterol. The corresponding pathway hence is named Δ5. Progesterone is made from pregnenolone and differs by the position of the double bond (4-5). Hence, it is the origin of the "Δ4 pathway." Additionally, the 3β-OH group is oxidized to an oxo function. Jointly, the 3-oxo-4-ene structure, characteristic to biologically active steroids, results. The Δ5 pathway proceeds via DHEA and ends with androst-5-ene-3β,17β-diol. Androst-5-ene-3β,17β-diol is converted to testosterone by the same enzyme that converts pregnenolone to progesterone. The Δ4 pathway features androst-4-ene-3,17-dione, the last immediate precursor of testosterone.

The intermediates downstream from pregnenolone and progesterone feature irreversible loss of two additional carbon atoms. As the way back is impossible, increase of the corresponding concentrations will result in an increased formation of testosterone. The immediate precursors (androst-5-ene-3β,17β-diol, androst-4-ene-3,17-dione) and DHEA are, therefore, often termed *prohormones*. Because of their testosterone-enhancing effects, their application is prohibited in sports. The rules applying to testosterone also apply to prohormones. Other well-recognized prohormones of anabolic steroids are 19-norandrostenedione (estr-4-ene-3,17-dione) and the 19-norandrostenediols (estr-4-ene-3β,17β-diol and estr-5-ene-3β,17β-diol), as well as androst-1-ene-3,17-dione and androsta-1,4-diene-3,17-dione. Several other steroids nowadays appear on the market as prohormones to circumvent current drug regulations. Also steroid esters may be considered as prohormones in a strict sense.

Esterification of the 17-hydroxy group enables prolonged liberation of testosterone in intramuscular preparations used as depot forms. Substances most often found on the market are propionate, enanthate, decanoate, undecanoate, and cypionate (cyclopentylpropanoate) esters. Others include acetate, laurate, undecylenate, phenylpropionate, isocaproate, and phenylpropionate. After liberation from the oily preparation, blood esterases rapidly hydrolyse these prodrugs into the active compound.

METABOLISM

Testosterone is extensively metabolized in the human body. The pathway towards its most abundant urinary metabolites is displayed in **Fig. 1**. The concentration of plasma testosterone is subject to precise homoeostatic regulation. Physiologically, this requires the possibility of rapid conversion of testosterone to inactive species. The

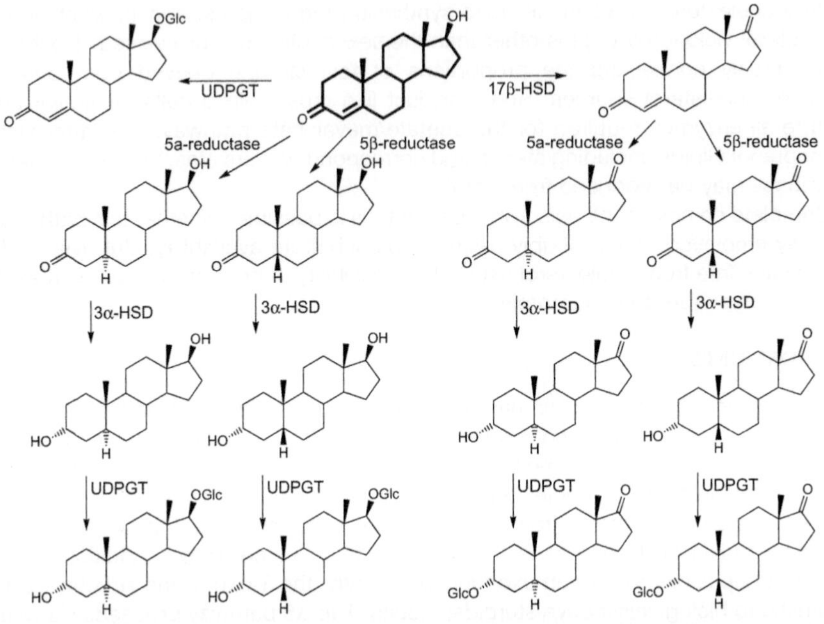

Fig. 1. Main urinary metabolites of testosterone in humans. HSD, hydroxysteroid dehydrogenase; OGlc, O glucuronide; UDPGT, uridine diphosphate glucuronyltransferase. (*Data from* Schänzer W. Metabolism of anabolic androgenic steroids. Clin Chem 1996;42(7):1001–20.)

biologic activity of steroids is often—but not always—bound to the presence of a 3-oxo-4-ene structure in the A-ring. It is therefore not surprising that the deactivation of testosterone starts with reduction at the 4-5 double bond. This reaction represents the initial and rate-limiting step of the testosterone catabolism. As the addition of hydrogen at C-5 may occur in positions α ("below" the molecular plane) or β ("above" the plane), two pathways are possible in principle. In fact, both do exist. Interestingly, they are promoted by different enzymes. The immediate metabolites are known as DHT and 5β-dihydrotestosterone. Although representing an inevitable intermediate of testosterone degradation, 5β-dihydrotestosterone itself is not detected in significant amounts. The 5α-isomer, DHT, is an important compound and much more abundant. To exert its effects, DHT is mostly derived from testosterone in the respective tissues.

DHT also features anabolic potential. It hence is also an attractive doping compound. Further testosterone metabolism mostly affects the oxygen atoms. Yielding androstanediols, the oxo function in position 3 is reduced. Again, α- and β-hydroxy isomers are possible. In the human, however, 3α forms dominate. The opposite situation may be found in other species. The 17β-hydroxy group may still be oxidized. This reaction yields 3α-hydroxy-5α-androstane-17-one (androsterone) and 3α-hydroxy-5β-androstane-17-one (etiocholanolone). These two compounds are the most abundant urinary metabolites of testosterone in the human. The respective concentrations in the urine amount to several mg*mL^{-1}, where the 5α-isomer typically dominates. Thus, the total testosterone production may easily be approximated to several milligrams per day. The fact that in plasma concentrations of merely several ng*mL^{-1} may be found illustrates the rapid turnover of testosterone and its rigorous homoeostatic regulation.

So far, only so-called "phase I metabolism" has been considered. It mostly occurs in the liver. A very large proportion of any drug that enters the human body perorally inevitably passes through this organ. The extensive metabolism associated with this is known as the *first-pass effect*. Therefore, the peroral administration of testosterone gives immediate and pronounced rise to the concentration of metabolites, while the increase of the plasma testosterone concentration is moderate in absolute terms.

The excretion of testosterone and its metabolites mostly occurs following conjugation to glucuronides. This step is generally known as phase II metabolism and largely increases the solubility in aqueous media. Thus, testosterone and its metabolites preferably leave the body in the urine. Because urine can be obtained easily and noninvasively, steroid analytical work in forensic and other sciences often is performed on this matrix. In doping control, a profile of a large set of endogenous steroids routinely is acquired to assess the possible administration of testosterone. As has been discussed above, so-called "prohormones" may also be abused to enhance testosterone levels. These eventually exert significant effects on the steroid profile. Still, the most relevant parameter here is the ratio of the concentrations of testosterone glucuronide to epitestosterone glucuronide (T/E ratio). Epitestosterone represents the 17-epimer of testosterone and does not seem to exhibit significant biologic activity. However, as has been elucidated only recently, there is a remarkable polymorphism concerning the underlying metabolism. A deletion of the UGT2B17 gene largely results in loss of testosterone glucuronidation.[4] This mutation appears to be especially abundant in parts of Asia. Heterozygous individuals already exhibit significantly reduced activity but the homozygous genotype effects a near complete loss. As a result, the urinary T/E is reduced because epitestosterone is glucuronized by a different enzyme. A relatively problematic consequence is that exogenous testosterone does not significantly alter the urinary T/E ratios anymore. Doping offenses may thus become difficult to detect.

Furthermore, several cytochrome P450 enzymes (CYP) also play a role in testosterone metabolism. The conversion of androgens to estrogens (**Fig. 2**) is initiated by 19-hydroxylation catalyzed by the enzyme complex aromatase (CYP19A1). Generated by CYP3A4, 4-hydroxy- and 6β-hydroxyandrostenedione are detectable in urine samples as minor metabolites. In in-vitro experiments employing either microsomes or recombinant enzymes, several additional hydroxylated metabolites of testosterone (1β-, 2α-, 2β-, 7α-, 11β-, 15β-, and 16β-hydroxytestosterones) were generated. These

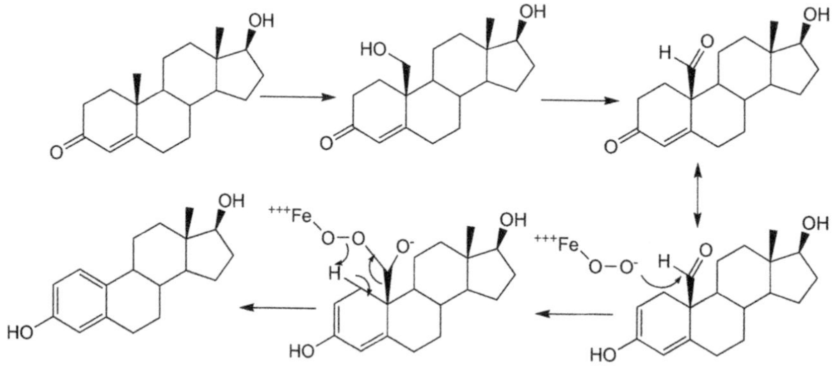

Fig. 2. Conversion of testosterone to estadiol by aromatase enzyme complex.

were mainly catalyzed by CYP 2C9, 2C19, and 3A4. In vivo detection of these metabolites has not yet been reported, however.[5–9]

SYNTHETIC ANABOLIC AGENTS

Since the 1940s, the testosterone molecule frequently has served as a template for chemical modifications of either the anabolic or the androgenic properties of steroid preparations. The enhancement of pharmacokinetic properties similarly has been subject to intense research. To enable effective oral administration, significant efforts have been spent to increase the metabolic stability. Scientists have found 17α-alkylation suitable to reduce the first-pass oxidation of the 17-hydroxy group. However, these steroids reveal a strong liver toxicity and have therefore been withdrawn from the list of licensed pharmaceuticals in many countries. Structural modifications, such as attachment of methyl groups at C-1, C-2, C-6, C-7, or C-11; chlorination or hydroxylation at C-4, C-6 or C-7; introduction of additional double bonds in ring A, B, and/or C; attachment of an additional ring at C-2/C-3 (mainly containing hetero atoms [eg, pyrazol]) shift the pharmacologic profile. The removal of the C-19 methyl group, by minimizing aromatization, enhances metabolic stability. Synthesis of these compounds and the investigation of their effects date back mainly to the period from the 1940s to the 1970s. Few of them have been legally marketed. Nowadays, they are found as ingredients of "dietary supplements," where these products often feature cryptic labeling concerning their steroid content. *Designer steroids* or *designer supplements* are typical terms, most likely employed to circumvent current drug-control legislation.

Metabolism of synthetic anabolic androgenic steroids in general follows analogous principles (3 and 17 reduction and oxidation, hydrogenation of Δ4 steroids, and hydroxylations) as described for testosterone. However, additional double bonds in ring A or B or additional substituents in position C-4 or C-6 push the reduction of the Δ4 double bond toward 5β orientation.[8] Exemptions for anabolic androgenic steroids that show a relatively high metabolic resistance with respect to phase I reactions are 3-oxo-4,9-diene, 3-oxo-4,9,11-triene, and 3-oxo-1,4,6-triene steroids.

Referring to the WADA list of prohibited substances, anabolic agents prohibited in sports are covered in section "S1. Anabolic Agents." Besides the anabolic androgenic steroids, this class also includes other anabolic agents, such as clenbuterol, selective androgen receptor modulators (SARMs), tibolone, zeranol, and zilpaterol. Tibolone is a 19-norsteroid therapeutically used for the treatment of menopausal disorders. Its therapeutic effects are based on its estrogenic activity. By contrast, zeranol is a nonsteroidal estrogen agonist synthesized as mycotoxine by *Fusarium* sp. Clenbuterol and zilpaterol represent beta-adrenergic agonists. Their anabolic effects are well documented but the mechanism is still poorly understood.

SARMs recently got the attention of the pharmaceutical industry and subsequently also of the sports community. They promote anabolic effects in muscle and bone, with very limited activation or sometimes even inhibition of reproductive organs, such as the prostate or seminal vesicles. Distinct genomic and nongenomic effects in cell lines derived from different tissues are mediated.

Explanations concerning the tissue-selective mechanism include specific expression and function of co-regulators, potential interactions with 5α-reductase and/or aromatase at the tissue level, selective intracellular signaling, and competition between SARM and DHT for binding to the androgen receptor. Conformation changes of androgen receptors in the presence of different ligands or phosporylation of androgen receptors or coactivators are reported to activate distinct combinations of intracellular signaling pathways. These changes may lead to completely different biologic effects in some androgen receptor target tissues.

In comparison to DHT, which stimulates proliferative extracellular signal-regulated kinase (ERK) in prostate cells, SARMs activate the antiproliferative p38 mitogen-activated protein kinase (MAPK). In bone cells, DHT and SARMs both activate ERK signaling. SARMs and DHT may recruit similar coactivator complexes in anabolic tissues but distinct different complexes in androgenic tissues.[10,11]

Currently, several classes of SARMs are under clinical investigation. These include analogs of quinolinone, aryl propionamide, hydantoin, and tetrahydroisoquinoline.[12,13] Compounds of major importance out of these classes are displayed in **Fig. 3**. However, some steroidal compounds (eg, 7α-methyl-19-nortestosterone and 19-norandrostenedione) have also been reported to exhibit SARM-like activity.

DIETARY SUPPLEMENTS

According to European legislation (Directive 2002/46/EC) dietary supplements are defined as "concentrated sources of nutrients or other substances with a nutritional or physiologic effect, alone or in combination, marketed in dose form and intended to supplement the normal diet." In the United States, the hormones DHEA, pregnenolone, and melatonin are also legally marketed as dietary supplements. Since 1996, prohormones of testosterone or 19-nortestosterone have been available on the United States sports supplement market. From the late 1990s on, the United States "nutritional supplement" company BALCO (Bay Area Laboratory Co-operative) marketed the designer steroids norbolethone, tetrahydrogestrinone (THG, "The Clear"), and

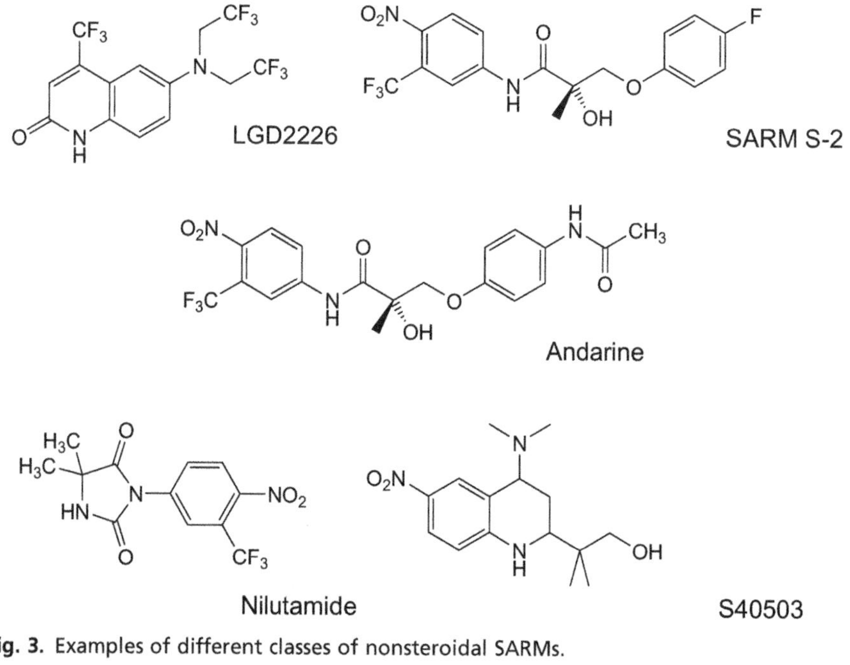

Fig. 3. Examples of different classes of nonsteroidal SARMs.

desoxymethyltestosterone (Madol, DMT) to sports people as "undetectable" steroids.[14–16]

In 2005, the Anabolic Steroids Control Act classified prohormones as Schedule III controlled substances. Subsequently, more and more products containing either "classical" anabolic androgenic steroids or steroids that were never marketed as approved drugs have appeared on the dietary supplement market. This mostly happens without proper labeling of the contents.[17] Little is known about the effects and side effects of these "new steroids" in humans. They are exclusively produced for the supplement market and are advertised as anabolic products and/or aromatase inhibitors. In several countries, the legal status of these supplements is not clear. In addition to the supplements containing steroids, products containing clenbuterol have also been labeled as dietary supplements.

Several studies have shown that the labeling of steroid-containing supplements does not reflect their actual content. These mislabelings indicate an insufficient surveillance and quality control of dietary supplements. The production evidently does not follow Good Manufacturing Practice guidelines. Triggered by some positive cases in doping control, several studies concerning possible contaminations of dietary supplements have been conducted. In fact, it has been revealed that nonhormonal nutritional supplements may also contain anabolic steroids, most likely because of cross-contamination in the production line. An international market study on 634 nonhormonal nutritional supplements revealed an overall steroid contamination rate of 15%. The consumption of such supplements has been shown to possibly lead to inadvertent positive doping cases.[18] Also, in 2006, cross-contaminations with the classical steroids metandienone and stanozolol were reported in vitamin and mineral supplements. Because products containing "new steroids" are made on the same production line as regular nutritional supplements, cross-contaminations with these compounds can be expected in the near future, leading possibly to accidental doping cases. Additionally the steroid contents of dietary supplements may cause health risks to the consumers, especially to women and adolescents.[17] To prevent athletes from unintentional doping offenses, the exclusive use of "low-risk supplements" is recommended. Available on the Internet are databases (eg, NZVT [Nederlands Zekerheidssysteem Voedingssupplementen Topsport] database and Kölner Liste) listing nutritional supplements from companies that perform quality control for anabolic steroids and stimulants or guarantee that they have no contact with these substances in the production and transportation processes.

Besides the above-mentioned steroids, other ingredients of dietary supplements can also alter the anabolic steroid profile in the body after consumption. Grapefruit is known to inhibit CYP 3A4 and thereby may increase some drugs' bioavailability. In contrast, an increased clearance of steroids was observed after administration of St John's wort extract because of increased metabolic conversion of steroids by CYP 3A4. Additionally, a modified steroid metabolite ratio (eg, increased T/DHT) was reported as a consequence of possible inhibition of the 5α-reductase.[19] Dietary zinc deficiency has been reported to result in lowered testosterone levels in humans. However, the effect of zinc supplementation on serum testosterone in nondeficient athletes was found controversial. Also the administration of preparations containing extracts from the plant *Tribulus terrestris* has been reported to release anabolic effects. Increased testosterone levels have been reported following administration in primates. However, for the human, data that indicate increased testosterone levels are available only from a company selling tribulus supplements. No cues are available from the scientific literature.

DOPING CONTROL

Testosterone and related compounds preferably leave the body via the urine. They can be detected in this matrix, mostly as glucuronized conjugates. A small proportion is excreted unconjugated. However, only some xenobiotics are exclusively found in "free" form. Mainly amongst Δ5 steroids, some compounds are found that preferably feature a sulfate moiety. This, analogous to glucuronides, enhances the solubility in aqueous media. For this and other reasons, urine represents an ideal material for doping-control purposes.

Most of the methods currently used for screening employ enzymatic deconjugation as an initial step. The cleaving enzyme often is β-glucuronidase from *Escherichia coli*. Its lack of specificity is a great advantage. A multitude of analytes thus becomes amenable to the subsequent preparative steps. Liquid-liquid extraction (t-butyl methyl ether [TBME]) separates lipophilic aglycons from the matrix. Solid phase extraction may serve the same need and is often employed as well.

Instrumental analysis still is predominantly performed by gas chromatography–mass spectrometry (GC-MS). To improve the chromatographic properties, the dried extract is derivatized by N-methyl-N-trimethylsilyl trifluoroacetamide (MSTFA). With this procedure, first introduced by M. Donike as early as 1969,[20] hydroxy groups are transformed to trimethylsilyl (TMS) ethers. The addition of trimethyliodosilane catalytically promotes the formation of enol-TMS derivatives. Thus, polar oxo functions are also converted. This results in largely reduced polarity, significantly improving the sensitivity of the whole assay. To cover a variety of anabolic substances, liquid chromatography–tandem mass spectrometry (LC-MS/MS) complements traditional GC-MS methods.[21]

For anabolic steroid testing in dietary supplements, solid products are generally extracted by organic solvents, such as methanol. For complete recovery of higher amounts of steroid ingredients, soxhlett extraction is quite often used with n-hexane. This typically yields clean extracts and thus facilitates reliable substance identification. Further purification is achieved by liquid-liquid or solid phase extraction, by column or high-performance liquid chromatography, and by crystallization. General strategies for the MS detection of "unknown" compounds focus on common steroid fragment ions or fragment losses.[17] The basic structure may thus be identified with relative ease. The elucidation of functional groups requires some additional efforts. Final identification of the molecule in question is performed by mass spectrometric comparison versus a multitude of reference compounds. Isomeric steroids, however, may yield virtually identical mass spectra. Separation by GC may then enable the assignment of the isomeric forms. For example, 3β-hydroxy isomers generally elute later than 3α congeners where analysis of per-TMS derivatives is presumed. The same applies to 17-hydroxy groups.[22] For confirmation, reference steroids are used that are either commercially available or are synthesized in house.

In addition to the above-mentioned techniques (GC-MS(/MS) and/or LC-MS/MS) the steroid analyst's toolbox contains nuclear magnetic resonance and x-ray structural analysis. The successful detection of contaminations requires the well-known methodology for trace analysis. In particular, elaborate (pre-)purification and concentration of the analytes are performed. Finally, most of the detection methods again rely on GC-MS(/MS) analysis following per-silylation.[23,24]

STABLE ISOTOPES

With the exception of phosphorous, the abundant bioelements (hydrogen, carbon, nitrogen, oxygen, sulfur) naturally possess isotopes. Among them, are several stable (ie, nonradioactive) nuclides. These inevitably contribute to the formation of all biomass, and hence also to steroids. As an example, roughly 1.1% of the earth's carbon is ^{13}C whereas the rest is mostly ^{12}C.[25] Due to its potential to facilitate dating of organic material, ^{14}C is well known as radiocarbon. However, it is present only in traces and is of no interest here. With few exceptions, heavy isotopes of a given element are less abundant than lighter ones. Usually, the lightest species is also the most abundant one.

The substitution of a light isotope by a heavier one may exert remarkable effects. Typically, the corresponding bonds become slightly but significantly more stable.[26] As a consequence, the isotopic molecule ("isotopologue") at this position will tend to react more slowly. Finally, incomplete reactions of this molecule will result in an overall depletion of heavy isotopes on the product side. This phenomenon is known as *isotope fractionation*. The restriction "incomplete" is of utmost importance here.[27] Biochemical processes are strongly controlled and directed. Thus, substrates may be exhausted completely, at least in specific compartments. This may prevent observable isotope fractionation, though the respective reaction rates may differ physically.

Nonetheless, the analysis of stable isotope ratios may be very instructive.[28] In many cases, these parameters are characteristic of classes of compounds, of different sources, or of specific processes. Biologists for a long time observed anatomic differences between certain groups of plants. Later on it turned out that these differences correspond to different mechanisms of carbon dioxide (CO_2) fixation. These mechanisms fractionate ^{13}C in ambient CO_2 to different degrees.[29] Note that the CO_2 pool in ambient air is virtually unlimited. As a consequence, the distribution of ^{13}C/^{12}C-ratios in nature features two maxima, depending on the proportion of so-called "C-3" (low ^{13}C/^{12}C) and "C-4" plants (high ^{13}C/^{12}C) contributing to the respective biomass production. Both types of plants contribute to human diet. In the United States, C-4 plants (corn) dominate. In other parts of the world, their contribution is smaller. The proportion of both types is roughly reflected also in the ^{13}C/^{12}C ratio of endogenous steroid hormones. Some isotope fractionation during the biosynthesis and metabolism of testosterone seems to occur. But the signal is pronounced enough to allow for the discrimination between synthetic and endogenous testosterone. Synthetic testosterone exclusively appears to be made from C-3 plant sterols. The ^{13}C/^{12}C ratio of pharmaceutical testosterone is very constant and this suggests the existence of few primary sources. Possibly there is only one.

The investigation of this phenomenon ("stable isotope analysis" [SIA]) has provided a major breakthrough in doping control. Though still bound to some quantitative reasoning, the different ^{13}C/^{12}C ratios often enable unequivocal identification of the primary testosterone source.[30] The classical T/E criterion nonetheless still has its merits. It is foremost used to identify suspicious samples. This parameter, however, exhibits considerable natural variation. Finally, the stable isotope analysis of testosterone and mainly of its metabolites is much more significant. One of the biggest advantages of ^{13}C/^{12}C analysis is that it nicely detects also the administration of prohormones. Exogenous DHEA, as an example, often influences the steroid profile merely within the natural variation. Nonetheless, an experienced steroid analyst often will then observe characteristic patterns. The corresponding samples in turn then will be submitted to SIA for confirmatory purposes.[31]

These achievements required major advancements in analytical instrumentation. The core device is known as an *isotope ratio mass spectrometer* (IRMS). Its basic design has not changed in decades. Originally employed by geoscientists, this instrument was first used mainly to analyze large amounts of bulk material. As it increasingly became of interest to investigate the isotope ratios of specific compounds, major efforts were performed to connect IRMSs to chromatographic devices. The breakthrough has been achieved by linking GC with IRMSs.[32] This, however, turned out to be much more demanding than the well-known GC-MS combination. As IRMSs work on simple gases only, an additional step is required. Known as GC-C-IRMS, current instrumentation employs quantitative combustion of the GC effluent before IRMS analysis. Meanwhile, the technique has been extended to the isotope analysis of hydrogen, nitrogen, and oxygen. With respect to testosterone and to the detection of its abuse, analysis of $^2H/^1H$ in particular offers interesting new perspectives.

SUMMARY

This article has offered a brief introduction to the physiology, biochemistry, and mechanisms of anabolic agents. The latter encompass testosterone, its prohormones, its chemical modifications, SARMs, and some β2-agonists. The article has provided an outline of the relevance of this diverse group of potential doping agents to sports, and has sketched the corresponding analytical strategies.

ACKNOWLEDGMENTS

The authors acknowledge the Federal Ministry for the Interior of the Federal Republic of Germany and the Manfred Donike Institute for Doping Analyses e.V., Cologne, for their support.

REFERENCES

1. Mohler ML, Bohl CE, Jones A, et al. Nonsteroidal selective androgen receptor modulators (SARMs): dissociating the anabolic and androgenic activities of the androgen receptor for therapeutic benefit. J Med Chem 2009;52(12):3597–617.
2. Payne AH, Hales DB. Overview of steroidogenic enzymes in the pathway from cholesterol to active steroid hormones. Endocr Rev 2004;25(6):947–70.
3. Goldstein JL, Brown MS. Regulation of the mevalonate pathway. Nature 1990; 343(6257):425–30.
4. Schulze JJ, Lundmark J, Garle M, et al. Doping test results dependent on genotype of uridine diphospho-glucuronosyl transferase 2B17, the major enzyme for testosterone glucuronidation. J Clin Endocrinol Metab 2008;93(7):2500–6.
5. Cawley AT, Trout GJ, Kazlauskas R, et al. The detection of androstenedione abuse in sport: a mass spectrometry strategy to identify the 4-hydroxyandrostenedione metabolite. Rapid Commun Mass Spectrom 2008;22(24):4147–57.
6. Sunde A, Tveter K, Eik-Nes KB. Hydroxylation of testosterone in the human testis. Identification of 4-androstene, 7 alpha,17 beta-diol-3-one (7 alpha-hydroxytestosterone) as a metabolite of testosterone. Acta Endocrinol (Copenh) 1980;93(2): 243–9.
7. Choi MH, Skipper PL, Wishnok JS, et al. Characterization of testosterone 11 beta-hydroxylation catalyzed by human liver microsomal cytochromes P450. Drug Metab Dispos 2005;33(6):714–8.
8. Schänzer W. Metabolism of anabolic androgenic steroids. Clin Chem 1996;42(7): 1001–20.
9. Rendic S, Nolteernsting E, Schänzer W. Metabolism of anabolic steroids by recombinant human cytochrome P450 enzymes: gas chromatographic-mass spectrometric determination of metabolites. J Chromatogr B Biomed Sci Appl 1999;735(1):73–83.

10. Narayanan R, Coss CC, Yepuru M, et al. Steroidal androgens and nonsteroidal, tissue-selective androgen receptor modulator, S-22, regulate androgen receptor function through distinct genomic and nongenomic signaling pathways. Mol Endocrinol 2008;22(11):2448–65.

11. Gao W, Dalton JT. Ockham's razor and selective androgen receptor modulators (SARMs): Are we overlooking the role of 5alpha-reductase? Mol Interv 2007; 7(1):10–3.

12. Jakobsson J, Ekstrom L, Inotsume N, et al. Large differences in testosterone excretion in Korean and Swedish men are strongly associated with a UDP-glucuronosyl transferase 2B17 polymorphism. J Clin Endocrinol Metab 2006;91(2): 687–93.

13. Thevis M, Schanzer W. Mass spectrometry of selective androgen receptor modulators. J Mass Spectrom 2008;43(7):865–76.

14. Catlin DH, Ahrens BD, Kucherova Y. Detection of norbolethone, an anabolic steroid never marketed, in athletes' urine. Rapid Commun Mass Spectrom 2002;16(13):1273–5.

15. Catlin DH, Sekera MH, Ahrens BD, et al. Tetrahydrogestrinone: discovery, synthesis, and detection in urine. Rapid Commun Mass Spectrom 2004;18(12). 1245–9.

16. Sekera MH, Ahrens BD, Chang YC, et al. Another designer steroid: discovery, synthesis, and detection of 'madol' in urine. Rapid Commun Mass Spectrom 2005;19(6):781–4.

17. Geyer H, Parr MK, Koehler K, et al. Nutritional supplements cross-contaminated and faked with doping substances. J Mass Spectrom 2008;43(7): 892–902.

18. Geyer H, Parr MK, Mareck U, et al. Analysis of non-hormonal nutritional supplements for anabolic-androgenic steroids—Results of an international study. Int J Sports Med 2004;25(2):124–9.

19. Donovan JL, DeVane CL, Lewis JG, et al. Effects of St John's wort (Hypericum perforatum L.) extract on plasma androgen concentrations in healthy men and women: a pilot study. Phytother Res 2005;19(10):901–6.

20. Donike M. N-Methyl-N-trimethylsilyl-trifluoroacetamide a new silylating agent from series of Silylated amides. J Chromatogr 1969;42(1):103–4.

21. Mareck U, Thevis M, Guddat S, et al. Comprehensive sample preparation for anabolic steroids, glucocorticosteroids, beta-receptor blocking agents, selected anabolic androgenic steroids and buprenorphine in human urine. In: Schänzer W, Geyer H, Gotzmann A, et al, editors. Recent advances in doping analysis (12). Köln: Sport und Buch Strauß; 2004. p. 65–9.

22. Parr MK, Zapp J, Becker M, et al. Steroidal isomers with uniform mass spectra of their per-TMS derivatives: synthesis of 17-hydroxyandrostan-3-ones, androst-1-, and -4-ene-3, 17-diols. Steroids 2007;72(6–7):545–51.

23. Van Thuyne W, Delbeke FT. Validation of a GC-MS screening method for anabolizing agents in solid nutritional supplements. Biomed Chromatogr 2004;18(3): 155–9.

24. Parr MK, Geyer H, Reinhart U, et al. Analytical strategies for the detection of non-labelled anabolic androgenic steroids in nutritional supplements. Food Addit Contam 2004;21(7):632–40.

25. Coplen TB, Bohlke JK, De Bievre P, et al. Isotope-abundance variations of selected elements—(IUPAC Technical Report). Pure Appl Chem 2002;74(10): 1987–2017.

26. Hoeffs J. Stable isotope geochemistry. 4th edition. Berlin, Heidelberg, New York: Springer; 1997.
27. Hayes JM. Fractionation of the isotopes of carbon and hydrogen in biosynthetic processes. Rev Min Geochem 2001;43:225–78.
28. Flenker U. Stable isotope analysis of the bioelements: an introduction. Bioanalysis 2009;1(6):1119–29.
29. O'Leary M. Carbon isotope fractionation in plants. Phytochemistry 1981;20(4): 553–67.
30. Becchi M, Aguilera R, Farizon Y, et al. Gas chromatography/combustion/isotope-ratio mass spectrometry analysis of urinary steroids to detect misuse of testosterone in sport. Rapid Commun Mass Spectrom 1994;8:304–8.
31. Mareck U, Geyer H, Flenker U, et al. Detection of dehydroepiandrosterone misuse by means of gas chromatography–combustion-isotope ratio mass spectrometry. Eur J Mass Spectrom (Chichester, Eng) 2007;13(6):419–26.
32. Brand W. High precision isotope ratio monitoring techniques in mass spectrometry. J Mass Spectrom 1996;31:225–35.

Endogenous Steroid Profiling in the Athlete Biological Passport

Pierre-Edouard Sottas, PhD*, Martial Saugy, PhD, PD,
Christophe Saudan, PhD

KEYWORDS

- Androgen • Doping • Steroid • Profiling
- Athlete biological passport

Anabolic–androgenic steroids (AAS) represent a class of steroidal hormones affiliated with the hormone testosterone. Testosterone is produced naturally in the human body and conjugated mainly with glucuronide and sulfate before excretion in urine (phase 2 metabolism). The androgenic effects of testosterone and its prohormones generally are associated with masculanization and virilization, while its anabolic effects are associated with protein building in the body.[1] In power sports, exogenous AAS primarily are used as myotrophic agents to promote muscle mass and strength. Although their efficacy in terms of improved physical function has been debated during decades,[1,2] a comprehensive study by Bhasin and colleagues demonstrated in 1996 that testosterone can act as a performance-enhancing substance when supraphysiological doses are administered.[3] Exogenous AAS also are known to be used in endurance sports for improved recovery. Endurance athletes favour low (to limit myotrophy) but frequent doses for replacement levels. Indeed, overtraining-induced stress can upset the balance between anabolic and catabolic states of the hormones of the endocrine system.[4] Some endurance athletes may find in synthetic AAS an ergogenic supercompensating agent for sustained testosterone concentrations and, in turn, a performance-enhancing substance to allow more intense training sessions. In addition, it has been shown that testosterone not only plays an important role in muscle metabolism during the regeneration phase after physical exercise, but also seems to increase the ability of the muscle to refill its glycogen storage through an increased activity of the muscle glycogen synthetase.[4,5]

This work was supported by Grant Number R07D0MS from the World Anti Doping Agency.
Swiss Laboratory for Doping Analyses, University Center of Legal Medicine, West Switzerland, Chemin des Croisettes 22, 1066 Epalinges, Switzerland
* Corresponding author.
E-mail address: Pierre-Edouard.Sottas@chuv.ch (P.-E. Sottas).

Endocrinol Metab Clin N Am 39 (2010) 59–73
doi:10.1016/j.ecl.2009.11.003
0889-8529/10/$ – see front matter © 2010 Elsevier Inc. All rights reserved.

endo.theclinics.com

Intake of exogenous AAS is not the only way to produce a sustained rise in testosterone levels. Various indirect steroid doping strategies produce the same effect. This includes, among others, estrogen blockade by estrogen receptor antagonists (antiestrogens) or aromatase inhibitors.[6] Although these two classes of estrogen blockers differ in their pharmacologic action, both are known to stimulate sustained increases in endogenous luteinizing hormone secretion, and, successively, increases in blood testosterone concentrations. In particular, estrogen blockade in men is known to produce elevations of testosterone concentrations at a level sufficient to produce ergogenic and performance-enhancing effects.[6]

MARKERS OF STEROID DOPING

As of today, triple quadrupole mass spectrometry cannot distinguish between pharmaceutical and natural testosterone based on the mass spectrum. In the 1980s, pursuant to the work of Donike and colleagues, an authorized upper limit of 6.0 for the testosterone over epistestosterone (T/E) ratio was introduced to deter testosterone administration.[7] Because epistestosterone is only a minor product of the metabolism of testosterone and does not increase after exogenous testosterone administration, the net effect of the latter is an increase in the T/E ratio.[8] Testosterone and epistestosterone levels in urine specimens commonly are measured in antidoping laboratories by gaz chromatography–mass spectrometry (GC/MS) after deconjugating the glucuronide moiety by enzymatic hydrolysis (β-glucuronidase) and derivatization (trimethylsilylation).[9,10] Alternatively, testosterone and epistestosterone can be measured directly using high-performance liquid chromatography (HPLC)/tandem MS.[11]

The T/E has been the first widely used indirect marker of doping with anabolic steroids, with a discrimination principle not based on the distinction between the exogenous substance and its endogenous counterpart, but rather on the effect induced by the intake of the exogenous substance on some selected biological markers. Although the value of evidence provided by population-based limits on biomarkers generally can be considered as being not useful from a forensic perspective,[12] a T/E ratio greater than 6.0 nevertheless was adopted as proof of steroid doping in 1982. Unsurprisingly enough, it was put forth a few years later that some individuals were shown to produce naturally elevated T/E.[13] Since then the T/E ratio mainly has been used as a screening test, with any positive result requiring a subsequent confirmation analysis by GC/C/IRMS. GC/C/IRMS allows measurement of slight differences in $^{13}C/^{12}C$ ratio of testoserone metabolites. Discrimination between pharmaceutical and natural testosterone is possible, because hemisynthetic testosterone is known to display a different ^{13}C content than its human counterpart produced by means of cholesterol metabolism.[14] GC/C/IRMS has become an indispensable tool in antidoping laboratories for the determination of synthetic AAS in urine samples, despite the fact that the method is not sensitive to indirect androgen doping.

LONGITUDINAL STEROID PROFILING

Whereas it already was known in the 1990s that subject-based reference ranges are much reliable than population-based reference ranges for androgens[15] and that individual T/E values do not deviate from the mean value by more than 30%,[8] it has only been recently that a method was proposed to take into account formally these characteristics.[16] Based on empirical Bayesian inferential techniques for longitudinal profiling that also are used for cancer screening,[17] the test progressively switches the focus from comparison with a population to the determination of individual values. Interestingly, this test is neither a purely population-based nor a purely subject-based approach, but an intermediate approach that makes the best decision in function of the between- and within-subject variance components of the marker and actual individual test results. At each moment in the course of data acquisition, it is possible to predict expected values for the markers and to define individual limits for a desired specificity (assuming a nondoped population). From a mathematical point of view, individualization of the expected values of the marker corresponds to the nullification of its between-subject variance component. Using the athlete as his own reference is particularly interesting when the marker presents a low ratio of within-subject to between-subject variations. In a population composed of male Caucasian athletes, this ratio has been estimated to be as low as 0.04 for the T/E.[18] Such a low ratio already questions the pertinence of a population-based threshold (fixed at 4.0 today)[19] for the T/E ratio.

In addition to general descriptive statistics, the sensitivity and specificity of various methods of interpretation applied to the T/E marker also have been evaluated empirically.[20] In detail, the specificity was estimated from 432 urine samples withdrawn from 28 control subjects, the sensitivity from 88 urine samples collected in a clinical trial at a maximum of 36 hours after administration of a pill of 80 mg of undecanoate testosterone. A population-based limit fixed at 4.0 for the T/E ratio returned 24 false positives (24/432 = 5.6%) for 34 true positives (34/88 = 39%), that is a positive predictive value (PPV) of only 59% on that set of data. A high PPV is particularly important in antidoping, because the PPV indicates the true probability of an athlete doped in case of a positive outcome. A PPV of 59% indicates that when the test returns a positive result, there is 41% chance of a false positive. On the same T/E data, the empiric Bayesian test for longitudinal data returned two false positives (2/432 = 0.5%, for a theoretical specificity of 99%) for 51 true positives (51/88 = 58%), that is a PPV of 96%. Still better results were obtained when some heterogenous and external factors were taken into account. In conclusion, these numbers confirmed the inefficiency of a unique and inflexible threshold for the marker T/E. Actually, from a forensic perspective, it can be shown that the value of the evidence given by the rule "T/E > 4.0" can be considered as being not useful.[12,21]

Every year, the World Anti-Doping Agency (WADA) publishes some statistics on the number of adverse analytical findings (AAFs) and atypical findings (ATFs) reported by antidoping laboratories. AAS represent by far the family of substances that lead to the highest number of AAFs and ATFs. For example, for 2007, the numbers are the following: 223,898 A samples were analyzed, for a total of 4,402 AAFs (1.97%), from which 2,322 (47.9% of all AAFs, 1% of all tests) were for AAS. Accordingly, it often is claimed that AAS, and testosterone in particular, represent the most abundant misused substances in elite sports. However, because all tests returning a T/E value higher than 4.0 are reported as an AAF (as an ATF since 2008) and knowing that a significant proportion of male athletes should present naturally higher values than 4.0,[20] one cannot exclude that most AAFs (or ATFs) obtained with the "T/E > 4.0" rule are false positives. This happens when the prevalence of steroid doping is low and when the test has been applied many times. Given that GC/C/IRMS analysis is particularly costly, the financial waste to apply a "T/E > 4.0" rule can be estimated at about $1 million. This unnecessary financial burden does prejudice expenditure on other more efficient investigations and the credibility of the antidoping movement in general.

STEROID PROFILE

While the terminology steroid profiling is used in the literature to denote a follow-up over time, a steroid profile encompasses concentration levels of endogenous steroids in urine and their respective ratios. Steroid profiles are employed widely in endocrinology to detect enzyme deficiencies or adrenal problems.[22] In antidoping laboratories, the urinary steroid profile usually includes the concentration levels of

Testosterone
Testosterone's inactive epimer, epistestosterone
Four testosterone metabolites, androsterone, etiocholanolone (Etio), 5α-androstane-3α,17β-diol (α-diol), and 5β-androstane-3α,17β-diol (β-diol)
A testosterone precursor, dehydroepiandrosterone (DHEA)

The following cut-off concentration levels of endogenous steroids equivalent to the glucuronide: testosterone >200 ng/mL, epistestosterone >200 ng/mL, androsterone >10'000 ng/mL, Etio >10'000 ng/mL and DHEA >100 ng/mL are considered as putative markers of steroid doping.[19] In contrast to absolute steroid concentrations, ratios such as T/E, androsterone (A)/Etio, A/T, α-diol/E and α-diol/β-diol are robust to circadian rhythm or changes in physiologic conditions such as exercise workload for athletes.[23] On the other hand, these parameters may be altered significantly according to the administered steroid and its application mode.

Although glucuronide conjugates up to now have been the preferred means of evaluating excretion of androgens, there is a high potential of improvement in the development of additional markers of steroid doping through other phase 2 metabolites, such as testosterone sulfate. Methods based on HPLC/MS have been developed for that purpose.[11,24,25] Introduction of sulfoconjugates, with biomarkers such as the ratio testosterone sulfate/ epistestosterone sulfate (Ts/Es), or testosterone glucuronide/testosterone sulfate (Tg/Ts), or (Tg+Ts)/(Eg+Ts) may help develop a more sensitive test for AAS abuse in the future.

HETEROGENEOUS FACTORS

Heterogeneous factors refer to the factors specific to an individual that are known to have an influence on a biomarker. For example, sex and age are well-known heterogenous factors used in the evaluation of a steroid profile.

It long has been known that urinary testosterone glucuronides present a bimodal distribution,[9] this effect being particularly marked between Caucasian and Asian populations.[26–28] It only was recently, however, that it was demonstrated that the significant differences observed in testosterone glucuronide excretion are associated with a deletion mutation in the UDP-glucuronide transferase 2B17 (UGT2B17) gene.[29] This discovery has important implications for doping tests. For example, when subjects deficient in the UGT2B17 gene (del/del) receive exogenous testosterone, it has been shown that their T/E ratio does not rise significantly, remaining well below current threshold at 4.0.[20,30] This suggests that the knowledge of genetic differences in metabolism and excretion is important in the evaluation of urinary steroid profiles.[2]

The understanding of the genetics of androgen disposition has grown quickly. Recent studies have shown, among others, that the cytochrome P-450c17alpha (CYP17) promoter polymorphism may partly explain high natural T/E ratios.[31] Also, the lack of the UGT2B17 enzyme may be compensated for by an increase in UGT2B15 transcription.[31] In addition, it has been shown that epistestosterone does not present a bimodal distribution because UGT2B17 does not glucuronidate E while

UGT2A1 conjugates testosterone and epistestosterone similarly,[25] and, finally, that testosterone is primarily glucuronidated by UGT2B17 while epistestosterone is primarily glucuronidated by UGT2B7.[25] The latter result is particularly interesting to understand the large between-subject variations of the T/E ratio, with low values of T/E (significantly < 1) expressed by subjects deficient in the UGT2B17 gene, and high values of T/E (significantly > 1) expressed by subjects deficient in the UGT2B7 gene. Additional discoveries in the genetics of androgen disposition are expected in the coming years, with genes involved in phase 1 drug metabolism, such as the P450 gene (CYP) family, and in phase 2 metabolism, such as the glucuronosyltransferases (UGT) and sulfotransferases (SULT) gene families.

A recent study by Xue and colleagues has shown that the UGT2B17 gene presents an unusually high degree of geographic variation, with a high frequency of the gene in most African populations, intermediate frequency in Europe/West Asia, and low frequency in East Asia.[32] Interestingly, an impressive worldwide map of the distribution of the UGT2B17 gene has been published for more than 30 ethnic groups. This high variability in the frequency of the UGT2B17 also has been confirmed in sports, in a study with five different ethnic groups of professional soccer players.[33]

All these studies have shown a large heterogeneity in androgen disposition. From a mathematical point of view, a large heterogeneity is expressed through a large between-subject variance of the marker. Introduction of genotyping information of the athlete, or of the frequencies of the genes in function of the ethnic origin of the athlete, can remove the part in the between-subject variance that originates from these differences.[34] These studies confirm, again, that unique and nonspecific thresholds on markers of steroid doping are not fit for indicating AAS misuse.

EXTERNAL CONFOUNDING FACTORS

Several confounding factors must be considered when a longitudinal steroid profile has to be interpreted. For that purpose, it is worth mentioning the review of Mareck and colleagues describing the factors known to exert an influence on the steroid profile.[23] The influence of some pharmaceutical preparations and the potential influence of microorganisms and bacterial activities in urine samples were reviewed. In particular, it is relevant to outline that the consumption of ethanol at dosages higher than 1 g/kg bodyweight may lead to a significant increase of the T/E ratio.[35] Similarly, the elevation of this ratio also can be observed upon application of oral contraceptives owing to suppression of epistestosterone excretion.[36] In contrast, the application of ketoconazole is known to lead to an inhibition of steroidogenesis and subsequently to result in a suppressed urinary profile and significant variation of the T/E ratio.[37]

STANDARDIZED PROTOCOLS FOR STEROID PROFILE DATA

In a medico–legal setting, it is the burden of the testing officials to demonstrate the validity of the presented evidence. In that context, the measurement of a steroid profile must follow standardized procedures based on justifiable protocols. Such compliance is necessary to control analytical uncertainties. This is particularly important in steroid profiling, because it is essential to quantify the expected variations of the markers. For GC/MS in particular, the effects of some technical parameters such as inhibition of hydrolysis, incomplete derivatization, or matrix issues must be under control.[23] For example, if two laboratories do not have the same limit of quantification (LOQ) for the concentration of a steroid, the analytical uncertainty will be different for the measurement of a concentration close to the LOQ, with, in turn, a within-subject variance of the markers that may change from one sample to the next. Therefore, a standardization of the protocols with all laboratories hanging to an external quality control system is an essential condition for a forensic evaluation of steroid data.

BAYESIAN INFERENCE FOR THE EVALUATION OF INDIRECT EVIDENCE

The causal relationship between doping (the cause) and the induced modification in the steroid profile (the effect) can be formalized and graphically represented by a causal network (**Fig. 1A**). The goal is to establish whether an athlete is doped by examining his steroid profile. This type of problem goes against the causal direction, and the only logic that may apply here is Bayesian reasoning.[38] For example, if an athlete takes a oral dose of synthetic testosterone (the cause), the value of his T/E ratio

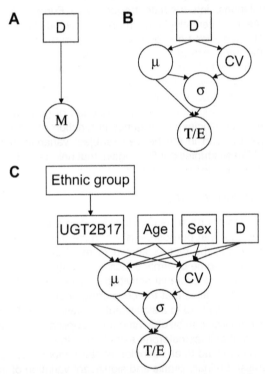

Fig. 1. Bayesian networks for the evaluation of the evidence with markers of steroid doping. Each rectangle presents a discrete variable, each circle a continuous variable, each arrow a causal relationship. (*A*) D represents the doping state of the athlete, M the marker. Doping (the cause) has an effect on the marker (the effect), and the goal is to know in which doping state the athlete is in light of the result of the marker M. This problematic goes against the causal direction, and only Bayes' theorem handles this point. (*B*) A longitudinal approach for the T/E can be modeled by making explicit the expected mean and coefficient of variation of the sequence of T/E values. A log-normal distribution is assumed for these two variables. (*C*) Addition of the heterogeneous factors age, sex, and UGT2B17 genotype. If the athlete's genotype is unknown, the prevalence of the UGT2B17 gene can be used instead in function of the ethnic origin of the athlete. Similar causal networks are used in genetics to represent so-called genotype-phenotype maps. (*Data from* Xue Y, Sun D, Daly A, et al. Adaptive evolution of UGT2B17 copy-number variation. Am J Hum Genet 2008;83:337–46. Rockman MV. Reverse engineering the genotype–phenotype map with natural genetic variation. Nature 2008;456:738–44.)

will increase (the effect). If a model that links cause and effect is available, Bayes' theorem can be used to follow the direction that is opposite to that of causality and to determine whether an increase in the T/E may be the result of doping or is caused by natural variations. In such a Bayesian network (see **Fig. 1A**), D is a discrete variable describing the doping state of the athlete, and M a continuous variable representing the result of a measurement of a marker of steroid doping (such as the T/E). According to Bayes' theorem, the causal relationship between M and D can be written as follows:

$$P(D|M) = \frac{P(M|D) \cdot P(D)}{P(M)}$$
(1)

where the formulations are given as probabilities. $P(D|M)$ represents the probability of being in state D as a function of the value of marker M, $P(M|D)$ the probability to measure the result M knowing that the athlete is in state D. For example, if M is T/E and $D = 0$ represents the nondoped state, $P(T/E|D = 0)$ is well described by a log-normal distribution with geometric mean of 1.40 and geometric standard deviation of 1.78 for a population of male athletes not deficient in the UGT2B17 gene. The advantage of a Bayesian approach resides in the possibility to use the conditional probability function $P(M|D)$ to determine $P(D|M)$, because a cause-to-effect relationship is much easier to establish than the reverse effect–cause relationship. The cause-to-effect relationship is typically built from data obtained in clinical trials, with control subjects to obtain samples of class $D = 0$, and volunteers to which a doping product has been administered to obtain samples of class $D \neq 0$. Dealing with reference populations of doped athletes requires, however, some assumptions on the type of doping (eg, type of substance or method, doses, toxicocinetics of the substance). Formally, this can be taken into account by means of multiple states of doping $D \in \{1, 2, 3...\}$, with the state $D = i$ specific to the type of substance and type of treatment used to obtain the data on which $P(M|D = i)$ has been developed. Assuming for the sake of simplicity and without loss of generality a unique state of doping $D = 1$, the conditional probability $P(M|D = 1)$ plays an important role in the odds form of Bayes' theorem:

$$\frac{P(D = 1|M)}{P(D = 0|M)} = \frac{P(M|D = 1)}{P(M|D = 0)} \cdot \frac{P(D = 1)}{P(D = 0)}$$
(2)

in which the first ratio in the right side of the equation is the so-called likelihood ratio, also known as the weight of evidence in forensics.[21] A likelihood ratio with a value greater than 1 leads to an increase in the odds (to favor the state $D = 1$), while a likelihood ratio with a value less than 1 leads to decrease in the odds (to favor the state $D = 0$).

In antidoping, it is not uncommon to have a decision rule based on a high threshold of specificity of a test or marker, with the underlying assumption that the athlete is part of a population composed of nondoped athletes only. This amounts to defining $\Pr(D = 0) = 1; \Pr(D \neq 0) = 0$ and this removes the true essence of a Bayesian approach. In that situation, only models for nondoped control athletes are required, not for doped athletes. To use a decision rule based on the specificity of the marker has large implications on the logic to evalute the value of evidence. In particular, if proper precautions are not taken, this logic can lead to the so-called false-positive fallacy,[21] a special case of the more general prosecutor's fallacy that results from misunderstanding the notion of multiplicity of tests. An increase in the number of tests on a population composed of nondoped athletes causes an increase in the probability of obtaining a false positive. For example, the limit at 6.0 introduced in 1982 for the T/E ratio was founded on the fact that nobody from a large number (say N) of control subjects had presented a so high T/E value at that time. It was thus believed that the specificity of this rule was close to 100%. It can be shown by Bayesian statistics, however, that if a number N of control subjects did not present a T/E greater than 6.0, the mean of the distribution of the expected specificity of the classification rule "T/E > 6.0" is $2N/(2N+1)$. Consequently, one can expect one false positive in average if the test is applied twice (ie, $2N$) as many times the number (ie, N) it was applied during its validation. Even though these are only theoretical considerations and that it remained possible at that time that no athlete would have ever presented a T/E greater than 6.0 (only empirical evidence is discussed here), care should have been taken because of the multiplicity of antidoping tests. Mathematically, the false-positive fallacy generally results from the fallacious transposition of the conditional distributions:

$$P(D = 1|M) = 1 - P(M|D = 0)$$

To base the decision solely on a threshold of specificity is not necessary if an estimate of the prevalence of doping is available. Although it may be thought at first sight that only a test able to easily identify drug cheats can be used to estimate the prevalence of doping, it has been shown recently that it can be accurately determined if several conditions are met.[12,39] The idea is to compare the test results of a population of athletes, such as when all athletes participating to the same competition are tested just before that competition, with reference populations of nondoped and doped athletes. For example, if the number of athletes is sufficiently large, the maximal difference between the empirical cumulative distribution function (ECDF) constructed from the values of the marker M on the tested population and the CDF of a reference population of nondoped athletes (ie, the CDF computed from $P(M|D = 0)$), represents a minimal estimate of the prevalence of doping in the tested population. This estimate then can be used as prior distribution $P(D)$ in Equation 1 (or via prior odds in Equation 2) for all athletes who participated to that competition. Then, for each athlete individually, it is possible with Bayes' rule to change the prior $P(D)$ in receipt of the individual test result M and the model $P(M|D)$ to obtain the posterior distribution $P(D|M)$ that represents the true probability that the athlete doped. The same logic is possible with the odds form of Bayes' theorem, with the likelihood ratio computed from the individual test result M updating the prior odds estimated from the group of athletes, to obtain the posterior odds on which a decision rule can be implemented.

Independent of the probability distribution on which the decision rule is applied, a Bayesian logic remains essential to take into account other variables (other than doping) in a natural manner. The Bayesian network of **Fig. 1**B is a graphical representation of the model described previously for longitudinal steroid profiling. In more detail, in this empirical two-level hierarchical Bayesian model, the variables μ and CV are unobservable variables with prior distributions assumed to be log-normal. These distributions are updated progressively on receipt of new test results. Bayesian inference permits the move from prior (pretest) to posterior (post-test) distributions, based on the outcome of the test result (this process goes against the causal direction). Then, the posterior distribution of the variables μ and CV can be used to define the expected values of the marker M for a next test (following this time the causal direction). The whole process is repeated, with posterior distributions obtained from the previous test becoming the prior distributions for a new test. When the number of tests is large, the distributions of μ and CV degenerate to the parameters specific to the athlete. Also, further techniques have been proposed to handle the lack of independence between two successive values,[17,40] a situation that may occur when two urine samples are collected in a too short a period of time.

Similarly, both heterogenous and confounding factors can be modeled in a natural manner in that framework. **Fig. 1C** shows a Bayesian network with heterogenous factors age, sex, UGT2B17 genotype, and ethnic origin for the evaluation of longitudinal T/E data. The strength of that approach relies in its flexibility to integrate sound scientific knowledge. For example, the relationships between the variables ethnic origin and UGT2B17, and between UGT2B17 and μ can be obtained from literature data.[20,25,29,34]

ATHLETE STEROIDAL PASSPORT

The use of indirect markers of doping has a long history, but it is only recently that this testing paradigm has matured into what is called today the Athlete Biological Passport (ABP). An ABP is an individual electronic document that stores any information valuable for the interpretation of indirect evidence of doping. The fundamental principle of the ABP is the monitoring over time of selected biomarkers to reveal the effects of doping. The more elaborated module of the ABP is the Athlete Haematological Passport,[39] which aims to identify blood doping with biologic markers of an altered erythropoiesis.

All ideas and concepts discussed in the precedent paragraphs on the markers of steroid doping can form the basis of an Athlete Steroidal Passport (ASP). Steroid profiling in an ASP appears especially appropriate, because all of these markers are known to present a low ratio of within-subject to between-subject variations.

Fig. 2 shows the results of an ASP for a male adult Caucasian athlete not deficient in the gene UGT2B17, for the marker T/E, T/A, A/Etio and α-diol/β-diol. This athlete has been tested 10 times, with all measurements performed in the authors' laboratory. The center lines represent the actual test results, the upper and lower lines the limits found for a specificity of 99% with the Bayesian network of **Fig. 1C**. For the T/E, initial limits are [0.24 6.88], meaning that only one individual out of a population of 100 male adult athletes not deficient in the gene UGT2B17 should present a value out of this range in average. The knowledge of the UGT2B7 genotype (unknown for this athlete) may still lead to more specific limits, in particular to avoid false positives (with a result higher than 6.88) if the athlete is shown to be deficient in that gene. With the first test result equal to 0.94, the reference range for the second test become 0.34 to 2.44, meaning that only one individual out of a group of 100 male adulte athletes not deficient in the gene UGT2B17 who have shown an initial value of 0.94 must fall out of this range in average. The last range of 0.51 to 1.28 represents the expected range for that athlete if tested an 11th time. With an upper value of 1.28, the athlete has an insignificant margin to monitor his profile with low doses of testosterone.

Fig. 3 shows the T/E sequence of a professional athlete tested 13 times in 1 year. In the upper left insert are represented the limits found with the empirical Bayesian approach without any other knowledge than the athlete is a Caucasian male. The sequence has 11 tests with T/E values significantly inferior to 1.0, and two outliers at 1.2 and 1.5. For example, the value at 1.2 is at the 99.9996 percentile of the distribution of expected values (this is a theoretical consideration, because the approach has not been validated empirically for a specificity higher than 99.9%). The value at 1.2 is abnormal at a level similar to the level that would have been achieved with an initial T/E value at around 22. If the two values at 1.2 and 1.5 are removed from the interpretation (upper right insert of **Fig. 3**), the sequence does not present any suspect

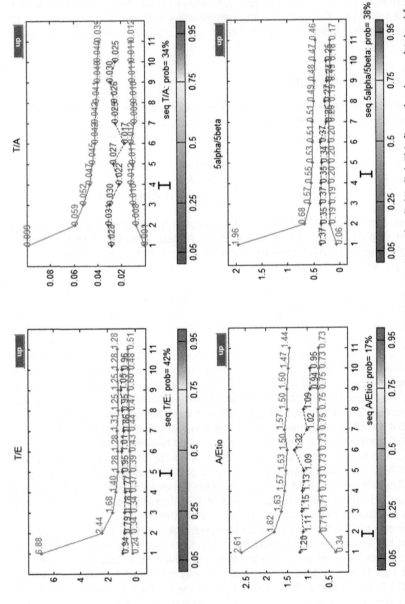

Fig. 2. Steroid profiling for a male Caucasian athlete for the markers T/E, T/A, A/Etio, and α-diol/β-diol. This figure has been obtained from the software Athlete Biological Passport (LAD, Lausanne, Switzerland). This software is available upon request to any antidoping organization.

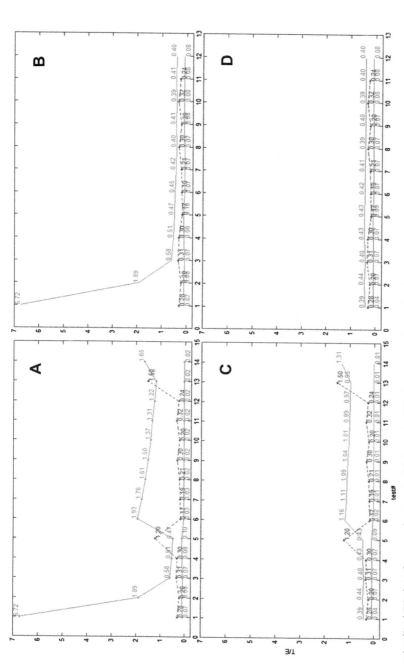

Fig. 3. Longitudinal T/E data for a professional athlete tested 13 times, as well as individual limits for a specificity of 99%. There are 11 tests with values significantly inferior to 1.0, and two outliers at 1.2 (fifth test) and 1.5 (13th test). Even though the athlete's UGT2B17 genotype is unknown, it can be inferred from his phenotype, with a probability of 99% of a full deletion in the UGT2B17 gene (see text). (A) All 13 test results are represented with individual limits obtained without any a priori on the UGT2B17 genotype. (B) Without the two outliers and without any a priori on the UGT2B17 genotype. (C) All 13 tests results and assuming a full deletion in the UGT2B17 gene. (D) Without the two outliers and assuming a full deletion in the UGT2B17 gene.

value anymore. With the Bayesian network of **Fig. 2C**, it is possible to infer the posterior probability (or posterior odds) that this athlete is deficient in the UGT2B17 gene in function of his test results, that is to infer the athlete's genotype from his phenotype.[41] With parameters given elsewhere,[16] the likelihood ratio is equal to 0.00092 (odds 1:1080) in favor of a deficiency of the gene. With prior odds of 9:1 in favor of the presence of at least one allele for Caucasians,[20,32] the posterior odds are 1:120 in favor of a deficiency of the UGT2B17 gene for that athlete, that is a probability higher than 99%. The results obtained when it is assumed a priori that this athlete is deficient in the UGT2B17 gene are shown in the lower left (full sequence) and lower right (without the two outliers) for comparison. Interestingly, in that case, the amount of between-subject variance removed by the (assumed) knowledge that this athlete has a full deletion of the UGT2B17 gene is similar to the amount of variance removed by the knowledge of about four basal values.

OUTLOOK OF AN ATHLETE STEROIDAL PASSPORT

The ASP represents the mature product of the development of biological markers of steroid doping. Much progress has been accomplished from the discovery and implementation of the T/E ratio at the beginning of the 1980's to the understanding of the implications of genetic differences in the steroid profile of an athlete. In particular, steroid profiling remains the fundamental principle of the ASP, allowing the removal of the largest part of the variations of the markers. Also, because the compliance to different analytical protocols leads to different expected variations, it is essential that these protocols are an integral part of the ASP.

The benefits of adopting the ASP concept are far-reaching, with multiple applications possible. First, the ASP can be used to target athletes for the GC/C/IRMS test with much better efficiency than it is performed today. Secondly, unusually large disparities found in an ASP may alert officials of doping or a medical condition requiring closer examination. In both cases, the sports authorities have a good reason to withdraw the athlete from competing for a short period, typically 2 weeks. Because fair play and athletes' health protection are fundamental in any antidoping program, the authors strongly believe that the benefits of adopting such a no-start rule would be huge. Also, with a no-start rule, an athlete can use his passport to attest his fair play by means of normal longitudinal profiles of biomarkers. Indeed, whereas a negative outcome of an antidoping test does not necessarily prove that the athlete is clean (because of the low sensitivity of some tests performed at one unique moment in time), the presentation of a passport at the beginning of a competition can ensure that the athlete will participate close to his natural, unaltered physiologic condition. It may be argued that today markers of doping do not have a perfect discrimination aptitude, but the limits set by the passport let a small margin for doping, so that finally the advantages to dope become outnumbered by the risks. Also, contrary to direct tests that must be developed and validated for each new doping substance, a marker is validated and introduced in the ABP once and for all. This means that today's markers only can gain in sensitivity in the future. In particular, it is probable that today's markers are already sensitive to future generations of doping substances (for example to all future substances that will aim to increase testosterone concentrations), whereas the sensitivity of today's direct tests to future substances is far from being guaranteed. Third, when unusually large disparities have been found, the ASP should be reviewed by a panel of experts to determine their origin. When it is much more likely that the detected abnormality originates from doping than from a medical condition or other external cause (eg, confounding factor, multiple testing), the information stored in an ASP can be sufficient to launch a disciplinary procedure against the athlete. This reviewing process typically can be performed during the short withdrawal of the athlete if a no-start rule has been implemented.

REFERENCES

1. Kicman AT. Pharmacolocy of anabolic steroids. Br J Pharmacol 2008;154:502–21.
2. Bowers LD. Testosterone doping: dealing with genetic differences in metabolism and excretion. J Clin Endocrinol Metab 2008;93:2469–71.
3. Bhasin S, Storer TW, Berman N, et al. The effects of supraphysiologic doses of testosterone on muscle size and strength in normal men. N Engl J Med 1996; 335:1–7.
4. Urhausen A, Kindermann W. The endocrine system in overtraining. In: Arren MP, Constantini NW, editors. Sports endocrinology. Totowa (NJ): Humana Press; 2000. p. 347–70.
5. Gillespie CA, Edgerton VR. The role of testosterone in exercise-induced glycogen supercompensation. Horm Metab Res 1970;2:364–6.
6. Handelsman DJ. Indirect androgen doping by oestrogen blockade in sports. Br J Pharmacol 2008;154:598–605.
7. Donike ML, Bärwald KR, Klosterman K, et al. Nachweis von exogenem Testosteron. In: Heck H, Hollmann H, Liesen H, et al, editors. Sport: Leistung and Gesundheit. Köln (Germany): Deutscher Artze Verlag; 1982. p. 293.
8. Catlin DH, Hatton CK, Starcevic SH. Issues in detecting abuse of xenobiotic anabolic steroids and testosterone by analysis of athletes' urine. Clin Chem 1997;43:1280–8.
9. Ayotte C, Goudreault D, Charlebois A. Testing for natural and synthetic anabolic agents in human urine. J Chromatogr B Biomed Appl 1996;687:3–25.
10. Catlin DH, Cowan DA, de la Torre R, et al. Urinary testosterone (T) to epitestosterone (E) ratios by GC/MS.I. Initial comparison of uncorrected T/E in six international laboratories. J Mass Spectrom 1996;31:397–402.
11. Borts DJ, Bowers L. Direct measurement of urinary testosterone and epitestosterone conjugates using high-performance liquid chromatography/tandem mass spectrometry. J Mass Spectrom 2000;35:50–61.
12. Sottas PE, Robinson N, Saugy M, et al. A forensic approach to the interpretation of blood doping markers. Law Probab Risk 2008;7:191–210.
13. Ofterbro H. Evaluating an abnormal urinary steroid profile. Lancet 1992;339:941–2.
14. Southan G, Mallat A, Jumeau J, et al. In: Program and abstracts of the Second International Symposium on Applied Mass Spectrometry in the Health Sciences. Barcelona (Spain), April 17, 1990. p. 306.
15. Donike M, Rauth S, Mareck-Engelke U, et al. Evaluation of longitudinal studies, the determination of subject-based reference ranges of the testosteorne/epitestosterone ratio. In: Donike M, Geyer H, Gotzmann A, et al, editors. Recent advances in doping analysis, proceedings of the 11th Cologne workshop on dope analysis. Köln (Germany): Sport und Buch Strausse Edition Sport; 1994. p. 33–9.
16. Sottas PE, Saudan C, Schweizer C, et al. Bayesian detection of abnormal values in longitudinal biomarkers with an application to T/E ratio. Biostatistics 2007;8:285–96.
17. McIntosh MW, Urban N. A parametric empirical Bayes method for cancer screening using longitudinal observations of a biomarker. Biostatistics 2003;4:27–40.
18. Donike M, Mareck-Engelke U, Rauth S. Statistical evaluation of longitudinal studies, part 2: the usefulness of subject based reference ranges. In:

Donike M, Geyer H, Gotzmann A, et al, editors. Proceedings of the 12th Cologne workshop on dope analysis. Köln (Germany): Sport und Buch Strausse Edition Sport; 1995. p. 157–65.

19. World Anti-Doping Agency Technical Document TD2004EAAS. Reporting and evaluation guidance for testosterone, epitestosterone, T/E ratio and other endogenous steroids. Montreal (Canada); 2004.

20. Sottas PE, Saudan C, Schweizer C, et al. From population- to subject based limit of T/E ratio to detect testosterone abuse in elite sports. Forensic Sci Int 2008;174: 166–72.

21. Aitken C, Taroni F. Statistics and the evaluation of evidence for forensic scientists. 2nd edition. Chichester (UK): Wiley & Sons; 2004.

22. Honour JW. Urinary steroid profile analysis. Clin Chim Acta 2001;313:45–50.

23. Mareck U, Geyer H, Opfermann G, et al. Factors influencing the steroid profile in doping control analysis. J Mass Spectrom 2008;43:877–91.

24. Strahm E, Kohler I, Rudaz S, et al. Isolation and quantification by high-performance liquid chromatography-ion-trap mass spectrometry of androgen sulfoconjugates in human urine. J Chromatogr A 2008;1196:153–60.

25. Sten T, Bichlmaier I, Kuuranne T, et al. UDP-glucuronosyltransferases (UGTs) 2B7 and UGT2B17 display converse specificity in testosterone and epitestosterone glucuronidation, whereas UGT2A1 conjugates both androgens similarly. Drug Metab Dispos 2009;37:417–23.

26. Ellis L, Nyborg H. Racial/ethnical variations in testosterone levels: a probable contributor to group differences in health. Steroids 1992;57:72–5.

27. De la Torre X, Segura J, Yang Z, et al. Testosterone detection in different ethnic groups. In: Donike M, Geyer H, Gotzmann A, et al, editors. Recent advances in doping analysis (4), proceedings of the Manfred Donike workshop, 14th Cologne workshop on dope analysis. Köln (Germany): Sport und Buch Strauß; 1997. p. 71–83.

28. Santner SJ, Albertson B, Zhang G-Y, et al. Comparative rates of androgen production and metabolism in Caucasian and Chinese subjects. J Clin Endocrinol Metab 1998;83:2104–9.

29. Jakobsson J, Ekström L, Inotsum N, et al. Large differences in testosterone excretion in Korean an Swedish men are strongly associated with a UDP-Glucuronosyl transferase 2B17 polymorphism. J Clin Endocrinol Metab 2006;91(2):687–93.

30. Jakobsson-Schulze JJ, Lundmark J, Garle M, et al. Doping test results dependent on genotype of UGT2B17, the major enzyme for testosterone glucoronidation. J Clin Endocrinol Metab 2008;93:2500–6.

31. Schulze JJ, Lorentzon M, Ohlsson C, et al. Genetic aspects of epitestosterone formation and androgen disposition: influence of polymorphisms in CYP17 and UGT2B enzymes. Pharmacogenet Genomics 2008;18:477–85.

32. Xue Y, Sun D, Daly A, et al. Adaptive evolution of UGT2B17 copy-number variation. Am J Hum Genet 2008;83:337–46.

33. Strahm E, Sottas PE, Schweizer C, et al. Steroid profiles of professional soccer players: an international comparative study. Br J Sports Med 2009;43:1126–30.

34. Schulze JJ, Lundmark J, Garle M, et al. Substantial advantage of a combined Bayesian and genotyping approach in testosterone doping tests. Steroids 2009;74:365–8.

35. Falk O, Palonek E, Björkhem I. Effect of ethanol on the ratio between testosterone and epitestosterone in urine. Clin Chem 1988;34:1462–4.

36. Mareck-Engelke U, Flenker U, Schänzer W. Stability of steroid profiles. In: Schänzer W, Geyer H, Gotzmann A, et al, editors. Recent advances in doping

analysis (4), proceedings of the Manfred Donike workshop, 13rd Cologne workshop on dope analysis. Köln (Germany): Sport und Buch Strauß; 1996. p. 139–57.
37. Saugy M, Cardis C, Robinson N, et al. Test methods: anabolics. Baillieres Best Pract Res Clin Endocrinol Metab 2000;14:111–33.
38. Gelman A, Carlin JB, Stern HS, et al. Bayesian data analysis. 2nd edition. Boca Raton (FL): Chapman & Hall; 2004.
39. Sottas PE, Robinson N, Saugy M. The athlete's biological passport and indirect markers of blood doping. In: Thieme D, Hemmersbach P, editors. Doping in sports (handbook of experimental pharmacology), vol. 195. Berlin: Springer; 2010.
40. Sottas PE, Lavoué J, Bruzzi R, et al. An empirical hierarchical Bayesian unification of occupational exposure assessment methods. Stat Med 2009;28:75–93.
41. Rockman MV. Reverse engineering the genotype–phenotype map with natural genetic variation. Nature 2008;456:738–44.

Ergogenic Effects of Inhaled β2-Agonists in Non-Asthmatic Athletes

Bernd Wolfarth, MD[a],*, Jan C. Wuestenfeld, MD[b],
Wilfried Kindermann, MD, PhD[c]

KEYWORDS

- β2-agonists • Asthma • Ergogenic potential
- Performance • Competitive athletes

Asthma is defined as a chronic inflammatory disorder of the airways with bronchial hyperresponsiveness and variable bronchoconstriction.[1] It is well recognized that physical exercise itself may cause asthmatic symptoms, described by the term exercise-induced asthma (EIA).[2] Numerous athletes suffer from EIA. The pharmacologic treatment is based on antiinflammatory drugs (eg, inhaled glucocorticosteroids [GCS]) and bronchodilators (eg, β2-agonists). These drugs are preferably administered by inhalation. Short-acting, inhaled β2-agonists are used prophylactically before exercise, when bronchoconstriction occurs with exercise, or other conditions. Long-acting β2-agonists are often used in combination with inhaled GCS as a basic treatment for severe cases.[3]

The use of β2-agonists is forbidden in athletes according to the "Prohibited List of the World Anti-Doping Agency" (WADA).[4] However, EIA in athletes is common and requires, in some cases, the use of inhaled β2-agonists before exercise. The proof of asthma by means of lung function and provocation tests requires a special medical examination to obtain a therapeutic use exemption (TUE).[5] The TUE process includes a complicated administrative process for the athletes and for the physicians who are responsible for the treatment. In addition, the responsibility to cover the cost for these additional tests remains unclear. Based on these considerations, the purpose of this article, as a follow-up of a recent review from 2007,[6] is to clarify whether inhaled β2-agonists have a performance-enhancing effect justifying the prohibition of these substances from the ergogenic point of view.

[a] Department of Preventive and Rehabilitative Sports Medicine, Technical University Munich, Connollystr. 32, 80809 Munich, Germany
[b] Department of Sports Medicine, Institute for Applied Training Science (IAT), Leipzig, Germany
[c] Institute of Sports and Preventive Medicine, University of Saarland, Saarbruecken, Germany
* Corresponding author.
E-mail address: wolfarth@sport.med.tum.de (B. Wolfarth).

Endocrinol Metab Clin N Am 39 (2010) 75–87
doi:10.1016/j.ecl.2009.10.005
0889-8529/10/$ – see front matter © 2010 Elsevier Inc. All rights reserved.

EPIDEMIOLOGY OF ASTHMA IN ATHLETES

Exercise-induced asthma is common in highly trained athletes. More than 10% of competitive athletes suffer from EIA. More elite athletes suffer from asthma, compared with the general population.[7] A maximum prevalence for EIA of 45% was reported in cyclists.[8] Up to 22% of Olympic athletes from the United States and Italy (Olympic Games 1996, 1998, and 2000) had asthma.[8–11] The prevalence of asthma in other highly trained athletes was reported to be between 10% to 23%,[12–14] and in adolescent athletes between 12% and 38%.[15,16] The prevalence of EIA is high in summer and winter sports. Studies show a high prevalence of EIA especially in cross-country skiers, other so-called cold-weather-athletes,[17,18] and summer endurance athletes.[14,19] Asthma also seems more common among female athletes.[8,11,14] However, this has not been entirely confirmed in other studies.[9]

Since 1984, the percentage of athletes using inhaled β2-agonists at the Olympic Games has slightly risen.[20–24] The percentage of German Olympic athletes using β2-agonists varied between 5.1% in Athens, 12.4% in Torino, and 8% in Beijing.[25–27] The question of whether this is a real increase because of EIA or a misuse because of potential ergogenic effects remains open. The increase in the use of inhaled β2-agonists has led to more stringent anti-doping rules regarding these substances.[4]

The type of training and the kind of sport can influence the prevalence of asthma.[28] The risk for developing asthmatic symptoms is higher in endurance athletes and swimmers than in other athletes.[8–12,14,19,29–34] Asthma is particularly more common in winter-sport athletes.[10,11,31,32,35] A remarkably high prevalence of asthma was reported in Swedish cross-country skiers.[31,32] Furthermore, asthma was also more frequent in athletes who participated in Nordic-combined events, short-track events,[10,11] figure skating,[36,37] and ice hockey.[37]

The highly increased ventilation during exercise and inhalation of cold, dry air are thought to be important triggers for EIA.[38] The risk for asthma seems to be higher in athletes training more than 20 hours per week when compared with training levels below 10 hours per week.[14] Atopic disposition and exposure to pollutants are risk factors for a marked bronchoconstriction during exercise.[12,34,37,39] Finally, respiratory tract infections transiently increase the bronchial hyperresponsiveness in athletes compared with non-active subjects during exercise.[40]

The more common occurrence of asthma in swimmers[19,29,30] can be explained by a number of sport-specific issues. For example, 36% of the swimmers in the 2008 German Olympic team had asthmatic symptoms and applied for a TUE to use β2-agonists by inhalation.[27] The water in swimming pools is usually chlorinated for disinfection purposes. Because of the inhalation of air floating just above the water surface, swimmers are exposed to high concentrations of chlorine.[29] In athletes with preexisting bronchial hyperreactivity, a bronchoconstriction is the logical result of chloride-gas inhalation. Furthermore, it is assumed that the repeated exposure to chlorine gas may promote the development of asthma. Based on the results of recent studies,[41–44] it was assumed that chlorination products may provoke an increase in lung-epithelium permeability in susceptible swimmers, so that the risk for developing asthma seems to be elevated.

RECOMMENDATIONS FOR THE TREATMENT OF EXERCISE-INDUCED ASTHMA

According to the guidelines,[3,45,46] baseline therapy for asthma in athletes should be anti-inflammatory, preferably with inhaled corticosteroids. Short-acting β2-agonists should be given before exercise to prevent attacks of EIA. In athletes with only rare episodes of EIA, the prophylactical application of inhaled short-acting β2-agonists may be sufficient. In all other athletes, a combined therapy with inhaled corticosteroids and long-acting β2-agonists is recommended.[3,45,46] Surprisingly there is no study published showing a positive effect of inhalative corticosteroids preventing EIA in elite athletes.

The efficiency of inhaled β2-agonists was demonstrated with several substances.[47,48] The positive effects for long-term acting β2-agonists, such as salmeterol and formoterol, were also shown.[49,50] Formoterol had a significant protective effect against EIA, compared with placebo, and a long duration of its effect was obtained.

Randomized and controlled studies for other substances, such as cromoglycate and nedocromil sodium, have not been conducted concerning the effects of inhaled β2-agonists on EIA in elite athletes, although there is evidence of a benefit in preventing EIA with leukotriene antagonists.[51–55]

RELEVANT SIDE EFFECTS OF INHALED β2-AGONISTS

Athletes can have fatal asthma exacerbations during and immediately after participating in sport activities, especially high-intensity training sessions or competition.[56] Therefore, sufficient diagnosis and therapy are necessary. On the other hand, adverse effects of β2-agonists can occur. The most frequent adverse effects from inhalation of β2-agonists are tachycardia and muscle fascillation/tremor, which are more pronounced with short-acting agents.[57] Further possible and relevant adverse effects are headaches and irritability, and at very high doses, hyperglycemia and hypokalemia.[57] Furthermore, the regular administration of β2-agonists may be associated with the development of tolerance to their effects and increased airway inflammation.[50,58–60] Tachyphylaxis develops with short- and long-acting β2-agonists, and the daily use of long-acting β2-agonists attenuates the bronchodilator effect of short-acting substances.[58,59,61] A combination with inhaled corticosteroids does not necessarily reduce tolerance.

TOLERANCE AGAINST INHALED β2-AGONISTS

The development of tolerance could influence the success of rescue therapy for severe EIA.[58–60] The increased tolerance is associated with downregulation of peripheral β2-receptors and desensitization of the receptors.[59] Tachyphylaxis to β2-agonists could be modulated by β2-adrenoceptor gene polymorphisms.[62]

In a recent review of the problems of inhaled long-acting β2-agonists,[63] a minor degree of tolerance to the bronchodilator activity was seen with formoterol, but not with salmeterol. However, there is a partial loss of protection against exercise-induced bronchoconstriction with regular use of either of these long-acting β2-agonists. Cardiac risks were not documented. In the same review, it was pointed out that the frequent administration of short-acting β2-agonists induces some loss of bronchodilatation and decrease in bronchoprotective action. However, it is the consensus, and scientifically proven, that the regular use of inhaled GCS and inhaled β2-agonists is state-of-the-art in the prevention of the bronchial system from chronic damage related to asthma.[45,46]

LEUKOTRIENE ANTAGONISTS

Leukotriene antagonists and cromolyn compounds (sodium cromoglycate and nedocromil) may provide an additional benefit and could be useful for athletes with asthma.[51–55] Leukotriene antagonists reduce asthma-related bronchoconstriction and inflammation. No relevant adverse effects have been reported.[52,53] Effects in the prevention of EIA in athletes were demonstrated for montelukast[52,53] and nedocromil.[54,55] On the other hand, montelukast was also shown to be of no benefit in the treatment of asthma like symptoms in elite ice-hockey players.[64] The performance

Table 1
Effects of inhaled β2-agonists on performance in elite athletes

Authors	Year	Subjects	Substance	Performance
McKenzie et al[69]	1983	Middle/long distance runners, 9 M, 10 F	Salbutamol	Performance unchanged
Bedi et al[68]	1988	Cyclists and triathletes, 14 M,1 F	Salbutamol	Endurance performance unchanged, final sprint improved
Meeuwisse et al[79]	1992	Cyclists, 7 M	Salbutamol	Performance unchanged
Morton et al[89]	1992	Middle/long distance runners, 16 M, 1 F	Salbutamol	Performance unchanged
Signorile et al[67]	1992	Recreational athletes, 8 M, 7 F	Salbutamol	Increased peak power in Wingate test
Fleck et al[90]	1993	Cyclists, 21 M	Salbutamol	Performance unchanged
Morton et al[91]	1993	Power athletes, 17 M	Salbutamol	Performance unchanged
Heir and Stemshaug[77]	1995	Cross-country skiers, marathon runners, orienteers, 17 M	Salbutamol	Running time until exhaustion decreased
Lemmer et al[92]	1995	Cyclists, 14 M	Salbutamol	Performance unchanged
Norris et al[93]	1996	Cyclists, 15 M	Salbutamol	Performance unchanged
Morton et al[94]	1996	Cyclists and triathletes, 16 M	Salmeterol	Performance unchanged
Carlsen et al[70]	1997	Cross-country skiers, biathletes, long dist. runners, 18 M	Salbutamol/salmeterol	Running time until exhaustion decreased

McDowell et al[95]	1997	Cyclists, 11 M	Salmeterol	Performance unchanged
Larsson et al[78]	1997	Cross-country skiers, middle/long distance runners, cyclists, 20 M	Terbutaline	Performance unchanged
Sandsund et al[72]	1998	Cross-country skiers, 8 M	Salbutamol	Performance unchanged
Sue-Chu et al[76]	1999	Cross-country skiers, 8 M	Salmeterol	Performance unchanged
Carlsen et al[96]	2001	Cross-country skiers, orienteers, others, 24 M	Formoterol	Performance unchanged
Goubault et al[71]	2001	Triathletes, 12 M	Salbutamol	Performance unchanged
Stewart et al[97]	2002	Highly trained athletes, 10 M	Salbutamol/formoterol	Performance unchanged
van Baak et al[73]	2004	Cyclists and triathletes, 16 M	Salbutamol	Time trial performance increased (+1.9%)
Riiser et al[74]	2006	Cross-country skiers, 20 M	Formoterol	Performance unchanged
Tjörhom et al[75]	2007	Cross-country skiers, 20 M	Formoterol	Performance unchanged
Sporer et al[98]	2008	Cyclists and triathletes, 37 M	Salbutamol	Performance unchanged

Abbreviations: F, female; M, male.

of highly trained non-asthmatic athletes is not affected by montelukast.[65] Different testing methods could have contributed to these varying results. In the study of Rundell and colleagues,[52] eucapnic voluntary hyperventilation was used for the identification of EIA, whereas other authors tested only baseline lung function or clinical aspects. In conclusion, cromolyn was less effective than β2-agonists.[66]

EFFECTS OF β2-AGONISTS ON PERFORMANCE IN ATHLETES

All studies investigating the effects of inhaled β2-agonists on physical performance in highly trained athletes are summarized in **Table 1**. The athletes were tested in randomized, double-blind, and mostly crossover placebo-controlled design. The studies by Signorile and colleagues[67] and Bedi and colleagues[68] are included, although these studies investigated recreational athletes and elite athletes in mixed cohorts. These studies are the only two published so far demonstrating a positive effect of therapeutic doses of inhaled β2-agonists on performance in athletes. All subjects were non-asthmatic, competitive athletes and had normal pulmonary function. The subjects were mainly endurance athletes such as cyclists, middle- and long-distance runners, cross-country skiers, and triathletes; in one study, power athletes were the subjects.

Differing test results, mainly ergometer and treadmill trials, were conducted by assessing, in numerous studies, the performance time until exhaustion, total exercise time, and time-trial performances. Also, sport-specific tests in ambient environments were conducted proving the laboratory results.

In most of the studies, the β2-agonists were inhaled 15 to 30 minutes before exercise. In one study, salbutamol was administered four times per day for 1 week.[69] The inhaled substances were salbutamol, salmeterol, formoterol, and terbutaline. High doses of salbutamol (800–1200µg) were given in four studies.[70–73] Proving the effects of extreme ambient conditions, five studies were conducted at an ambient temperature of $-10\,°C$, $-15\,°C$, and $-20\,°C$ and one study was conducted under hypobaric conditions.[72,74–76] In the presented studies, inhaled β2-agonists were without effect on VO2max, anaerobic threshold, alactic and lactic anaerobic power, strength performance, blood lactate, rate of perceived exertion, and psychomotor performance. In two studies, the performance in running time until exhaustion was even reduced under salbutamol[70,77] and salmeterol.[70] Even high doses of salbutamol had no ergogenic effect in four of five studies.[70–72] Furthermore, inhaled β2-agonists did not change physical performance under the stress of cold temperatures or hypobaric conditions.[72,76,78]

On the other hand, ergogenic effects were demonstrated in three studies.[67,68,73] Bedi and colleagues[68] found an increased performance in ride time in an exhaustive final sprint after salbutamol inhalation. However, two recreational cyclists were included in their study. In a subsequent study, with a similar study design, these results could not be confirmed.[79] In the study by van Baak and colleagues,[73] the inhalation of a supratherapeutic dose of salbutamol (800µg) improved the cycling performance in a time trial by 2%. The largest improvements were found in those subjects with lower performance. After inhalation of salbutamol, a better performance was seen in 11 of 16 subjects; however, this effect was minimal in five of these subjects. In the frequently cited study by Signorile, an increase in peak power during a 15 second Wingate test was observed after inhalation of salbutamol before performance. In contrast to all other studies cited here, Signorile and colleagues[67] observed only recreational athletes assuming that there might be an ergogenic effect of β2-agonists in recreational athletes.

Despite unchanged performance-related variables, the lung function was improved after inhalation of β2-agonists in most studies (measured by an increase in the forced expiratory volume in 1 second [FEV1]). Apparently, inhaled β2-agonists also induce a small bronchodilation in healthy athletes. However, the increase in lung function does not induce enhancement in performance.

In contrast to inhaled β2-agonists, oral administration of salbutamol can induce ergogenic effects.[80–86] Oral administration of salbutamol can improve muscle strength,[80,85,86] anaerobic power,[83,84] and endurance performance in men.[81] In addition, concomitant hormonal and metabolic changes were demonstrated.[82,83] The dose needed to obtain this effect is higher than that used for therapeutic purposes in asthma. The oral administration dose of salbutamol is 10- to 20-fold greater than the dose used by inhalation.

In conclusion, inhaled β2-agonists seem to be without relevant effect on physical performance in highly trained non-asthmatic athletes. The improved lung function, as demonstrated in the majority of studies, cannot be regarded as ergogenic. The ventilation is generally considered as non-limiting during maximal exercise in young non-asthmatic subjects.[87] During maximal exercise, pulmonary ventilation is not as high as the maximal achievable ventilation. Specific inspiratory muscle training does not improve aerobic capacity.[88] There is no evidence for anabolic effects of inhaled β2-agonists.

WORLD ANTI-DOPING CODE AND THERAPEUTIC USE EXEMPTIONS

The so-called "Prohibited List" was first published in 1963 under the leadership of the International Olympic Committee (IOC). Since 2004, as mandated by the World Anti-Doping Code (WADA Code), WADA is responsible for the preparation and publication of this list.[4] In the current WADA list (2009), all β2-agonists are prohibited, in and out of competition. As an exception, formoterol, salbutamol, salmeterol, and terbutaline are permitted by inhalation to prevent or treat asthma and EIA. In these cases, a TUE is necessary. A specific form for this must be completed and signed by the physician and the athlete. A clinical history of the athlete and results of lung-function tests are mandatory. The complete form package, including the signed forms and the medical file, has to be sent to the responsible anti-doping organization (eg, National Anti Doping Organization [NADO], International Federation [IF]). Each anti-doping organization has to establish a TUE committee (TUEC) of at least three people experienced in sports medicine who are in charge to review the applications and to decide whether an approval for the use of β2-agonists will be granted or not.[5]

The IOC was the first anti-doping body who established concrete limits for diagnostic methods aimed to prove EIA and asthma for the 2002 Salt Lake City Olympic Winter Games in the United States. The following tests were accepted[20]: (1) bronchodilator test (increase in FEV1 of at least 12% from baseline FEV1 after the administration of a β2-agonist by inhalation); (2) bronchial provocation with either exercise challenge in the laboratory or field, or eucapnic voluntary hyperpnea test ($\geq$10% fall in FEV1, respectively); or (3) bronchial provocation with methacholine (diagnostic limits: Provocative Concentration (PC20) FEV1 <4 mg/ml or Provocative Dose (PD20) $\leq$400μg in steroid naive subjects. If subjects inhaled steroids >3 months: PC20 FEV1$\leq$16mg/ml or PD20 $\leq$1600μg).

At the printing time of this article WADA released new regulations becoming effective from January 2010. The new reglament allows the use of two β2-agonists (salbutamol and salmeterol) by inhalation without the need for a full TUE. In these cases a so called declaration of use is sufficient. However, for the use of other inhalative substances like formoterol or terbutaline the formerly described TUE process remains the same.

SUMMARY

Empiric data suggests that some non-asthmatic athletes use β2-agonists believing this could potentially enhance their performance. However, on the basis of scientific evidence, inhaled β2-agonists do not have a relevant performance-enhancing effect in non-asthmatic competitive athletes. To prevent an overuse of non-performance–enhancing medication in general, education and prevention programs seem to be more appropriate compared to prohibition and sanctioning. For these reasons and from the ergogenic point of view, inhaled β2-agonists should not be prohibited for athletes. Considering the possibility for quantitative analysis of salbutamol, the recently implemented threshold regulation is sufficient to detect misuse of this substance. From this point of view, it would make sense to include the β2-agonists in the so-called monitoring list of the WADA anti-doping program. This inclusion would enable the anti-doping bodies to control for a possible increase in the use of β2-agonists, and in this case to bring back the substance to the list without greater efforts, if needed. On the other hand, it would significantly reduce the administrative expenses for the handling of these substances. With the announced changes of the WADA list 2010, the first step in that direction is done. Considering the limited financial and personal resources, the fight against doping should concentrate on substances and methods that have performance-enhancing effects, and therefore, lead to unfair competition conditions.

REFERENCES

1. Reddel HK, Taylor DR, Bateman ED, et al. An official American Thoracic Society/European Respiratory Society statement: asthma control and exacerbations: standardizing endpoints for clinical asthma trials and clinical practice. Am J Respir Crit Care Med 2009;180:59–99.
2. Carlsen KH, Anderson SD, Bjermer L, et al. Exercise-induced asthma, respiratory and allergic disorders in elite athletes: epidemiology, mechanisms and diagnosis: part I of the report from the Joint Task Force of the European Respiratory Society (ERS) and the European Academy of Allergy and Clinical Immunology (EAACI) in cooperation with GA2LEN. Allergy 2008;63:387–403.
3. Carlsen KH, Anderson SD, Bjermer L, et al. Treatment of exercise-induced asthma, respiratory and allergic disorders in sports and the relationship to doping: part II of the report from the Joint Task Force of European Respiratory Society (ERS) and European Academy of Allergy and Clinical Immunology (EAACI) in cooperation with GA(2)LEN. Allergy 2008;63:492–505.
4. World Anti-Doping Agency. Available at: http://www.wada-ama.org. Accessed 2009.
5. International Standard for Therapeutic Use Exemptions. World anti-doping agency. Available at: http://www.wada-ama.org/rtcontent/document/TUE_Standard_2009_en.pdf. Accessed 2009.
6. Kindermann W. Do inhaled beta(2)-agonists have an ergogenic potential in non-asthmatic competitive athletes? Sports Med 2007;37:95–102.
7. Rundell KW, Jenkinson DM. Exercise-induced bronchospasm in the elite athlete. Sports Med 2002;32:583–600.
8. Weiler JM, Layton T, Hunt M. Asthma in United States Olympic athletes who participated in the 1996 summer games. J Allergy Clin Immunol 1998;102:722–6.
9. Maiolo C, Fuso L, Todaro A, et al. Prevalence of asthma and atopy in Italian Olympic athletes. Int J Sports Med 2004;25:139–44.

10. Weiler JM, Ryan EJ III. Asthma in United States Olympic athletes who participated in the 1998 Olympic winter games. J Allergy Clin Immunol 2000;106: 267–71.
11. Wilber RL, Rundell KW, Szmedra L, et al. Incidence of exercise-induced bronchospasm in Olympic winter sport athletes. Med Sci Sports Exerc 2000;32: 732–7.
12. Helenius IJ, Tikkanen HO, Sarna S, et al. Asthma and increased bronchial responsiveness in elite athletes: atopy and sport event as risk factors. J Allergy Clin Immunol 1998;101:646–52.
13. Langdeau JB, Turcotte H, Thibault G, et al. Comparative prevalence of asthma in different groups of athletes: a survey. Can Respir J 2004;11:402–6.
14. Nystad W, Harris J, Borgen JS. Asthma and wheezing among Norwegian elite athletes. Med Sci Sports Exerc 2000;32:266–70.
15. Mannix ET, Roberts MA, Dukes HJ, et al. Airways hyperresponsiveness in high school athletes. J Asthma 2004;41:567–74.
16. Rupp NT, Guill MF, Brudno DS. Unrecognized exercise-induced bronchospasm in adolescent athletes. Am J Dis Child 1992;146:941–4.
17. Karjalainen EM, Laitinen A, Sue-Chu M, et al. Evidence of airway inflammation and remodeling in ski athletes with and without bronchial hyperresponsiveness to methacholine. Am J Respir Crit Care Med 2000;161:2086–91.
18. Helenius IJ, Tikkanen HO, Haahtela T. Occurrence of exercise induced bronchospasm in elite runners: dependence on atopy and exposure to cold air and pollen. Br J Sports Med 1998;32:125–9.
19. Helenius I, Haahtela T. Allergy and asthma in elite summer sport athletes. J Allergy Clin Immunol 2000;106:444–52.
20. Anderson SD, Fitch K, Perry CP, et al. Responses to bronchial challenge submitted for approval to use inhaled beta2-agonists before an event at the 2002 Winter Olympics. J Allergy Clin Immunol 2003;111:45–50.
21. McKenzie DC, Stewart IB, Fitch KD. The asthmatic athlete, inhaled beta agonists, and performance. Clin J Sport Med 2002;12:225–8.
22. Pierson WE, Voy RO. Exercise-induced bronchospasm in the XXIII summer Olympic games. N Engl Reg Allergy Proc 1988;9:209–13.
23. Tsitsimpikou C, Tsiokanos A, Tsarouhas K, et al. Medication use by athletes at the Athens 2004 Summer Olympic Games. Clin J Sport Med 2009;19:33–8.
24. Fitch KD. beta2-agonists at the Olympic Games. Clin Rev Allergy Immunol 2006; 31:259–68.
25. Kindermann W, Engelhardt M, Eder K. Sportmedizinische Betreuung bei Olympia 2004. Leistungssport 2005;35:1–4.
26. Huber G, Kreutzer P, Eder U, et al. Olympische Winterspiele Turin - eine besondere Herausfórderung für die medizinische Betreuung. Leistungssport 2006;36: 25–8.
27. Wolfarth B, Engelhardt M, Eder K, et al. Sportmedizinische Betreuung bei den Olympischen Spielen 2008. Leistungssport 2009;39:1–4.
28. Belda J, Ricart S, Casan P, et al. Airway inflammation in the elite athlete and type of sport. Br J Sports Med 2008;42:244–8.
29. Drobnic F, Freixa A, Casan P, et al. Assessment of chlorine exposure in swimmers during training. Med Sci Sports Exerc 1996;28:271–4.
30. Langdeau JB, Boulet LP. Prevalence and mechanisms of development of asthma and airway hyperresponsiveness in athletes. Sports Med 2001;31:601–16.
31. Larsson K, Ohlsen P, Larsson L, et al. High prevalence of asthma in cross country skiers. BMJ 1993;307:1326–9.

32. Sue-Chu M, Larsson L, Bjermer L. Prevalence of asthma in young cross-country skiers in central Scandinavia: differences between Norway and Sweden. Respir Med 1996;90:99–105.
33. Thole RT, Sallis RE, Rubin AL, et al. Exercise-induced bronchospasm prevalence in collegiate cross-country runners. Med Sci Sports Exerc 2001;33:1641–6.
34. Tikkanen H. Helenius I Asthma in runners. BMJ 1994;309:1087.
35. Mannix ET, Farber MO, Palange P, et al. Exercise-induced asthma in figure skaters. Chest 1996;109:312–5.
36. Provost-Craig MA, Arbour KS, Sestili DC, et al. The incidence of exercise-induced bronchospasm in competitive figure skaters. J Asthma 1996;33:67–71.
37. Rundell KW, Spiering BA, Evans TM, et al. Baseline lung function, exercise-induced bronchoconstriction, and asthma-like symptoms in elite women ice hockey players. Med Sci Sports Exerc 2004;36:405–10.
38. Bougault V, Turmel J, St-Laurent J, et al. Asthma, airway inflammation and epithelial damage in swimmers and cold-air athletes. Eur Respir J 2009;33: 740–6.
39. Pierson WE, Covert DS, Koenig JQ, et al. Implications of air pollution effects on athletic performance. Med Sci Sports Exerc 1986;18:322–7.
40. Heir T, Aanestad G, Carlsen KH, et al. Respiratory tract infection and bronchial responsiveness in elite athletes and sedentary control subjects. Scand J Med Sci Sports 1995;5:94–9.
41. Bernard A, Carbonnelle S, Michel O, et al. Lung hyperpermeability and asthma prevalence in schoolchildren: unexpected associations with the attendance at indoor chlorinated swimming pools. Occup Environ Med 2003;60:385–94.
42. Bernard A, Nickmilder M, Voisin C. Outdoor swimming pools and the risks of asthma and allergies during adolescence. Eur Respir J 2008;32:979–88.
43. Bernard A, Carbonnelle S, De BC, et al. Chlorinated pool attendance, atopy, and the risk of asthma during childhood. Environ Health Perspect 2006;114: 1567–73.
44. Lagerkvist BJ, Bernard A, Blomberg A, et al. Pulmonary epithelial integrity in children: relationship to ambient ozone exposure and swimming pool attendance. Environ Health Perspect 2004;112:1768–71.
45. Kelly HW. What is new with the beta2-agonists: issues in the management of asthma. Ann Pharmacother 2005;39:931–8.
46. Sears MR, Lotvall J. Past, present and future–beta2-adrenoceptor agonists in asthma management. Respir Med 2005;99:152–70.
47. Shapiro GG, Kemp JP, DeJong R, et al. Effects of albuterol and procaterol on exercise-induced asthma. Ann Allergy 1990;65:273–6.
48. Anderson SD, Rodwell LT, Du TJ, et al. Duration of protection by inhaled salmeterol in exercise-induced asthma. Chest 1991;100:1254–60.
49. Ferrari M, Balestreri F, Baratieri S, et al. Evidence of the rapid protective effect of formoterol dry-powder inhalation against exercise-induced bronchospasm in athletes with asthma. Respiration 2000;67:510–3.
50. Nelson JA, Strauss L, Skowronski M, et al. Effect of long-term salmeterol treatment on exercise-induced asthma. N Engl J Med 1998;339:141–6.
51. Leff JA, Busse WW, Pearlman D, et al. Montelukast, a leukotriene-receptor antagonist, for the treatment of mild asthma and exercise-induced bronchoconstriction. N Engl J Med 1998;339:147–52.
52. Rundell KW, Spiering BA, Baumann JM, et al. Effects of montelukast on airway narrowing from eucapnic voluntary hyperventilation and cold air exercise. Br J Sports Med 2005;39:232–6.

53. Steinshamn S, Sandsund M, Sue-Chu M, et al. Effects of montelukast and salme-terol on physical performance and exercise economy in adult asthmatics with exercise-induced bronchoconstriction. Chest 2004;126:1154–60.

54. Todaro A, Faina M, Alippi B, et al. Nedocromil sodium in the prevention of exer-cise-induced bronchospasm in athletes with asthma. J Sports Med Phys Fitness 1993;33:137–45.

55. Valero A, Garrido E, Malet A, et al. Exercise-induced asthma prophylaxis in athletes using inhaled nedocromil sodium. Allergol Immunopathol (Madr) 1996; 24:81–6.

56. Becker JM, Rogers J, Rossini G, et al. Asthma deaths during sports: report of a 7-year experience. J Allergy Clin Immunol 2004;113:264–7.

57. Abramson MJ, Walters J, Walters EH. Adverse effects of beta-agonists: are they clinically relevant? Am J Respir Med 2003;2:287–97.

58. Anderson SD, Brannan JD. Long-acting beta 2-adrenoceptor agonists and exer-cise-induced asthma: lessons to guide us in the future. Paediatr Drugs 2004;6: 161–75.

59. Salpeter SR, Ormiston TM, Salpeter EE. Meta-analysis: respiratory tolerance to regular beta2-agonist use in patients with asthma. Ann Intern Med 2004;140: 802–13.

60. Anderson SD, Caillaud C, Brannan JD. Beta2-agonists and exercise-induced asthma. Clin Rev Allergy Immunol 2006;31:163–80.

61. Salpeter SR, Buckley NS, Ormiston TM, et al. Meta-analysis: effect of long-acting beta-agonists on severe asthma exacerbations and asthma-related deaths. Ann Intern Med 2006;144:904–12.

62. Taylor DR, Drazen JM, Herbison GP, et al. Asthma exacerbations during long term beta agonist use: influence of beta(2) adrenoceptor polymorphism. Thorax 2000;55:762–7.

63. Nelson HS. Is there a problem with inhaled long-acting beta-adrenergic agonists? J Allergy Clin Immunol 2006;117:3–16.

64. Helenius I, Lumme A, Ounap J, et al. No effect of montelukast on asthma-like symptoms in elite ice hockey players. Allergy 2004;59:39–44.

65. Sue-Chu M, Sandsund M, Holand B, et al. Montelukast does not affect exercise performance at subfreezing temperature in highly trained non-asthmatic endur-ance athletes. Int J Sports Med 2000;21:424–8.

66. Anderson SD. Single-dose agents in the prevention of exercise-induced asthma: a descriptive review. Treat Respir Med 2004;3:365–79.

67. Signorile JF, Kaplan TA, Applegate B, et al. Effects of acute inhalation of the bronchodilator, albuterol, on power output. Med Sci Sports Exerc 1992;24: 638–42.

68. Bedi JF, Gong H Jr, Horvath SM. Enhancement of exercise performance with inhaled albuterol. Can J Sport Sci 1988;13:144–8.

69. McKenzie DC, Rhodes EC, Stirling DR, et al. Salbutamol and treadmill perfor-mance in non-atopic athletes. Med Sci Sports Exerc 1983;15:520–2.

70. Carlsen KH, Ingjer F, Kirkegaard H, et al. The effect of inhaled salbutamol and sal-meterol on lung function and endurance performance in healthy well-trained athletes. Scand J Med Sci Sports 1997;7:160–5.

71. Goubault C, Perault MC, Leleu E, et al. Effects of inhaled salbutamol in exercising non-asthmatic athletes. Thorax 2001;56:675–9.

72. Sandsund M, Sue-Chu M, Helgerud J, et al. Effect of cold exposure (-15 degrees C) and salbutamol treatment on physical performance in elite nonasthmatic cross-country skiers. Eur J Appl Physiol Occup Physiol 1998;77:297–304.

73. van Baak MA, de Hon OM, Hartgens F, et al. Inhaled salbutamol and endurance cycling performance in non-asthmatic athletes. Int J Sports Med 2004;25:533–8.
74. Riiser A, Tjorhom A, Carlsen KH. The effect of formoterol inhalation on endurance performance in hypobaric conditions. Med Sci Sports Exerc 2006;38: 2132–7.
75. Tjorhom A, Riiser A, Carlsen KH. Effects of formoterol on endurance performance in athletes at an ambient temperature of -20 degrees C. Scand J Med Sci Sports 2007;17:628–35.
76. Sue-Chu M, Sandsund M, Helgerud J, et al. Salmeterol and physical performance at -15 degrees C in highly trained nonasthmatic cross-country skiers. Scand J Med Sci Sports 1999;9:48–52.
77. Heir T, Stemshaug H. Salbutamol and high-intensity treadmill running in nonasthmatic highly conditioned athletes. Scand J Med Sci Sports 1995;5:231–6.
78. Larsson K, Gavhed D, Larsson L, et al. Influence of a beta2-agonist on physical performance at low temperature in elite athletes. Med Sci Sports Exerc 1997;29: 1631–6.
79. Meeuwisse WH, McKenzie DC, Hopkins SR, et al. The effect of salbutamol on performance in elite nonasthmatic athletes. Med Sci Sports Exerc 1992;24: 1161–6.
80. Caruso JF, Signorile JF, Perry AC, et al. The effects of albuterol and isokinetic exercise on the quadriceps muscle group. Med Sci Sports Exerc 1995;27: 1471–6.
81. Collomp K, Candau R, Collomp R, et al. Effects of acute ingestion of salbutamol during submaximal exercise. Int J Sports Med 2000;21:480–4.
82. Collomp K, Candau R, Lasne F, et al. Effects of short-term oral salbutamol administration on exercise endurance and metabolism. J Appl Phys 2000;89: 430–6.
83. Collomp K, Le PB, Portier H, et al. Effects of acute salbutamol intake during a Wingate test. Int J Sports Med 2005;26:513–7.
84. Le PB, Collomp K, Portier H, et al. Effects of short-term salbutamol ingestion during a Wingate test. Int J Sports Med 2005;26:518–23.
85. Martineau L, Horan MA, Rothwell NJ, et al. Salbutamol, a beta 2-adrenoceptor agonist, increases skeletal muscle strength in young men. Clin Sci (Lond) 1992;83:615–21.
86. van Baak MA, Mayer LH, Kempinski RE, et al. Effect of salbutamol on muscle strength and endurance performance in nonasthmatic men. Med Sci Sports Exerc 2000;32:1300–6.
87. Stromme SB, Boushel R, Ekblom B. Cardiovascular and respiratory aspects of exercise: endurance training. In: Kjaer M, Krogsgaard M, Magnusson P, editors. Textbook of sports medicine. Oxford (UK): Blackwell Science; 2003. p. 11–29.
88. Inbar O, Weiner P, Azgad Y, et al. Specific inspiratory muscle training in well-trained endurance athletes. Med Sci Sports Exerc 2000;32:1233–7.
89. Morton AR, Papalia SM, Fitch KD. Is salbutamol ergogenic? The effects of slabutamol on physical performance in the high-performance non-asthmatic athlete. Clin J Sport Med 1992;2:93–7.
90. Fleck SJ, Lucia A, Storms WW, et al. Effects of acute inhalation of albuterol on submaximal and maximal VO2 and blood lactate. Int J Sports Med 1993;14: 239–43.
91. Morton AR, Papalia SM, Fitch KD. Changes in anaerobic power and strength performance after inhalation of salbutamol in non-asthmatic athletes. Clin J Sport Med 1993;3:14–9.

92. Lemmer JT, Fleck SJ, Wallach JM, et al. The effects of albuterol on power output in non-asthmatic athletes. Int J Sports Med 1995;16:243–9.
93. Norris SR, Petersen SR, Jones RL. The effect of salbutamol on performance in endurance cyclists. Eur J Appl Physiol Occup Physiol 1996;73:364–8.
94. Morton AR, Joyce K, Papalia SM, et al. Is salmeterol ergogenic? Clin J Sport Med 1996;6:220–5.
95. McDowell SL, Fleck SJ, Storms WW. The effects of salmeterol on power output in nonasthmatic athletes. J Allergy Clin Immunol 1997;99:443–9.
96. Carlsen KH, Hem E, Stensrud T, et al. Can asthma treatment in sports be doping? The effect of the rapid onset, long-acting inhaled beta2-agonist formoterol upon endurance performance in healthy well-trained athletes. Respir Med 2001;95:571–6.
97. Stewart IB, Labreche JM, McKenzie DC. Acute formoterol administration has no ergogenic effect in nonasthmatic athletes. Med Sci Sports Exerc 2002;34:213–7.
98. Sporer BC, Sheel AW, McKenzie DC. Dose response of inhaled salbutamol on exercise performance and urine concentrations. Med Sci Sports Exerc 2008;40:149–57.

Stimulants and Doping in Sport

Mario Thevis, PhD*, Gerd Sigmund, MSc, Hans Geyer, PhD,
Wilhelm Schänzer, PhD

KEYWORDS

- Doping • Sport • Amphetamine • Ephedrine
- 4-methylhexan-2-amine • Mass spectrometry

Stimulants represent one of the oldest classes of doping agents and have been used to increase performance, endurance, and stamina for centuries. According to reports on the habits of the indigenous people in the Peruvian Andes, the consumption of coca leaves (and thus cocaine) was widespread and mostly uncontrolled in the pre-Inca period.[1] It became also part of religious Inca rituals, which were hardly related to athletic challenges; however, cocaine's potential to reduce pain and hunger as well as to enhance or prolong physical work was recognized, and it was used during long and energy-demanding marches under hypoxic conditions.[2]

The first documents demonstrating a doping offense with cocaine according to modern regulations were found in racewalking competitions in the eighteenth century. Racewalking, a British invention, potentially arose from the job of "footmen" accompanying wealthy travelers in the sixteenth and seventeenth centuries and later became a competitive sporting event with the goal to complete 100 miles (or more) in 24 hours without breaking into a run. In the late nineteenth century, various astonishing achievements in racewalking were reported and the use of cocaine was frequently mentioned, which further outlined the performance-enhancing properties of the stimulating and fatigue-reducing drug.[3]

The continuous research on active ingredients of plants in the nineteenth century; the constantly improving possibilities to isolate, purify, and characterize substances from complex mixtures; and the options to chemically modify these compounds have led to the detection, production, and use of various additional stimulating agents for clinical and nonclinical purposes (eg, strychnine,[4] ephedrine,[5,6] and related synthetic derivatives).[7–9] The efficiency of stimulating drugs such as strychnine, cocaine, ephedrines, and amphetamines on performance was hardly systematically evaluated; only a few studies allowed an estimation of performance enhancement in selected sport disciplines, which ranged from 0.6% to 4% for amphetamines.[10–19]

Institute of Biochemistry, Center for Preventive Doping Research, German Sport University Cologne, Am Sportpark Müngersdorf 6, 50933 Cologne, Germany
* Corresponding author.
E-mail address: m.thevis@biochem.dshs-koeln.de (M. Thevis).

Endocrinol Metab Clin N Am 39 (2010) 89–105
doi:10.1016/j.ecl.2009.10.011
0889-8529/10/$ – see front matter © 2010 Elsevier Inc. All rights reserved.

Although these numbers appear comparably low, such small improvements might represent the competitive edge in elite sport. A great variety of stimulating drugs have been detected in human routine doping control samples since systematic sports drug-testing programs were installed in 1967, and stimulants in general have been among the most frequently found prohibited compounds since.

In the following sections, a selection of stimulants, their prevalence in sports, particular challenges, and detection strategies are described. It is noteworthy that sports drug testing, especially with regard to alkaloid-based stimulants, was first introduced in animal doping controls in the early twentieth century, and much effort was necessary to establish and continuously improve detection methods that sensitively and selectively measure banned compounds in bodily specimens.

CHEMISTRY AND PHARMACOLOGY OF STIMULANTS
Categories of Stimulants

The class of stimulants prohibited by the World Anti-Doping Agency (WADA)[20] contains various agents with different structural features. Many of these compounds are derived from phenethylamine or phenylpropanolamine core structures (Fig. 1) and represent drugs such as amphetamine (1), methamphetamine (2), methylenedioxymethamphetamine (MDMA, ecstasy, 3), or cathine (4), ephedrine (5), and metamfepramone (6). Additional alkaloids with stimulating properties are cocaine (7) and strychnine (8), which bear entirely different structures based on tropane and indole nuclei. Moreover, alkylamines such as tuaminoheptane (9) or 4-methylhexan-2-amine (10) as well as designer substances such as the hybrid of amphetamine and piracetam referred to as carphedone (11), were considered relevant for doping controls. In contrast to most prohibited stimulants, ephedrine, methylephedrine, and cathine are currently banned only when they exceed a urinary threshold level of 10 μg/mL (ephedrine and methylephedrine) or 5 μg/mL (cathine).

Mechanisms of Action

Detailed studies on the mechanisms of action of selected central nervous system (CNS) stimulants have been conducted for more than 3 decades, and at least 3 major modes of influencing the process of neurotransmission at the nerve terminal were elucidated. The modes include (1) an elevated release of neurotransmitters (eg, dopamine, noradrenaline, and serotonin) into the synaptic cleft, (2) the direct stimulation of postsynaptic receptors, and (3) the inhibition of neurotransmitter reuptake.[21–24]

One of the most widely studied topics in stimulants is amphetamine (see Fig. 1, 1) and its effect on dopaminergic neurons, although numerous articles on the influence of amphetamine on noradrenergic and serotonergic systems have been published also. In the case of dopamine, amphetamine was shown to exert mechanism (1), ie, causing an increased secretion of the neurotransmitter, through manipulation of the Na^+/Cl^- dependent dopamine transporter (DAT). The function of the DAT to clear extracellular dopamine from the synaptic cleft is reversed in the presence of extracellular amphetamine, and bursts of dopamine are released into the synaptic cleft in a channel-like mode,[25] which intensifies the dopaminergic neurotransmission significantly. Moreover, the inhibitory effect of amphetamine on monoamine oxidase (MAO) was reported, which further interferes with the metabolism and thus elimination of dopamine. Direct interaction of amphetamine with the neurotransmitter receptors and its potential to counteract reuptake were also hypothesized.[21] In contrast to amphetamine and related drugs, the CNS stimulant cocaine (7) (see Fig. 1) does not increase the release of dopamine from nerve terminals but elevates concentrations of dopaminergic and

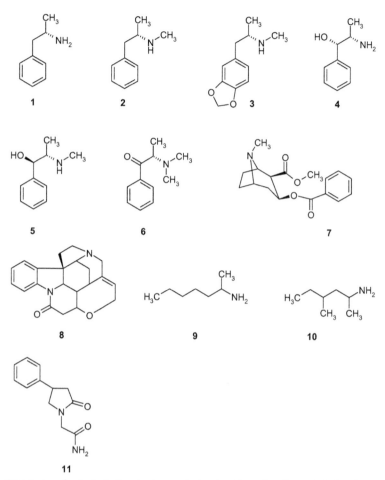

Fig. 1. Structures of selected stimulants: amphetamine (**1**, molecular weight [mol wt] = 135), methamphetamine (**2**, mol wt = 149), MDMA/ecstasy (**3**, mol wt = 193), cathine (**4**, mol wt = 151), ephedrine (**5**, mol wt = 165), metamfepramone (**6**, mol wt = 177), cocaine (**7**, 303), strychnine (**8**, mol wt = 334), tuaminoheptane (**9**, mol wt = 115) or 4-methylhexan-2-amine (**10**, mol wt = 115), and carphedone (**11**, mol wt = 218).

noradrenergic transmitters at the neuronal synapse, predominantly by binding to the DAT and efficiently blocking dopamine reuptake.[2] In a similar fashion, the sympathomimetic compounds tuaminoheptane (**9**) and 4-methylhexan-2-amine (**10**) (see **Fig. 1**) were shown to hamper the noradrenaline reuptake.[26] The mechanism underlying the stimulating activity of ephedrine (**5**) (see **Fig. 1**) is reported to be based on the displacement of neurotransmitters from respective storage sites. Extracellular ephedrine is transferred into the presynaptic neuron and stored in vesicles, where it exhibits considerable resistance against MAOs because of the methylated amino function and further prolongs the effect of released neurotransmitters. In addition to its indirect mechanism of action, ephedrine was also shown to possess weak direct effects on alpha- and beta-adrenergic receptors. It affects primarily the adrenergic receptor system that is a part of the sympathetic nervous system rather than the CNS due to its reduced lipophilicity, which results from the β-positioned hydroxyl function.

The peripheral effects of the sympathomimetic amines commonly include an elevated blood pressure, increased pulse rate, and bronchodilatation, which is complemented by diminished fatigue and improved alertness. These beneficial effects are considered the major reasons for athletes to abuse stimulants in sports, and numerous doping rule violations have been recorded ever since systematic doping controls have been conducted.

PREVALENCE OF STIMULANTS IN SPORT

Stimulants have been a major problem in elite sports and numerous adverse analytical findings (AAFs) have been annually reported by doping control laboratories worldwide. In **Table 1**, the WADA statistics of 2003 to 2007 are summarized,[27] indicating that constantly more than 10% of all AAFs were related to drugs belonging to the class of stimulating agents. In 2003, more than 50% of doping offenses with stimulants were because of ephedrine and its stereoisomer pseudoephedrine. The latter was removed, together with caffeine, from the prohibited list at the end of 2003 and was no longer a subject of sanctions when detected in doping control urine samples. In the following 4 years, amphetamine was constantly the most frequently detected stimulant, representing up to 54% of all AAFs resulting from stimulant misuse, complemented predominantly by findings of cocaine and ephedrine applications; however, it must be considered that various drugs categorized as stimulating agents metabolize to give amphetamine,[22] which might contribute to and explain the prominent occurrence of amphetamine cases.

Pseudoephedrine—Prevalence Before and After Lifting the Ban

Until the end of 2003, pseudoephedrine, the stereoisomer of ephedrine (**Fig. 2**), was prohibited in sports when a threshold value of 25 μg/mL of urine was exceeded. The threshold level for pseudoephedrine was initially set to 10 μg/mL, then increased to 25 μg/mL in 2000, and since January 2004 the presence of this drug in doping control urine samples and its use in sports were no longer sanctioned. Hence, pseudoephedrine represents an interesting object to outline a possible effect of lifting a ban for a drug, the ergogenic properties of which are controversially discussed.[24]

Data generated and recorded in the doping control laboratory of Cologne between 1996 and 2003 that included a total of 52,347 in-competition analyses yielded 33 and 93 AAFs for pseudoephedrine and ephedrine, respectively, which accounts for an average of 4.1 (0.06%) and 11.6 (0.18%) positive controls per year. In 2007 and 2008, that is, 3 years after pseudoephedrine was removed from the prohibited list, the prevalence of pseudoephedrine and ephedrine was determined in 16,335 in-competition doping control samples. The analyses resulted in 102 (0.62%) and 9 (0.06%) cases of pseudoephedrine and ephedrine use or misuse, respectively, representing a considerable increase of findings for pseudoephedrine at concentrations higher than the formerly valid threshold. One of the major contributors to these samples were cyclists, who provided 53 positive test results in 1343 specimens, including 44 (3.28%) and 9 (0.67%) cases of pseudoephedrine and ephedrine, respectively. This is particularly interesting because only 10 findings were reported in cycling in the period between 1996 and 2003 (4 samples containing pseudoephedrine and 6 samples containing ephedrine exceeding their respective threshold levels). These observations are confirmed by data of the Belgian sports drug-testing laboratory, which reported a significant increase in urine samples containing pseudoephedrine in concentrations higher than 25 μg/mL.[28] Over a 3-year period, only 0.2% of all urine specimens were tested positive for pseudoephedrine, which increased to 1.4% AAFs

Table 1
Prevalence of stimulants in elite sports from 2003 to 2007

Year	Total Number of A-Samples	Total Number of AAF with Stimulants	Percent of Total Number of AAFs Worldwide	Top 5 of The Detected Compounds	Percent of Total Number of AAFs with Stimulants
2003	151,210	516	19.0	Pseudoephedrine	36.6[a]
				Ephedrine	19.4
				Cocaine & metabolites	9.3
				Amphetamine	8.3
				Caffeine	7.6[a]
2004	169,187	382	11.6	Amphetamine	29.3
				Ephedrine	26.7
				Cocaine & metabolites	19.6
				MDMA	3.9
				Phentermine	3.4
2005	183,337	509	11.8	Amphetamine	38.1
				Ephedrine	18.3
				Cocaine & metabolites	16.7
				Methylphenidate	3.3
				Cathine	2.8
2006	198,143	490	11.3	Amphetamine	40.6
				Cocaine & metabolites	17.3
				Ephedrine	13.5
				Methylphenidate	6.5
				Cathine	4.5
2007	223,898	793	16.4	Amphetamine	54.2
				Cocaine & metabolites	12.7
				Ephedrine	6.3
				Methylphenidate	4.8
				Cathine	4.2

[a] Removed from prohibited list in 2004.
Data from WADA. Laboratory statistics. 2008. Available at: http://www.wada-ama.org/en/dynamic.ch2?pageCategory.id=594. Accessed February 15, 2008.

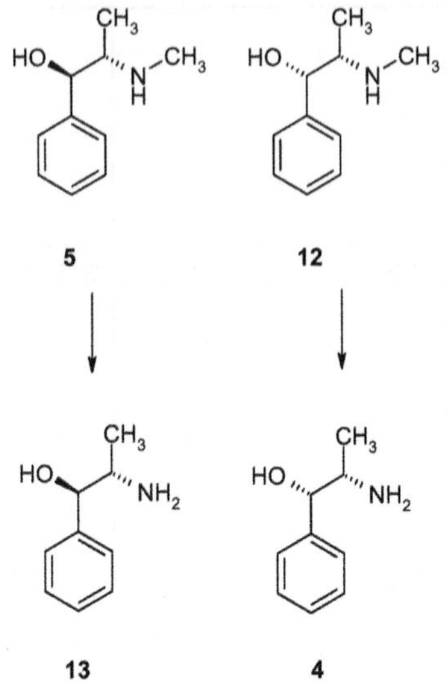

Fig. 2. Structures of ephedrine (**5**, mol wt = 165), pseudoephedrine (**12**, mol wt = 165), and their major metabolites phenylpropanolamine (**13**, mol wt = 151) and cathine (**4**, mol wt = 151).

in 2007/2008. Also here, the major reason was the considerably elevated numbers of pseudoephedrine findings in samples collected during cycling events. While only 0.2% of specimens measured between 2001 and 2003 yielded pseudoephedrine levels greater than 25 μg/mL, 3.9% of all samples analyzed in 2007/2008 were found to contain more than the formerly existing threshold value.

These data suggest that the misuse of the stimulating agent pseudoephedrine was rather limited as long as the substance was prohibited and that lifting the ban resulted in a much more frequent use aiming for performance enhancement. Consequently, it has been suggested to reconsider the implementation of a threshold value to control the nontherapeutic ingestion of the drug, especially since the major metabolite of pseudoephedrine, cathine (**4**) (see **Fig. 1**), has remained prohibited when exceeding a urinary threshold level of 5 μg/mL despite decontrolling pseudoephedrine. An athlete might thus produce an AAF with cathine, although no banned substance was administered. Amongst others, these facts have led to the installation of a new threshold value for urinary pseudoephedrine of 150 μg/mL becoming effective in January 2010.

DETECTION METHODS FOR STIMULANTS IN DOPING CONTROLS
Gas Chromatography, Mass Spectrometry/Nitrogen–Phosphorus Specific Detection

Stimulants and alkaloids in general were among the first analytes to be tested in systematic doping controls. In the late 1950s, based on chemistry that provided characteristic and more or less quantitative data by means of color reactions, the capability of gas chromatography (GC) to separate compounds relevant for doping controls was recognized and introduced into sports drug testing to measure various classes of analytes, predominantly sympathomimetic amines.[29–33] Analyzers such as flame ionization and nitrogen–phosphorus detectors (FID and NPD, respectively) as well as ionization β-ray (strontium 90) or electron capture detectors were used, and sample extraction and concentration methodologies were mostly adapted from earlier purely "chemical" procedures. The need to improve GC properties of target analytes and to obtain supporting information that would provide additional confidence in analytical results led to the development of various derivatization strategies, which improved chromatographic peak shapes and yielded additional data characterizing a substance. A strategy to identify a compound by its retention times obtained from the native and derivatized analyte or 2 different derivatives was termed the "peak-shift technique"[34] and was used as a common standard in confirmatory analyses. Trimethylsilylation (using, for example, N-methyl-N-trimethylsilyltrifluoroacetamide [MSTFA][35]); acylation (using, for example, acetic or heptafluorobutyric anhydride, bis[acylamide]); alkylation; formation of several Schiff-bases (eg, acetone-, propionaldehyde-, benzyl methyl ketone-Schiff-bases)[36]; or preparation of mixed derivatives were used to modify the physicochemical nature of substances and thus enhance their traceability in sports drug testing. Seminal assays for doping controls were finally based on trimethylsilylation or acylation as established by Donike and coworkers,[37–41] and they were used for the comprehensive doping control program undertaken at the 1972 Olympic Games in Munich and at the subsequently conducted great sporting events.[42–44] The enormous complexity of biologic matrices and the continuously increasing number of therapeutics have, however, necessitated more specific and unequivocal analyzers than for instance NPD and FID alone. This resulted in the frequent use of GC equipped with NPD plus mass spectrometry (MS), a combination that allows the exploitation of advantages provided by both analytical techniques simultaneously. MS is commonly operated using electron ionization (EI), which frequently results in comprehensive fragmentation of analytes and thus hardly yields information on the molecular weight; however, the obtained EI mass spectra contain diagnostic ions and provide detailed information that enables the characterization and identification of target compounds. Moreover, various derivatives of stimulants have been shown to produce stable molecular ions also under EI conditions. An example of a recent AAF (4-methylhexan-2-amine) as detected by means of GC-EI/MS is presented in Case Vignette 1.

Liquid Chromatography–(Tandem) MS

The considerable proton affinity of amines, which constitute an important structural feature of most stimulants, has also enabled the use of robust and sensitive instruments composed of liquid chromatography (LC) combined with (tandem) mass spectrometers (LC-MS/MS) to detect and quantify stimulants in doping controls.[45] The analytes are commonly ionized by means of electrospray ionization (ESI) or atmospheric pressure chemical ionization that yields a protonated molecule $[M+H]^+$. Subsequent collision-induced dissociation (CID) of $[M+H]^+$ gives rise to product ion mass spectra that allow the sensitive and specific analysis of numerous stimulants with the advantages that the intact molecular ion is recorded in addition to diagnostic product ions and that no derivatization is required even in case of heavy volatile or thermolabile analytes (eg, phase I or phase II metabolites). The specificity of ion transitions (ie, the direct correlation of precursor and product ions) has been used to establish fast and sensitive detection assays that complement GC-MS/NPD-based procedures, and case vignettes of the finding of 4-methylhexan-2-amine and methoxyphenamine abuse as proved by LC-MS/MS are described in the following sections.

Case Vignette 1—4-methylhexan-2-amine

4-Methylhexan-2-amine (geranamine, **10**) (see **Fig. 1**) is a natural product produced to a minor extent in *Pelargonium graveolens* (also referred to as geranium or Pelargonium), a plant that is indigenous particularly to South Africa. *Pelargonium* is largely cultivated because of the great interest in its foliage that is used for the preparation of various different scents, which are derived from an oily distillate that contains approximately 0.7% of 4-methylhexan-2-amine. The oil has been approved as a food additive, and "geranium extracts" are frequently declared as ingredients of nutritional supplements and so-called party pills. In addition to its natural occurrence, 4-methyl-hexan-2-amine is synthetically obtained by the reaction of 4-methylhexan-2-one and hydroxylamine followed by reduction using, for example, hydrogen in the presence of Raney nickel catalyst.[46] As such, a pharmaceutical product was prepared and patented in 1944, which was marketed as a nasal decongestant (Forthane sulfate [Eli Lilly, Indianapolis, IN]) and as a therapeutic agent for the treatment of hypertro-phied gums. Although it was supposed to be less stimulating than drugs such as amphetamine or ephedrine typical sympathomimetic effects, tremor, excitement, or insomnia were reported. Its advantages over amphetamine and ephedrine were greater volatility and reduced toxicity, and its efficacy was greater than that of heptyl-amine derivatives such as tuaminoheptane (**9**) (see **Fig. 1**).[47]

In January 2007, WADA expanded the list of prohibited substances by adding tuaminoheptane to the list, which has since been monitored in all in-competition samples. In 2009, doping control urine specimens were found suspicious for a drug closely related to tuaminoheptane according to GC-MS and LC-MS/MS data, but retention times did not match the reference of tuaminoheptane. Further studies led to the identification of 4-methylhexan-2-amine using authentic refer-ence material, and detection assays based on GC-MS and LC-MS/MS were established.

The approach based on LC-MS/MS consisted of an alkaline liquid-liquid extraction of the target analyte, followed by concentration and subsequent measurement using diagnostic product ions obtained from the protonated molecule at m/z 116 (mass-to-charge ratio) after CID.[48] By means of this assay, a detection limit of approximately 50 ng/mL was accomplished, and an AAF with 4-methylhexan-2-amine was reported for an in-competition doping control urine sample that contained about 15 μg/mL of the banned substance, indicating an application shortly before the contest. The test result was further confirmed by GC-MS after derivatization of 4-methylhexan-2-amine to the corresponding Schiff-base using cyclohexanone.

Almost simultaneously, 4-methylhexan-2-amine was found in a doping control sample in Germany using an entirely GC-MS–based procedure, which was initially es-tablished for the detection and confirmation of tuaminoheptane (**9**) (see **Fig. 1**).[49] In brief, the analytes of interest are extracted from urine into methyl tert-butyl ether under alkaline conditions and subsequently derivatized to Schiff-bases by adding a metha-nolic solution of benzaldehyde. After 30 minutes without further treatment, the samples are injected into a GC-EI/MS/NPD system equipped with a HP-5MS analyt-ical column (Agilent Technologies, Inc, Santa Clara, CA, USA). The extracted ion chro-matograms of a mixture containing 4-methylhexan-2-amine and tuaminoheptane are illustrated in **Fig. 3**A along with respective EI mass spectra. Notably, tuaminoheptane (retention time of 4.49 min) yielded 1 signal, and 4-methylhexan-2-amine gave rise to 2 peaks at 4.27 and 4.32 min, indicating the presence of diastereomers as also reported earlier.[48] The blank urine sample did not yield any signal (see **Fig. 3**B), whereas the AAF in a doping control sample included 2 baseline-resolved peaks of 4-methylhex-an-2-amine isomers (see **Fig. 3**C). In the same context, a nutritional supplement (NOX PUMP [Ultralife, Aylesbury, UK]) declaring to contain "geranium root extract" was analyzed and found to contain 4-methylhexan-2-amine at approximately 1 mg/g. A single administration of the product according to the recommended dosage (1 portion of 17 g/d) resulted in the presence of the banned substance in urine samples with nearly identical appearance of diastereoisomers (see **Fig. 3**D) as observed with the reference compound and the doping control urine sample.

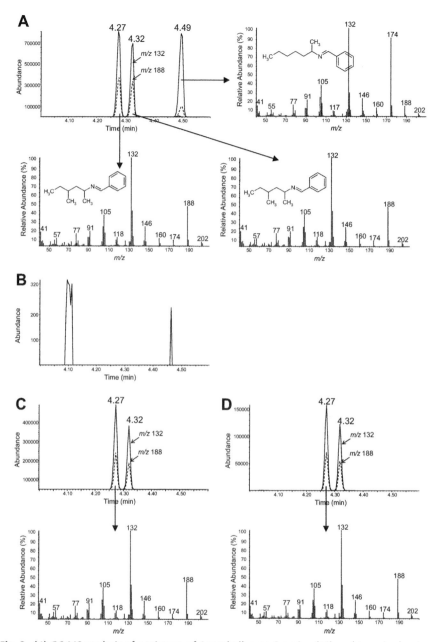

Fig. 3. (*A*) GC-MS analysis of a mixture of 4-methylhexan-2-amine (**10**) and tuaminoheptane (**9**) derivatized with benzaldehyde yielding respective Schiff-bases with a molecular weight of 203 Da; 2 baseline-separated stereoisomers of **10** are observed at 4.27 and 4.32 min, which yield identical EI-MS spectra (*bottom left and right*). The constitutional isomer **9** differs in retention time (4.49 min) and relative abundances of diagnostic fragment ions such as *m/z* 188 and 174 (*top right*). (*B*) GC-MS analysis of a blank urine sample for compounds **9** and **10**. No signals are detected. (*C*) GC-MS analysis of a doping control urine sample tested positive for 4-methylhexan-2-amine; appearance of 2 diastereomers and EI mass spectrum are identical with those measured from reference substances. (*D*) GC-MS analysis of a urine sample collected after administration of a nutritional supplement labeled to contain "geranium root extract." Also here, 4-methylhexan-2-amine was detected with diastereomers.

The mass spectrometric fragmentation of 4-methylhexan-2-amine as benzaldehyde derivative is in accordance with earlier reported dissociation pathways.[49] Imines such as the derivatized target analytes are likely ionized by EI at the nitrogen atom because of the electron-donating nature of the amino function.[50] The resulting radical cations can subsequently undergo isomerization triggered by intramolecular hydrogen abstraction and formation of so-called distonic ions.[51] Hence, besides the commonly observed and characteristic α-cleavage products,[52] complex cascades of rearrangements were described to precede the dissociation of amines, which allowed for the explanation of frequently detected additional fragment ions in EI mass spectra of aliphatic amines. The molecular ion of the condensation product of 4-methylhexan-2-amine at m/z 203 is hardly visible, which is a well-known issue of EI-MS–based assays for primary and secondary amines. However, abundant diagnostic ions originating from α-cleavages are found at m/z 188 and 132 (**Fig. 4**), which are suggested to represent the cations of benzylidene-(3-methyl-pentyl)-amine and benzylidene-ethylamine, respectively. These are complemented by losses of alkyl radicals such as ethyl-, propyl- and butyl-residues from the molecular ion to yield the fragments at m/z 174, 160, and 146, which support the MS-based identification of 4-methylhexan-2-amine (see **Fig. 3**C, D).

Case Vignette 2—methoxyphenamine

Methoxyphenamine (**14**) (o-methoxy-N,α-dimethylphenethylamine, **Fig. 5**) was synthesized and clinically evaluated for the treatment of asthma bronchiale in the 1940s[53–55] and it demonstrated promising bronchodilator activity after oral administration with reduced influence on blood pressure and the CNS as compared with ephedrine.[56–58] It is metabolized to 3 major products that are derived from N- or O-demethylation and ring hydroxylation at position 5 (see **Fig. 5, 15–17**) with introduced hydroxyl functions further conjugated to glucuronic acid. Because of the structural analogy of methoxyphenamine to stimulants such as amphetamine (**1**) (see **Fig. 1**) and its β2-agonistic properties, it has been prohibited in sports according to the rules established by the WADA.[59] For clinical and forensic purposes, several methods were established allowing the detection of methoxyphenamine, its metabolites, and its designer analogues in plasma and urine using GC or GC-MS, and sports drug-testing procedures have commonly used the previously described GC-MS/NPD methods and, more recently, the methods that use LC-MS/MS.[45,60–63] Although stimulants

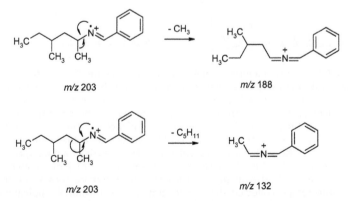

m/z 203 $-$ CH$_3$ m/z 188

m/z 203 $-$ C$_5$H$_{11}$ m/z 132

Fig. 4. Proposed fragmentation pathway of the Schiff-base benzaldehyde derivative of 4-methylhexan-2-amine (**10**) under EI conditions.

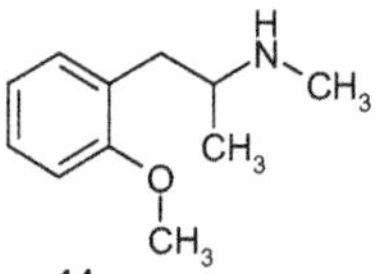

Fig. 5. Structures of methoxyphenamine (**14**, mol wt = 179), N-demethyl methoxyphen-amine (**15**, R = H: mol wt = 165, R = glucuronic acid: mol wt = 341), O-demethyl methoxyphenamine (**16**, R = H: mol wt = 165, R = glucuronic acid: mol wt = 341), 5-hydroxy-methoxyphenamine (**17**, R = H: mol wt = 195, R = glucuronic acid: mol wt = 371), and PMMA (**18**, mol wt = 179).

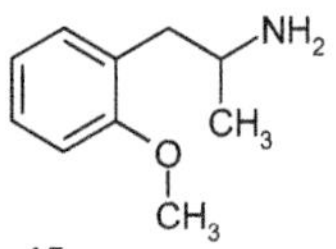

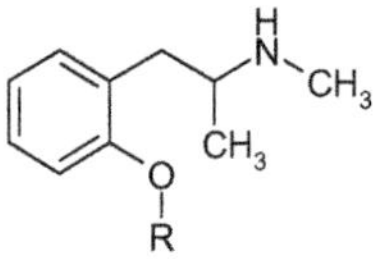

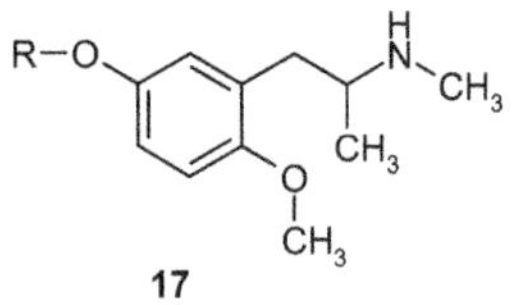

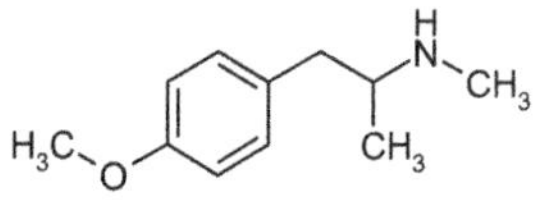

represent one of the most frequently detected classes of compounds in sports drug-testing samples, the prevalence of methoxyphenamine has been very low during the last 4 years with only 2 findings in doping controls.[64]

In early 2008, another doping control specimen yielded an AAF for methoxyphen-amine and because mono-methoxy positional ring isomers are possible,[65] an LC-MS/MS procedure was used to confirm the presence of the banned substance. The chromatographic separation of the active drug from isomeric compounds such as the designer drug p-methoxymethamphetamine (PMMA, **18**) (see **Fig. 5**) was of partic-ular interest. Product ion mass spectra of methoxyphenamine (**14**) and PMMA (**18**) were obtained from protonated molecules (**Fig. 6**A, B, respectively) using identical collision energies of 25 eV. Major product ions derived from the precursor at m/z 180 were found at m/z 149, 121, 93, and 91, and slightly different relative abundances were observed in particular for the ion at m/z 149. The proposed origin of the product ions is illustrated in **Fig. 7**, and supporting information for the suggested dissociation pathway was obtained from MS^3 experiments. The protonated molecule at m/z 180 yielded the ion at m/z 149 by the elimination of methylamine (31 Da), which subse-quently released ethylene (28 Da) to yield the product ion at m/z 121. Subsequently, m/z 121 liberated formaldehyde (30 Da) from the methoxy residue to yield the ion at m/z 91.

Besides methoxyphenamine, further analytes were found in the doping control sample and they are attributed to N-demethyl methoxyphenamine (**15**), O-demethyl methoxyphenamine (**16**) and its glucuronic acid conjugate, and 5-hydroxy-methoxy-phenamine (**17**) glucuronide (see **Fig. 5**).[66] The N-demethylation was characterized by the presence of a primary amine (**15**), which eliminated ammonia (17 Da) under ESI/CID conditions giving rise to m/z 149 (see **Fig. 6**C), which subsequently released ethylene (28 Da) to m/z 121 as observed also with methoxyphenamine (**14**). In contrast,

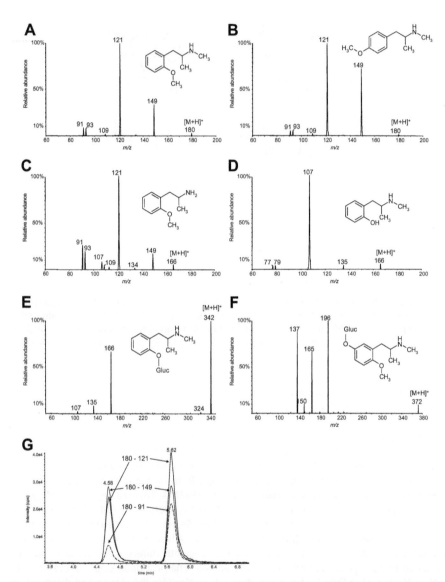

Fig. 6. ESI-MS/MS spectra obtained from protonated molecules of methoxyphenamine (*A*), *N*-demethyl methoxyphenamine (*B*), *O*-demethyl methoxyphenamine (*C*), 5-hydroxy-methoxyphenamine (*D*), glucuronide of *O*-demethyl methoxyphenamine (*E*), and glucuronide of 5-hydroxy-methoxyphenamine (*F*). Extracted ion chromatograms of a mixture containing methoxyphenamine and PMMA further demonstrate the chromatographic and mass spectrometric differentiation of both compounds (*G*).

the *O*-demethylated analogue (**16**) generated a product ion at *m/z* 135 instead of 149, indicating the loss of methylamine (31 Da) and the presence of an intact and methylated secondary amine (see **Fig. 6**D). Consequently, the following elimination of ethylene yielded a product ion at *m/z* 107, which corresponded to *m/z* 121 in case of **15** and **17**. Further to the phase I metabolism, the *O*-demethylated metabolite (**16**) and the 5-hydroxylated analogue to methoxyphenamine (**17**) are conjugated to

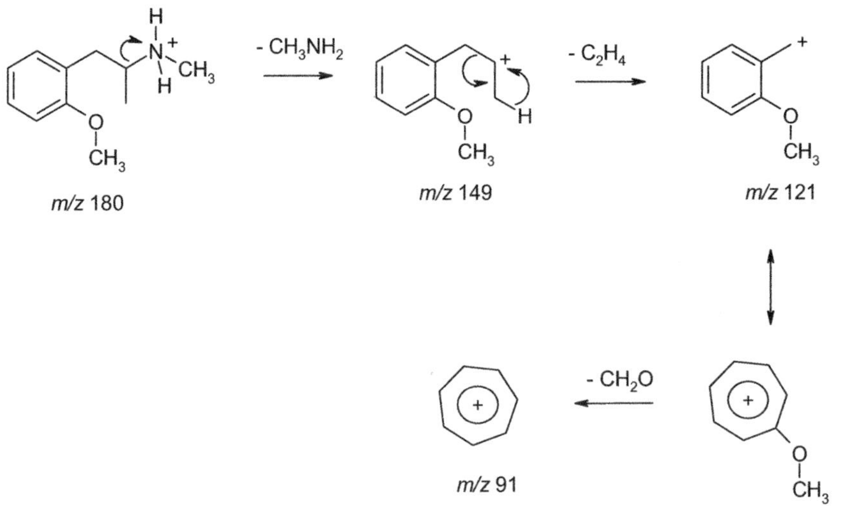

Fig. 7. Proposed dissociation pathway of the protonated molecule of methoxyphenamine under CID conditions.

glucuronic acid in phase II metabolic reactions. Respective product ion spectra were obtained from the doping control urine specimen containing methoxyphenamine as shown in **Fig. 6**E, F. The protonated molecule of *O*-demethylated and glucuronidated methoxyphenamine was observed at *m/z* 342 and yielded product ions at *m/z* 166, 135, and 107 (see **Fig. 6**E). These were attributed to the consecutive losses of the glucuronic acid moiety (176 Da) and the previously reported eliminations of methylamine (31 Da) and ethylene (28 Da), respectively. Accordingly, the precursor ion of 5-hydroxy-methoxyphenamine was detected at *m/z* 372, which gave rise to abundant product ions at *m/z* 196, 165, and 137 (see **Fig. 6**F).

Besides the mass spectrometric identification, chromatographic separation of methoxyphenamine (**14**) and PMMA (**18**) was aimed and accomplished using LC with isocratic elution of the analytes (see **Fig. 6**G). The para-substituted amphetamine derivative (**18**) eluted at 4.58 min, whereas methoxyphenamine (**14**) demonstrated a considerably longer retention, eluting at 5.62 min. In addition, the selected ion transitions (180–149, 180–121, and 180–91) yielded different relative abundances, which further supported the unambiguous differentiation of both compounds.[67]

SUMMARY

Stimulants play an important role in sports drug-testing programs. The great variety of compounds belonging to this class of prohibited substances represents a challenge for doping control laboratories, but the sensitive and selective nature of analytical instruments and detection assays has enabled comprehensive screening procedures that not only reveal the misuse but also the presumably unintended intake of banned compounds. Several instances of natural products illegally enriched with synthetic compounds were reported (eg, sibutramine in an herbal tea),[68] and the addition of synthetically produced natural stimulants (such as 4-methylhexan-2-amine) to nutritional supplements is conceivable.

Studies concerning the prevalence of the stimulating agent pseudoephedrine have highlighted its great misuse potential, that is, lifting the ban for pseudoephedrine in

2004 resulted in a significant increase of findings in doping control urine samples subjected to a monitoring program. Consequently, pseudoephedrine has been added to the list of prohibited compounds being valid from January 2010.

ACKNOWLEDGMENTS

The authors thank the Manfred Donike Institute for Doping Analysis, Cologne, for supporting the presented work.

REFERENCES

1. Van Dyke C, Byck R. Cocaine. Sci Am 1982;246(3):108–19.
2. Wadler GI, Hainline B. Drugs and the athlete. Philadelphia: F.A. Davis Company; 1989.
3. Karas M, Hillenkamp F. Laser desorption ionization of proteins with molecular masses exceeding 10,000 daltons. Anal Chem 1988;60(20):2299–301.
4. Pelletier PJ, Caventou JB. Note sur un Nouvel Alcali [Note on a new alkaloid]. Annales de chimie et de physique 1818;3:323–36 [in French].
5. Rasmussen N. Making the first anti-depressant: amphetamine in American medicine, 1929–1950. J Hist Med Allied Sci 2006;61:288–323.
6. Raza M. A role for physicians in ethnopharmacology and drug discovery. J Ethnopharmacol 2006;104(3):297–301.
7. Edeleano L. Ueber einige Derivate der Phenylmethacrylsäure und der Phenylisobuttersäure [On some derivatives of phenylmethacrylic acid and phenylisobutyric acid]. Berichte der Deutschen Chemischen Gesellschaft 1887;20(1):616–22 [in German]
8. Nagai N. Kanyaku maou seibun kenkyuu seiseki (zoku) [Research results on a component of ephedra in Chinese medicine]. Yakugaku zasshi 1893;13: 901–33 [in Japanese].
9. Freudenmann RW, Öxler F, Bernschneider-Reif S. The origin of MDMA (ecstasy) revisited: the true story reconstructed from the original documents. Addiction 2006;101(9):1241–5.
10. Wyndham CH, Rogers GG, Benade AJS, et al. Physiological effects of the amphetamines during exercise. S Afr Med J 1971;45:247–52.
11. Laties VG, Weiss B. The amphetamine margin in sports. Fed Proc 1981 Oct; 40(12):2689–92.
12. Ariens EJ. Centrally-active drugs and performance in sports. Schweiz Z Sportmed 1965;13(3):77–98.
13. Golding LA, Barnard JR. The effect of D-Amphetamine sulfate on physical performance. J Sports Med Phys Fitness 1963;44:221–4.
14. Karpovich PV. Effect of amphetamine sulfate on athletic performance. J Am Med Assoc 1959;170(5):558–61.
15. Magkos F, Kavouras SA. Caffeine and ephedrine: physiological, metabolic and performance-enhancing effects. Sports Med 2004;34(13):871–89.
16. Hodges K, Hancock S, Currell K, et al. Pseudoephedrine enhances performance in 1500-m runners. Med Sci Sports Exerc 2006;38(2):329–33.
17. Smith GM, Beecher HK. Amphetamine sulfate and athletic performance. I. Objective effects. J Am Med Assoc 1959;170(5):542–57.
18. Smith GM, Beecher HK. Amphetamine, secobarbital, and athletic performance. III. Quantiative effects on judgment. J Am Med Assoc 1960;172:1623–9.

19. Smith GM, Beecher HK. Amphetamine, secobarbital, and athletic performance. II. Subjective evaluations of performance, mood states, and physical states. J Am Med Assoc 1960;172:1502–14.
20. WADA. The 2009 prohibited list. Available at: http://www.wada-ama.org/rtecontent/document/2009_Prohibited_List_ENG_Final_20_Sept_08.pdf. Accessed February 1, 2009.
21. George AJ. Central nervous system stimulants. Baillieres Best Pract Res Clin Endocrinol Metab 2000;14(1):79–88.
22. Docherty JR. Pharmacology of stimulants prohibited by the World Anti-Doping Agency (WADA). Br J Pharmacol 2008;154(3):606–22.
23. Fleckenstein AE, Volz TJ, Riddle EL, et al. New insights into the mechanism of action of amphetamines. Annu Rev Pharmacol Toxicol 2007;47:681–98.
24. Jones G. Caffeine and other sympathomimetic stimulants: modes of action and effects on sports performance. In: Cooper CE, Beneke R, editors. Essays in biochemistry. London: Portland Press; 2008. p. 109–24.
25. Kahlig KM, Binda F, Khoshbouei H, et al. Amphetamine induces dopamine efflux through a dopamine transporter channel. Proc Natl Acad Sci U S A 2005;102(9):3495–500.
26. Delicado EG, Fideu MD, Miras-Portugal MT, et al. Effect of tuamine, heptaminol and two analogues on uptake and release of catecholamines in cultured chromaffin cells. Biochem Pharmacol 1990;40(4):821–5.
27. WADA. Laboratory statistics. Available at: http://www.wada-ama.org/en/dynamic.ch2?pageCategory.id=594. Accessed February 15, 2008.
28. Deventer K, Van Eenoo P, Baele G, et al. Interpretation of urinary concentrations of pseudoephedrine and its metabolite cathine in relation to doping control. Drug Test Analysis 2009;1:209–13.
29. Lloyd HA, Fales HM, Highet PF, et al. Separation of alkaloids by gas chromatography. J Am Chem Soc 1960;82:3791.
30. Parker KD, Fontan CR, Kirk PL. Separation and identification of some sympathomimetic amines by gas chromatography. Anal Chem 1962;34(10):1345–6.
31. Parker KD, Fontan CR, Kirk PL. Rapid gas chromatographic method for screening of toxicological extracts for alkaloids, barbiturates, sympathomimetic amines, and tranquilizers. Anal Chem 1963;35(3):356–9.
32. Brochmann-Hanssen E, Svendsen AB. Gas chromatography of sympathomimetic amines. J Pharm Sci 1962;51:393.
33. Brochmann-Hanssen E, Svendsen AB. Separation and identification of sympathomimetic amines by gas-liquid chromatography. J Pharm Sci 1962;51:938–41.
34. Langer SH, Pantages P. Peak-shift technique in gas-liquid chromatography: trimethylsilyl ether derivatives of alcohols. Nature 1961;191:141–2.
35. Donike M. N-Methyl-N-trimethylsilyl-trifluoracetamide, ein neues Silylierungsmittel aus der Reihe der silylierten Amide [N-Methyl-N-trimethylsilyltrifluoroacetamide, a new silylation agent of the series of silylated amides]. J Chromatogr 1969;42:103–4 [in German].
36. Capella P, Horning EC. Separation and identification of derivatives of biologic amines by gas-liquid chromatography. Anal Chem 1966;38:316–21.
37. Donike M. Stickstoffdetektor und Temperaturprogrammierte Gas-Chromatographie, ein Fortschritt für die Routinemäßige Dopingkontrolle [Nitrogen-specific detector and temperature-programmed gas chromatography, an improvement of routine doping controls]. Sportarzt und Sportmedizin 1970;21:27–30 [in German].
38. Donike M. Acylierung mit Bis(Acylamiden); N-Methyl-Bis(Trifluoracetamid) und Bis(Trifluoracetamid), zwei neue Reagenzien zur Trifluoracetylierung [N-methyl-

bis(trifluoroacetamide) and bis(trifluoroacetamide), two new reagants for trifluor-ocetylation]. J Chromatogr 1973;78:273–9 [in German].

39. Donike M, Jaenicke L, Stratmann D, et al. Gas chromatographic detection of nitrogen-containing drugs in aqueous solutions by means of the nitrogen detector. J Chromatogr 1970;52:237–50.
40. Donike M, Derenbach J. Die Selektive Derivatisierung Unter Kontrollierten Bedingungen: Ein Weg zum Spurennachweis von Aminen [Selective derivatization using controlled conditions: A way to detect trace amounts of amines]. Z Anal Chem 1976;279:128–9 [in German].
41. Donike M. Temperature programmed gas chromatographic analysis of nitrogen-containing drugs: the reproducibility of retention times (I). Chromatographia 1970;3:422–4.
42. Donike M, Stratmann D. Temperaturprogrammierte gas-chromatographische Analyse stickstoffhaltiger Pharmaka: Die Reproduzierbarkeiten der Retentions-zeiten und der Mengen bei automatischer Injektion (II) "Die Screeningprozedur für flüchtige Dopingmittel bei den Olympischen Spielen der XX. Olympiade München 1972" [Temperature-programmed gas chromatographic analysis of nitrogen-containing drugs: the reproducibility of retention times using automatic injection (II). "The screening procedure for volatile doping agents at the Olympic Games of the XX. Olympiade Munich 1972"]. Chromatographia 1974;7:182–9 [in German]
43. Schänzer W. Dem Doping keine Chance [No Chance for doping]. In: Kozel J, editor. 25 Jahre Trainerausbildung. Cologne (Germany): Sport & Buch Strauss; 1999. p. 59–94 [in German].
44. Hemmersbach P. History of mass spectrometry at the Olympic games. J Mass Spectrom 2008;43(7):839–53.
45. Thevis M, Schänzer W. Examples of doping control analysis by liquid chromatography-tandem mass spectrometry: ephedrines, beta-receptor blocking agents, diuretics, sympathomimetics, and cross-linked hemoglobins. J Chromatogr Sci 2005;43(1):22–31.
46. Shonle HA, Rohrmann E, Inventors; Eli Lilly & Company, Assignee. Aminoalkanes. US patent US 23503181944, 1944.
47. Marsh DF, Howard A, Herring DA. The comparative pharmacology of the isomeric nitrogen methyl substituted heptylamines. J Pharmacol Exp Ther 1951;103(3):325–9.
48. Perrenoud L, Saugy M, Saudan C. Detection in urine of 4-methyl-2-hexaneamine, a doping agent. J Chromatogr B 2009;877:3767–70.
49. Thevis M, Sigmund G, Koch A, et al. Determination of tuaminoheptane in doping control urine samples. Eur J Mass Spectrom (Chichester, Eng) 2007;13(3):213–21.
50. Gohlke RS, McLafferty FW. Mass spectrometric analysis - aliphatic amines. Anal Chem 1962;34(10):1281–7.
51. Hammerum S. Distonic radical cations in gaseous and condensed phase. Mass Spectrom Rev 1988;7(2):123–202.
52. Hammerum S, Norrman K, Solling TI, et al. Competing simple cleavage reactions: the elimination of alkyl radicals from amine radical cations. J Am Chem Soc 2005;127(17):6466–75.
53. Woodruff EH, Lambooy JP, Burt WE. Physiologically active amines. Secondary and tertiary β−phenylpropylamines and β−phenylisopropylamines. J Am Chem Soc 1940;62:922–4.
54. Curry JJ, Fuchs JE, Leard SE. Clinical and experimental studies with orthoxine in the treatment of bronchial asthma. J Allergy 1949;20(2):104–10.

55. Schiller IW, Lowell FC, Franklin W, et al. Orthoxine in bronchial asthma; a clinical evaluation. N Engl J Med 1949;241(6):231–3.
56. Heinzelman RV. Physiologically active secondary amines. β–(o-Methoxyphenyl)-isopropyl-N-methylamine and related compounds. J Am Chem Soc 1953;75:921–5.
57. Graham BE, Kuizenga MH. A pharmacologic study of ortho-methoxy-beta-phenylisopropyl methylamine hydrochloride, and thirteen related methoxy analogues. J Pharmacol Exp Ther 1948;94(2):150–66.
58. Ogden HD, Cullick L. Orthoxine in bronchial asthma. Ann Allergy 1952;10(3):335–8.
59. WADA. The 2008 prohibited list. 2008. Available at: http://www.wada-ama.org/rtecontent/document/2008_List_En.pdf. Accessed November 28, 2007.
60. Thevis M, Schänzer W. Current role of LC-MS(/MS) in doping control. Anal Bioanal Chem 2007;388:1351–8.
61. Deventer K, Van Eenoo P, Delbeke FT. Screening for amphetamine and amphetamine-type drugs in doping analysis by liquid chromatography/mass spectrometry. Rapid Commun Mass Spectrom 2006;20(5):877–82.
62. Thevis M, Sigmund G, Schänzer W. Confirmation of ephedrines - comparison between GC-MS and LC-MS/MS. In: Gotzmann A, Geyer H, Mareck U, et al, editors. Recent advances in doping analysis - 21st cologne workshop on doping analysis. Cologne (Germany): Sport & Buch Strauß; 2003. p. 303–7.
63. Thevis M, Opfermann G, Schänzer W. N-methyl-N-trimethylsilyltrifluoroacetamide promoted synthesis and mass spectrometric characterization of deuterated ephedrines. Eur J Mass Spectrom (Chichester, Eng) 2004;10(5):673–81.
64. WADA. Adverse analytical findings reported by accredited laboratories. 2008. Available at: http://www.wada-ama.org/en/dynamic.ch2?pageCategory.id=594. Accessed May 29, 2008.
65. Dal Cason TA. A re-examination of the mono-methoxy positional ring isomers of amphetamine, methamphetamine and phenyl-2-propanone. Forensic Sci Int 2001;119(2):168–94.
66. Midha KK, Cooper JK, McGilveray IJ, et al. Metabolism of methoxyphenamine in man and in monkey. Drug Metab Dispos 1976;4(6):568–76.
67. Thevis M, Sigmund G, Koch A, et al. Doping control analysis of methoxyphenamine using liquid chromatography-tandem mass spectrometry. Eur J Mass Spectrom 2008;14:145–52.
68. Geyer H, Parr MK, Koehler K, et al. Nutritional supplements cross-contaminated and faked with doping substances. J Mass Spectrom 2008;43(7):892–902.

Glucocorticoids: A Doping Agent?

Martine Duclos, MD, PhD[a,b,c,d],*

KEYWORDS

• Glucocorticoids • Exercise • Performance • Doping
• Adrenal insufficiency • Adverse effects

Certain international sports federations are requesting that glucocorticoids (GCs) be removed from the World Antidoping Agency's (WADA) list of banned products. This pharmacologic class is banned by WADA after systemic administration, but only in competition. Their arguments are based on the fact that GC are in widespread use in sports medicine and have no demonstrated ergogenic activity (ie, are not performance enhancers). To be included on the list of banned products a substance should meet any two of the following three criteria: (1) evidence that the substance improves athletic performance, (2) evidence that the substance represents a health risk for the athlete, and (3) the use of the substance violates the spirit of sports.

This article shows that, using appropriate testing based on physiologic effects, GCs have real and demonstrated ergogenic activity and that the use of GCs poses a real danger to athletes' health.

PHYSIOLOGIC EFFECTS OF GCS AND EXPECTED EFFECTS OF GC ABUSE

Cortisol is a steroid hormone secreted from the adrenocortical glands under hypothalamic and pituitary control defining the hypothalamic-pituitary-adrenal (HPA) axis. The activation of the HPA axis represents a physiologic response to the energetic, metabolic, vascular, neurophysiologic, or psychologic needs of exercise.[1–3] GCs, the end product of the HPA axis, exert many beneficial actions in exercising humans. GCs increase the availability of metabolic substrates for the need of energy of muscles (increased lipolysis and plasma free fatty acids [FFA], increased glycogen synthesis) and maintain normal vascular integrity and responsiveness during exercise. In

a Department of Sport Medicine and Functional Explorations, University-Hospital (CHU), Hôpital G. Montpied, Clermont-Ferrand, F-63003, France
b INRA, UMR 1019, 58 rue Montalembert, BP 321, Clermont-Ferrand, F-63009, France
c University Clermont 1, UFR Médecine, 58 rue Montalembert, Clermont-Ferrand, F-63009, France
d Centre de Recherche en Nutrition Humaine d'Auvergne, 58 rue Montalembert, BP 321, Clermont-Ferrand, F-63009, France
* Service de Médecine du Sport et d'Explorations Fonctionnelles, CHU Hôpital G. Montpied, BP 68, 63009 Clermont Ferrand Cedex 1, France.
E-mail address: mduclos@chu-clermontferrand.fr

Endocrinol Metab Clin N Am 39 (2010) 107–126
doi:10.1016/j.ecl.2009.10.001
0889-8529/10/$ – see front matter © 2010 Elsevier Inc. All rights reserved.

addition, GCs prevent an overreaction of the immune system as a result of exercise-induced muscle damage (immunosuppressive and anti-inflammatory effects).[3] Cortisol also prepares the organism for the next bout of exercise, explaining why when an acute bout of endurance-exercise is stopped, cortisol levels may return to pre-exercise values with a delay (≤ 2 hours postexercise).[3,4] At the central level (central nervous system), GCs may exert positive hedonic effects by an increase of dopamine release in the nucleus accumbens.[5] The interplay between central noradrenergic systems and GC is also involved in the physiology and physiopathology of GC-induced mood changes (euphoria, depression, and withdrawal syndrome).[6]

These physiologic properties of GCs suggest that GCs could enhance performance, and this explains why GCs are in such widespread use in the sporting world. Indeed, the expected effects of the use and abuse of GCs are numerous: neurostimulatory effects at cerebral GC receptors could attenuate central impressions of fatigue, and anti-inflammatory and analgesic effects could inhibit sensations of muscle pain on effort and raise the fatigue threshold. The metabolic effects of these compounds consolidate glycogen reserves in muscle tissue and accelerate lipolysis and glycolysis mechanisms induced by catecholamines and growth hormone, thereby leading to more efficient use of energy sources by the muscles in the course of exercise.[1,2]

GCs have pleiotropic effects, however, causing several adverse effects, especially at higher doses and for long periods, such as osteoporosis, insulin resistance, and cardiovascular effects (hypertension and atherosclerosis).[7] In addition to their presumed ergogenic effects, the salient question is whether these adverse effects may be counteracted by intensive and regular exercise or limited by intermittent intake.

ERGOGENIC ACTIVITY OF GCS: SCIENTIFIC EVIDENCE
Human Data

Few studies have been performed on GC administration and exercise performance. The main characteristics and results of these studies are summarized in humans (**Table 1**) and animals (**Table 2**).

Review of the scientific literature clearly shows two types of results: studies supporting the hypothesis that there is no relationship between performance and corticosteroid use in humans (negative studies)[8–13]; and studies supporting the hypothesis that there are relationships between performance and corticosteroid use in humans (positive studies).[14–16] A third, intermediate tendency, however, can also be found in studies with data showing relationships between performance and GC use in humans but interpreting these data as negative taking into account the initial hypothesis of the authors.[17]

It should be noted that inconsistencies found regarding the ergogenic effect of GC administrations in humans may be attributed to (1) the GC administration dosage, route, and mode (acute or short term); (2) the type, duration, and intensity (submaximal, maximal) of exercise tested; (3) the participants (highly trained or professional vs recreational trained); (4) the differences in diet, such as whether or not experiments are food-controlled and whether or not subjects fasted; and (5) GC intake coupled or not with intensive training.

Negative studies

Marquet and colleagues[8] and Petrides and colleagues[9] have evaluated the effects of GCs (dexamethasone, 4.5 or 13.5 mg; hydrocortisone, 100 mg) on performance in terms of GC effects either on maximal oxygen consumption (Vo_2max) (maximum exercise duration 10–12 minutes)[8] or on a short series of submaximal exertions (10 bouts of 30 seconds of exercise at 90% Vo_2max)[9] (see **Table 1**) and found no difference between the placebo and the treatment groups. Taking into account the physiologic effects of GCs, these results were foreseeable because it is difficult to hypothesize that GCs may increase Vo_2max[8] or maximal heart rate[9] during brief exercises. Respiratory exchange ratio was also considered in the study of Petrides and colleagues[9] but values of respiratory exchange ratio should be interpreted with caution because no respiratory steady-state can be reached in 30 seconds (duration of the measure in this study). Moreover, the metabolic state of their subjects (fasted, postprandial) and the time of exercise (GCs were taken 4 hours before exercise without notification of the exercise's timing) are unknown.

Considering the effects of GCs, studies conducted during a prolonged endurance test to exhaustion or using a series of brief high-effort exercises to exhaustion in which GCs might attenuate impressions of fatigue and pain are more appropriate to demonstrate an ergogenic effect of GCs. Using trials to exhaustion (cycling) at intensity varying from 70% to 75% Vo_2max[12] to 80% to 85% Vo_2max[13] or during a maximal exercise (steady-state exercise followed by a ramped test)[17] or a fatiguing sprint session followed by a time trial (time to complete 20 km),[10] however, no study has demonstrated any ergogenic effect of acute systemic adrenocorticotropic hormone (ACTH)[10] or GC administration.[12,13,17]

The main limitation of these studies is the dosage of GC used, which remained within the physiologic ranges of plasma cortisol levels (but at high-stress level). For example, Kuipers and colleagues[11] have tested the ergogenic effects of therapeutic GC inhalation (800 μg/day). Such local low-dose administration failed to improve performance probably because of the lack of significant systemic bioavailability of inhaled GC. The study of Baume and colleagues[10] is another good illustration of this limitation. The design of their study comprised injection of 0.25 mg ACTH (Synacthen), resulting in a doubling cortisol levels.[10] Although significantly increased compared with placebo, the ACTH-induced value of cortisol (900 vs 500 nmol/L in the placebo study) remained within physiologic high range (stress levels) of cortisol concentrations. The 0.25-mg dose of ACTH is the dose normally administered during studies of pituitary function. With this dose plasma cortisol generally peaked 30 to 60 minutes after injection, remaining at maximal values for 100 to 120 minutes and thereafter cortisol rapidly returned to control values. In the study by Baume and coworkers,[10] ACTH injection elevated cortisol (two times compared with placebo study) for 2 hours and the 20-km time trial was performed at the peak cortisol concentration with no difference in time to complete the 20-km trial compared with the placebo group. Moreover, as anticipated, on day 2 of the trials, there was no difference in ACTH and cortisol profiles between the placebo and ACTH groups indicating that the single intramuscular injection received 24 hours previously had no further influence on the HPA axis. The intense effort exhibited during the 20-km time trial on day 2 normally stimulated the production of cortisol in both groups without any significant difference between the groups.

Administration of Synacthen at a higher dose or for a longer time period inducing a permanent high cortisol concentration in the body is more near the real state of ACTH intake by athletes. As suggested by the authors, "in appropriate forums on Internet, it appeared that athletes from different levels take up to 2.5 mg of Synacthen." The authors also assumed that this substance is administered on a short time period to boost the cortisol production right before an event. The potential positive effects of cortisol "would allow a higher energetic state and better feelings for athletes during exercise." Real athletes would also use Synacthen during recovery of competition, for its anti-inflammatory and metabolic effects (favoring glycogen resynthesis and storage) to prepare for the next event in a situation of repeated intense challenges,

Table 1
GC administration and exercise performance: results of the studies in humans

Study	Methods	Participants	Interventions	Outcomes	Results
8	Double-blind Randomized Crossover	12 untrained ♂ 12 trained ♂	3 treatments for each subject: - Pla - Dex for 4.5 d (per os) ➤ Low dose: 0.5 mg/12 h (total: 4.5 mg) ➤ High dose: 1.5 mg/ 12 h (total: 13.5 mg) Last capsule ingested 1 h before EX 3 experimental sessions per subject 2-wk intervals between each session	Maximal incremental cycling exercise (12–18 min long)	No effect of GC on performance measured on: - Vo_2max - ventilatory threshold - perceived difficulty of the exercise bouts Other effects of GC: - ↑ blood G at rest vs pla - but lower G in post-EX vs pla
9	Double-blind Randomized Crossover	19 moderately trained ♂	3 treatments for each subject: - Dex 4 mg - Hydrocortisone 100 mg - Pla 4 h before EX 3 experimental sessions per subject 1-wk intervals between each session	Submaximal high-intensity exercise test (25 min) (treadmill): - 5 min warm-up: 50% Vo_2max - 10 min high-intensity intermittent run: 10 bouts of 30 s of exercise at 90% Vo_2max alternated with 30 s of rest at 10% grade - 10 min cool down of walking (3.3 mph)	No effect of GC on performance measured on: - Heart rate - RER - absolute Vo_2 - relative Vo_2 (%) - blood lactate (parameters averaged over the last 4 intermittent bouts of high intensity EX) Other effects of GC: - ↑ pre-EX and peak EX-induced G responses (Dex-hydrocortisone vs pla)

	Design	Subjects	Treatment	Protocol	Results
10	Double-blind Randomized Crossover	8 highly trained ♂ cyclists	2 treatments for each subject: ACTH (0.25 mg) or pla (saline) IM; 2 consecutive days: D1 and D2; S1: D1 pla or ACTH; D2: no injection; 2 experimental sessions (S1 and S2) per subject separated by 7–10 d; Diet controlled	- D1: 90 min fatiguing sprint period: (50% power max interspersed with multisprint sessions: 3×1 min sprints at 90% power max and 2×4 min sprints at 70% power max) followed by a maximal effort: 20 km time trial; - D2: 20 km time trial	No effect of GC on performance measured on: time to complete the 20 km time trial; No ≠ in resting perceived exertion on either day of the trials (vs pla)
11	Double-blind Placebo-controlled study No crossover (parallel groups)	28 well-trained ♂ endurance athletes (involved in cycling and rowing)	1 treatment for each subject: - Pla or budenoside Daily inhalation of 800 μg for 28 d; 1 experimental session per subject	3 incremental cycle ergometer tests until exhaustion Before and after 2 and 4 wk of pla or budenoside	No effect of inhaled GC on performance measured on: maximal power output (at 4 wk of treatment) (pla: 374 ± 26 vs budesonide: 378 ± 37 W); No ≠ in POMS score every week
12	Double-blind Randomized Crossover	14 recreationally trained ♂	2 treatments for each subject: - 20 mg pred per os (0.25 mg/kg BW); - Pla; 3 h before EX; 2 experimental sessions per subject; 3 weeks (of normal training) between the 2 sessions	Trial to exhaustion during submaximal exercise (cycling) at 70%–75% Vo_2max	No effect of GC on performance measured on: cycling time: 48.8 ± 2.9 (pla) vs 55.9 ± 5.2 min (pred); Other effects of GC: blood hormonal and metabolic parameters - ↑G under pred during rest, EX, and recovery - No ≠ in insulin - ↑basal levels of interleukin-6 during EX but this increase is significantly blunted at exhaustion and during recovery under GC vs pla

(continued on next page)

Table 1
(continued)

Study	Methods	Participants	Interventions	Outcomes	Results
13	Double-blind Randomized Crossover	7 recreationally trained ♂	3 treatments for each subject: - Pla - 20 mg pred per os (2 h before EX) - Pred-salb (4 mg) (3 h before EX for salb) 3 experimental sessions per subject 72-h intervals between the 3 sessions 1 h after ingesting a small meal (500 kcal) identical for each trial	Cycling until exhaustion at 80%–85% Vo_2max	No effect of GC on performance measured on: cycling time during intense submaximal EX: 21.5 ± 2.9 (pla), 22 ± 2.5 (pred), 24.2 ± 2.8 min (pred-salb) Other effects of GC: ↑G at rest and during recovery but not during EX, no ≠ in insulin (pred, pred-salb vs pla)
17	Double-blind Crossover	16 ♂ professional cyclists	2 treatments for each subject: - Injection of ACTH (Synacthen: 1 mg) IM - Pla 45 min before the start of each session 4 experimental sessions (S): S1 (day 1) and S2 (day 2) were conducted on consecutive days during the 1st week S3 (day 3) and S4 (day 4) were conducted on consecutive days during the second week. ACTH or pla at S1 (day 1) or S3 (day 3) and day 2 and 4 were included to examine the influence of ACTH on recuperation	Steady-state cycling followed by a ramped test: 1 h cycling at submax level (60% maximal performance) and after 1 h, load was increased by 10 W/min until exhaustion	No effect of GC on performance measured on: submaximal performance (in watts) Other effects of GC: - performance beneficial: sequential effect from the first to the second day of 2 consecutive days and the increase was larger for ACTH than for pla: day 1 vs day 2 Pla: 311 vs 322 W = +3.5% ACTH: 300 vs 325 W = +8.3% (day effect: $P<.01$; drug effect: $P>.05$) - ↓feeling of fatigue: fatigue score ACTH <pla ($P<.001$) on both days - POMS: ↑ total vigor score: ACTH > pla on S2 or S4 - ↑blood G and free fatty acids levels (ACTH > pla)

			Treatments	Protocol	Effects
14	Double-blind Randomized Crossover	10 recreationally trained ♂	2 treatments for each subject: - Pred: 60 mg per os at 7–8 AM for 7 d - 3-wk drug free - Pla for 7 d 2 experimental sessions per subject 4-wk intervals between each session 1 h after ingesting a small meal (500 kcal) identical for each trial	Trial to exhaustion during submax cycling at 70%–75% VO_2max - at the end of each treatment (2 h after a final capsule ingestion: (pla-pred) - after the drug washout period	Effect of GC on performance measured on: time of cycling to exhaustion: ↑ +54% (pla: 46.1 ± 3.3 vs pred: 74.5 ± 9.5 min; $P<.01$) Other effects of GC: - ↑G at rest and during exercise and recovery - ↑ insulin at rest and during the first 30 min of exercise
15	Double-blind Randomized Crossover	8 recreationally trained ♂	2 treatments for each subject: - Pred: 60 mg per os at 7–8 AM for 7 d - 3-wk drug free - Pla for 7 d + 1 wk of strenuous training 2 h/d 2 experimental sessions per subject 3-wk intervals between each session	Trial to exhaustion during submax cycling at 70%–75% VO_2max - before (pla1-pred1) - at the end of each ttt (3 h after a final capsule ingestion (pla2-pred2)	Effect of GC on performance measured on: time of cycling to exhaustion: ↑ +80%(pla1/pla2/pred1: 50.4 ± 6.2/64 ± 9.1/56.1 ± 9.1 min vs pred2: 107 ± 20.7 min; $P<.05$) Other effects of GC: - ↑ G basal and during EX (insulin no ≠)

(continued on next page)

Table 1
(continued)

Study	Methods	Participants	Interventions	Outcomes	Results
16	Double-blind Randomized Crossover	9 recreationally trained ♂	2 treatments for each subject: - 4 mg dex per d - 4 mg pla for 5 d 2 experimental sessions per subject 4-wk intervals between each session	One-legged knee extensor exercise with 3 EX periods separated by more than 45 min of rest 1. Low intensity EX (LI): 10 min 2. Moderate intensity EX (MI) 5 min MI + 2 min rest + MI EX until exhaustion (MI2) 3. High-intensity EX (HI) 1 min, 40 s HI + 2 min rest + HI EX until exhaustion (HI2)	Effect of GC on performance measured on: MI2: time to exhaustion tended to be prolonged in dex vs pla 393 ± 50 vs 294 ± 41 s ($P = .07$) No effect of GC on performance during HI2: dex = pla time to exhaustion: 106 ± 10 vs 108 ± 9 s
26	Double-blind Randomized Crossover	9 recreationally trained ♂	2 treatments for each subject: - 20 mg pred per os (0.25 mg/kg BW) - Pla 2 h before EX 2 experimental sessions per subject 72-h intervals between each session Overnight fasted	Steady-state exercise (cycling) at 60% Vo_2max for 1 h	Effect of GC during exercise: → Higher fat oxidation and lower G oxidation during submax EX - ↑ Total EX energy expenditure (+2.3%) - ↓ Total G oxidation (−23.2%) - ↑ Fat oxidation: +42.9% No effect of G at rest: no change in energy metabolism in fasting humans

Abbreviations: ACTH, adrenocorticotropic hormone; BW, body weight; dex, dexamethasone; EX, exercise; G, glucose; GC, glucocorticoids; IM, intramuscular; pla, placebo; POMS, positive influence of ACTH-induced increased cortisol on mood; pred, prednisolone; RER, respiratory exchange ratio (Vco_2/Vo_2); salb, salbutamol.

such as during international cycling competitions (eg, the 3 weeks of consecutive competitions of the Tour de France or the 3700 km covered in 22 stages over the 3-week period of Vuelta a España). No study has as yet examined whether it is actually possible to maintain a higher work intensity during several weeks of competition, however, when GC is ingested daily to favor recovery. Regarding article 25 of the UNESCO International Convention on the Fight against Doping,[18] which reads "When promoting anti-doping research...States parties shall ensure that such research will...b) Avoid the administration to athletes of prohibited substances and methods; c) Be undertaken only with adequate precautions in place to prevent the results of anti-doping research being misused and applied for doping," there is no authorization to administer GCs (and even less at high doses) to elite athletes during real competitive conditions. This attractive hypothesis will never be able to be tested.

Finally, Arlettaz and colleagues[12] reported that acute GC intake (20 mg prednisolone) does not improve performance during endurance exercise. This dose of GC is considered as a "relatively modest therapeutic dose." Actually, this dose of prednisolone is comparable with 80 mg hydrocortisone (a pharmaceutical reference for cortisol), but in conditions of maximal stress-induced endogenous cortisol production (such as seen in sepsis), approximately 150 to 300 mg hydrocortisone equivalents daily should be given to the subjects corresponding to 6 mg dexamethasone or 30 to 70 mg prednisolone.[19] This is much less than the acute dose used by Arlettaz and colleagues.[12] This hypothesis of too weak a dose to increase performance is corroborated by the fact that increased prednisolone dose (60 mg) for a longer duration significantly increased performance.[14]

The whole of these data suggest that to search for an ergogenic effect of GCs, high doses of GCs or longer periods should be used. This has been tested in the studies described next.

Positive studies
Contrary to acute intake, after short-term prednisolone administration (60 mg for 7 days) Arlettaz and colleagues[14] found a significant improvement of performance (+54% compared with placebo) measured by time to exhaustion at 70% to 75% Vo_2max in healthy, recreationally trained men. To determine if the effects of GC treatment could be extrapolated to elite athletes, Collomp and colleagues[15] investigated in a further study the influence of short-term prednisolone administration (60 mg for 7 days) combined with a standardized training (2 hours per day) on performance measured by time to exhaustion at 70% to 75% Vo_2max. Compared with the placebo condition, strenuous training associated with the GC treatment resulted in a marked improvement in endurance performance (average increase of about 80% compared with an average increase of 54% in their previous study without training).[14] Interestingly, the greatest increase in time to exhaustion with GCs was obtained in the subject performing the best trial with placebo, suggesting that elite male athletes may be more sensitive to the ergogenic effect of GCs during endurance exercise. Even if it seems necessary to verify whether elite athletes are more sensitive to the ergogenic effects of GCs than recreationally trained subjects, these results bring scientific evidence of an increased performance effect of GCs.

Using another exercise protocol (one-legged knee extension) in recreationally trained men, Nordsborg and colleagues[16] showed that time to exhaustion tended to be prolonged after dexamethasone treatment (393 $\pm$ 50 vs 294 $\pm$ 41 seconds; $P = .07$; dexamethasone vs placebo, respectively) during one-legged knee extension at moderate intensity exercise lasting 3 to 8 minutes. These differences were explained through the increased capacity of muscle to regulate (maintain) K+

Table 2

GC administration and exercise performance: results of the studies in animals

Study	Participants	Interventions	Outcomes	Results
22	Female Sprague-Dawley rats	Single sc injection of CA (100 mg/kg body weight) 21 h before treadmill running or NaCl (sal) Rats acquired treadmill familiarity (3 wk)	Treadmill running (30.8 m/min) (7% incline) until exhaustion To determine the effects of increasing substrate availability (glycogen, plasma free fatty acids) by GC on energy metabolism during EX to exhaustion	Effects of GC on performance ↑ EX time to exhaustion: 114 ± 5 vs 95 ± 6 min (approximately +20 min) (CA vs sal, $P<.05$) Other effects of GC - At the start of EX: ↑ glycogen in liver (+40%), ↑ glycogen in muscles: slow-twitch soleus: +61%, fast twitch white vastus: +38%, fast twitch red vastus: +85% and heart: +32% ↑ plasma free fatty acids: +40% with no ≠ during EX - At the time of exhaustion: no ≠ in glycogen concentration in liver and muscles - Vo_2 and RER: no ≠ in RER but ↓ in running economy (↑Vo_2 for a given work rate)

| 23 | Female Sprague-Dawley rats | 14 consecutive daily sc injections of CA 100 mg/kg or sal
Dosage selected because it is effective in producing skeletal wasting | - Vo_2max and maximal EX test run times
- prolonged treadmill running test (28.7 m/s up a 5.5% incline) until exhaustion | Effects of GC on performance
CA enhanced performance despite muscle atrophy (predominantly in white muscle: no ≠ in ventricular or soleus muscle weights but plantaris muscle weights were 27% less in the CA-treated group)
1. Maximal EX test:
  - ↑Vo_2 peak (CA: 95.6 ± 3.2 vs 79.5 ± 1.8 mL/kg/min)
  - ↑ total run times: 962 ± 61 vs 825 ± 33 s (CA vs sal, $P<.05$)
2. Prolonged endurance test: ↑ total run times: 158 ± 12 vs 116 ± 11 min (CA vs sal, $P<.05$)
Unchanged oxygen uptake by homogenates of all fiber types |

(continued on next page)

Table 2
(continued)

Study	Participants	Interventions	Outcomes	Results
25	Male Wistar rats	Daily intraperitoneal injection of dex (1 mg/kg) or sal for 12 d	Investigation of the effects of contraction (electric stimulation) on G uptake, insulin signaling, and glycogen synthesis in isolated skeletal muscles from dex-treated rats	- Insulin resistance but no impairment of G uptake during contraction in soleus or epitrochlearis muscle - ↑ glycogen content ($P<.02$) in rested muscles either incubated with or without insulin for epitrochlaeris (150 vs 200 mmol/kg dry weigh) and soleus (100 vs 150 mmol/kg dry weigh) (dex vs saline) - After contraction, insulin-stimulated glycogen synthesis was improved in soleus from dex-treated rats (20 vs 24 mmol/kg dry weigh/h)

| 20 | Male Lewis rats | Experiment 1: ad libitum fed rats
5 groups:
Sham-ADX (Sham) or ADX implanted with sc pellet containing 0 (ADX-0), 12.5 (ADX-12.5), 50 (ADX-50), or 100 mg (ADX-100) corticosterone (CORT) that continuously deliver a constant dosage of CORT for 10 d
Experiment 2: food-restricted rats (access to food 1.5 h/d): effects of chronic increase in corticosterone levels on wheel running activity
Same 5 groups than experiment 1
Experiment 3: effects of acute increase in corticosterone levels in ad libitum and food-restricted rats (access to food 1.5 h/d) on wheel running activity
Injection of corticosterone or vehicle sc once daily at 11 h on D2–D4 | Permanent access to a running wheel: determination of wheel activity (number of kilometers run per day)
Experiments 1 and 2: effects of chronic administration of increasing doses of CORT (implanted capsules) on wheel running activity
Experiment 3: effects of acute administration of CORT (injection of CORT) on wheel running activity | Effects of GC on performance (wheel activity)
Experiment 1: no effect of ≠ in CORT levels in ad libitum fed rats
Experiments 2 and 3: in food restricted rats
- Experiment 2:
↑ wheel running activity in a dose dependent-fashion ADX100>ADX50> ADX12.5>ADX0
- Experiment 3: acute ↑ wheel running activity after acute CORT injection ADX100>ADX50> ADX12.5>ADX0
- Experiment 3: acute ↑ wheel running activity after acute CORT injection |

Abbreviations: ADX, adrenalectomized; CA, cortisol acetate; dex, dexamethasone; EX, exercise; GC, glucocorticoids; RER, respiratory exchange ratio (V_{CO_2}/V_{O_2}); sal, saline; sc, subcutaneous.

homeostasis and muscle fatigue development because short-term dexamethasone increased the Na+, K+ pump $\alpha1$, $\alpha2$, $\beta1$, and $\beta2$ subunits protein expression in human skeletal muscle (with lower thigh K+ release during low and moderate one-legged knee extension). By contrast, dexamethasone did not affect performance of repeated high-intensity exercises lasting 1 to 3 minutes.

The results of the study of Soetens and colleagues[17] should also be considered. Although the authors concluded that their results demonstrate that there is no influence of an ACTH injection on maximal performance as measured with a standardized bicycle ergometer design, however, other data obtained from their experiment demonstrate positive effects of ACTH during submaximal exercise. Soetens and colleagues[17] injected a high dose of ACTH depot (1 mg). The use of a depot preparation gave them the opportunity to study recuperation on the second day because plasma cortisol concentration doubled for 2 consecutive days (day 1 and day 2 of the protocol) (see **Table 1**).

They reported four points: (1) Decreased feelings of fatigue with ACTH during submaximal performance (1 hour cycling at 60% maximal performance). The decrease is systematic over the whole interval of submaximal performance. As stated by the authors: "With ACTH, subjects seem to postpone the increase in feelings of fatigue as long as the load is low to moderate. It means that ACTH, for that matter, could help competitors in long races to bridge over the long and boring first hours of a competition more pleasantly or less wearily." That delay of fatigue in submaximal conditions is not translated, however, into increase of maximal performance during the ramped test that followed the steady-state exercise. (2) Positive influence of ACTH-induced increased cortisol on mood; on the second day of the protocol subjects indicate significantly more vigor after the test with ACTH than after placebo. (3) Metabolic effects; there was a significant supplementary increase of glucose after exercise, and the mobilization of extra FFAs was also notable after the test with ACTH (increased compared with placebo). (4) Recuperation on the second day of the protocol. After the test with ACTH, feelings of fatigue are suppressed during the submaximal exercise test realized on day 2 but, compared with the placebo group, there is no increase of maximal performance during the ramped test that followed the steady state exercise (day 2). The authors concluded that "despite all these impressive physiologic changes" under influence of ACTH (1 mg Synacthen depot), there was no performance enhancement during at least a ramped test.

These results also leave open the more important question as to what is the ergogenic significance of these reduced feelings of fatigue and increased vigor during submaximal performance in real conditions of competition, during the complex of events necessary to elicit a victory during a race. The absence of increased performance from a statistical point of view does not exclude the fact that this nonstatistical gain in performance (in terms of distance ran) may translate into a gain during a final sprint, and could make the difference between the winner and second place. The other question arising from these results is to what extent laboratory tests can be assimilated to real competition and what could be the effect of reduced feelings of fatigue and more vigor during long races lasting more than 3 to 4 hours (instead of the 1 hour protocol of Soetens and colleagues[17]) on the final sprint.

Data obtained in animal experiments clarify the mechanisms of the ergogenic effects of GCs adding insights into the central and peripheral (metabolic) effects of GCs.

Animal Data

Experiments conducted in rats also support the ergogenic effect of GCs with demonstrated positive effects of GCs on performance. In food-restricted rats with ad libitum access to a running wheel, wheel activity (number of kilometers run in 24 hours) was significantly increased (times two) when they had been given a subcutaneous injection of corticosterone (the rat natural GC hormone).[20] In addition to this stimulatory effect of acute corticosterone, the administration of increasing doses of corticosterone (by implanted capsules that continuously deliver a constant dosage of corticosterone for 10 days) to adrenalectomized rats increased wheel running activity in a dose-dependent fashion. The range of corticosterone achieved in the different experiments represented reference values from low to high (stress-induced) HPA axis activity. These observations show that GC can enhance physical activity in rats after both acute (injected corticosterone) and chronic (subcutaneous implants continuously delivering corticosterone) administration.[20] These effects are probably caused by central effects of GCs with the stimulation of dopamine production in the nucleus accumbens and, possibly, the activation of other parts of the brain involved in motor activity (M. Duclos, unpublished results, 2008).[21]

With regard to the peripheral (metabolic) effects of GC, Gorostiaga and colleagues[22] have reported in rats that a single injection of cortisol acetate 21 hours before treadmill running induced an increase in glycogen content in liver and muscles (slow-twitch, fast-twitch, white and red fibers) and increased plasma FFA. In these conditions where both carbohydrate (glycogen) and fatty acid availability were increased, endurance improved significantly with increased time during exercise (treadmill running) to exhaustion (+20 minutes compared with the placebo group).

After 14 consecutive daily injections of cortisol acetate[23] in rats at a dose selected to produce skeletal wasting, and despite muscle atrophy, cortisol acetate–treated groups showed enhanced performance with increased total run times during maximal exercise (Vo_2max) (962 $\pm$ 61 vs 825 $\pm$ 33 seconds, cortisol acetate vs placebo) and increased running time during endurance test (158 $\pm$ 12 vs 116 $\pm$ 11 minutes, cortisol acetate vs placebo).

With regard to the known metabolic effects of GCs, some of these results can seem intriguing. Indeed, GCs in excess induce insulin resistance. Skeletal muscles dispose of the major part of glucose during insulin stimulation and GCs impair metabolic regulation, at least in part, by reducing insulin-stimulated glucose uptake in skeletal muscles. Muscle contraction, however, like insulin, stimulates glucose uptake but by different mechanisms than insulin and contraction stimulates glucose uptake by an insulin-independent mechanism.[24] This has been well demonstrated by Ruzzin and Jensen[25] who investigated in muscles from dexamethasone-treated rats whether contraction (1) normally stimulates glucose uptake, (2) activates glycogen synthase, and (3) enhances insulin action, and whether insulin's ability to stimulate glycogen synthesis is improved after contraction. They demonstrated that glucose uptake is stimulated normally during contraction in insulin-resistant muscles from dexamethasone-treated rats. Moreover, following contraction, glycogen synthase activity increased to a similar extent in muscles from control and dexamethasone-treated rats. Finally, dexamethasone stimulated the resynthesis of muscle glycogen after exercise (dexamethasone more than placebo), whereas less glycogen was stored at rest than in placebo animals as a result of dexamethasone-induced insulin resistance.[25] This enhanced glycogen production following exercise promotes metabolic recuperation and is a crucial factor for optimal, high-intensity endurance performance explaining the previous results of Gorostiaga and colleagues[22] and Capaccio and colleagues.[23] It should be noted that similar metabolic effects (increased plasma glucose and FFA levels) have been reported in most of the previously cited studies in humans dealing with GC administration after both acute and short-term intake (see **Table 1**).[8,9,12–15,17,26]

Altogether, these studies clarify the effects of GC based on scientific evidence. They clearly demonstrate both in animals and humans that GCs have ergogenic effects (performance-enhancing effects). Many more questions have been raised, however, which demand answers:

Can GCs indirectly affect performance by helping athletes to recover from exhaustive competitions?

It is actually possible to maintain higher work intensity during several weeks of training when GC is ingested during the training sessions?

Are the results obtained in male athletes gender dependent?

Are the results obtained in recreationally trained athletes applicable to elite athletes?

Are highly trained athletes more sensitive to the ergogenic effects of GCs during endurance exercise than recreationally trained subjects?

GC DOPING AND THE DEMONSTRATED RISKS TO HEALTH

Long-term GC use has been shown incontrovertibly to lead to complications, notably on bone tissue (osteoporosis); metabolism (insulin resistance); and the cardiovascular system (hypertension and atherosclerosis).[7] Cases of GC dependence have been reported.[6] In addition to these well-characterized effects, other complications are beginning to emerge.

Short and colleagues[27] showed that, after a 6-day course of prednisone (0.5 mg/kg/d) in healthy, young adults, blood flow in the leg had dropped by 25%. This is consistent with the results of recent experiments in pigs that showed that a single pharmacologic dose of prednisone significantly reduced blood flow in the muscles, the skin, and hip bone tissue. This effect was of rapid onset, being detectable within 1 hour of administration and persisting for at least 24 hours, which suggests that it involves a nongenomic mechanism; it is probably mediated at endothelial cells by GC-induced inhibition of nitric oxide (NO)–dependent endothelial relaxation because in vitro experiments have shown that umbilical cord epithelial cells produce less NO when exposed to dexamethasone because of increased levels of free radicals. Reduced NO production inhibits endothelial vessel relaxation and leads to diminished blood flow. Iuchi and colleagues[28] defined the role of free radicals in this phenomenon and established the link with GC. When blood flow in the arm of a healthy subject was artificially inhibited using a tourniquet (a cuff inflated to 250 mm Hg for 5 minutes), increased blood flow was observed in the forearm 60 and 90 seconds after removal of the tourniquet as a result of NO-dependent vasodilatation of the vascular endothelium. When the same measurement was performed in subjects who had been prescribed GCs to treat autoimmune disease before and after the beginning of the course of treatment, a reduction of 43% was induced by the drug (on average, 28 days after the beginning of the course of treatment [range, 12–50 days]). This effect is dependent on dosage and the duration of exposure to the GCs. In parallel, the same researchers showed that GCs induced a dose-dependent increase in free radical production in cultured endothelial cells. Free radicals cut down the availability of NO by inducing the production of superoxide, which interacts with NO to generate peroxynitrites, which leads to an increase in NO consumption. Reduced NO availability can impair endothelial function leading to hypertension and atherosclerosis, both of which are major cardiovascular complications associated with excessive GC use.

GCs induce free radicals by interfering with mitochondrial electron transfer systems, pointing to impaired mitochondrial function. In previous experiments in rats, however,

Duclos and colleagues[29] have shown that excessive endogenous corticosterone (the equivalent of cortisol in rats) production induced by repetitive stress led to a reduction in mitochondrial density in muscle tissue. The mitochondrion is the main seat of energy production in cells and worries about potential adverse effects on mitochondrial metabolism in muscle tissue are justified if supraphysiologic doses of synthetic GC are being taken by athletes to enhance their performance.

Another series of experiments warrants attention. A number of studies have shown that increasing blood cortisol (by the infusion of cortisol or ACTH) to stress-related levels (880 and 1100 nmol/L) inhibited hyperglycemic hormone responses (adrenaline, noradrenalin, glucagon) and lowered glucose production in the liver in response to subsequent pharmacologically induced hypoglycemia.[30,31] In the course of prolonged exercise (lasting hours), blood glucose levels significantly fall, but not usually below 0.6 to 0.7 g/L (3.3–3.9 nmol/L) in healthy subjects, although a few cases of full-blown hypoglycemia have been reported in marathon and long-distance runners. In sports involving prolonged exertion or repetition over several days in a row (bicycle races, desert marathons, long-distance races), problems of blood glucose counterregulation could explain certain phenomena in subjects who had taken a pharmacologic dose of a GC the day before, such as sudden exhaustion forcing the athlete to withdraw from the event or to considerably drop in the race positioning.

Above and beyond chronic effects, a major (possibly life-threatening) complication can arise on the withdrawal of GCs: acute adrenal insufficiency. This risk is real and is not anecdotal. When top-level cyclists from the French Cycling Federation were surveyed, a nonnegligible number of cases of crude adrenal insufficiency (undetectable cortisol coupled with a negative ACTH test result) were identified.[32] Of 659 elite cyclists monitored during the 2001 and 2002 sporting seasons, 34 (5.2%) had low blood cortisol levels (at least two standard deviations below the mean of the test kit used). More seriously, of these 34 cyclists, 8 of the 15 who agreed to undergo an ACTH test had crude adrenal insufficiency (low cortisol levels and a negative ACTH test result).

The effects of long-term corticosteroid use on endogenous cortisol production are well characterized in the literature; this inhibition has been documented even at low doses. Henzen and colleagues[33] detected adrenal insufficiency in 45% of subjects who had been given a short (<1 month) course of a systemic GC at a dosage of greater than 25 mg of prednisone in 24 hours. Broide and colleagues[34] and Kannisto and colleagues[35] found respective incidences of impaired adrenal function of 25% and 35% in children with asthma being treated with inhaled GCs. The duration of HPA inhibition ranges from 2 to 4 weeks at doses of greater than 25 mg of prednisone per 24 hours (low doses), but can be sustained for a matter of months.

Limited data are available on the effect of biologic adrenal insufficiency on athletic performance. The most current signs of adrenal insufficiency in subjects taking inhaled corticosteroids are lethargy and nausea.[36] Other subjects (mainly children but cases in adults have been reported) presented with acute hypoglycemia and decreased levels of consciousness, coma, or coma and convulsions.[36,37] It is plausible that atypical forms of adrenal crisis (hypoglycemia, feeling of faintness) could explain some apparently unexplained decreased performances observed in some athletes. Whereas most adults presented with insidious onset of symptoms, the potential severity of the decompensation of subclinical adrenal insufficiency induced by corticosteroids is reported in sedentary subjects[36–38] and requires evaluation in a population exposed to other stresses than sedentary subjects. Indeed, competitive or intensive exercising may require intense and prolonged physical effort, sometimes in extreme conditions that can change suddenly (heat, cold, hypoxia). Moreover some athletes (eg, cyclists, rugby players, soccer players) are at risk of severe injuries that may require surgery and have a high risk of infections, affecting the upper respiratory tract in particular. Although biologic insufficiency did not seem to be always associated with clinical symptoms, in view of the severity of cases of adrenal crisis described in subjects taking corticosteroids,[36,37] in the event of some form of superimposed stress (eg, infection, physical injury entailing surgery), there is a real risk of life-threatening acute adrenal insufficiency in athletes abusing GCs.

SUMMARY

There is scientific evidence that GCs mediate ergogenic effects in animals and humans. It is difficult to understand why GCs are the type of product most commonly detected in doping tests if they had no beneficial effect on performance (or recuperation). Moreover, the health risks of using GCs are well characterized. GCs are doping agents and should remain on WADA's list of banned products. Moreover, it is necessary to prohibit systemic use of this class of drugs at all times (in- and out-of-competition) and not just with in-competition controls as in the current WADA legislation.

REFERENCES

1. Duclos M. Hypothalamo-pituitary-adrenal axis adaptation to repeated and prolonged exercise-induced cortisol secretion in endurance training: physiology is the first target. In: Selkirk TB, editor. Focus on exercise and health research. New York: NovaScience Publishers; 2005. p. 131–61.
2. Duclos M, Guinot M, Le BY. Cortisol and GH: odd and controversial ideas. Appl Physiol Nutr Metab 2007;32(5):895–903.
3. Sapolsky RM, Romero M, Munck AU. How do glucocorticoids influence stress responses? Integrating permissive, suppressive, stimulatory, and preparative actions. Endocr Rev 2000;21:55–89.
4. Duclos M, Gouarne C, Bonnemaison D. Acute and chronic effects of exercise on tissue sensitivity to glucocorticoids. J Appl Physiol 2003;94:869–75.
5. Piazza PV, Rouge-Pont F, Deroche V, et al. Glucocorticoids have state-dependent stimulant effects on the mesencephalic dopaminergic transmission. Proc Natl Acad Sci U S A 1996;93(16):8716–20.
6. Hochberg Z, Pacak K, Chrousos GP. Endocrine withdrawal syndromes. Endocr Rev 2003;24(4):523–38.
7. Buttgereit F, Burmester GR, Lipworth BJ. Optimised glucocorticoid therapy: the sharpening of an old spear. Lancet 2005;365(9461):801–3.
8. Marquet P, Lac G, Chassain AP, et al. Dexamethasone in resting and exercising men. I. Effects on bioenergetics, minerals, and related hormones. J Appl Physiol 1999;87(1):175–82.
9. Petrides J, Gold PW, Mueller GP, et al. Marked differences in functioning of the hypothalamic-pituitary-adrenal axis between groups of men. J Appl Physiol 1997;82(6):1979–88.
10. Baume N, Steel G, Edwards T, et al. No variation of physical performance and perceived exertion after adrenal gland stimulation by synthetic ACTH (Synacthen) in cyclists. Eur J Appl Physiol 2008;104(4):589–600.
11. Kuipers H, Van't Hullenaar GA, Pluim BM, et al. Four weeks' corticosteroid inhalation does not augment maximal power output in endurance athletes. Br J Sports Med 2008;42(11):568–71.
12. Arlettaz A, Collomp K, Portier H, et al. Effects of acute prednisolone administration on exercise endurance and metabolism. Br J Sports Med 2008;42(4):250–4.

13. Arlettaz A, Collomp K, Portier H, et al. Effects of acute prednisolone intake during intense submaximal exercise. Int J Sports Med 2006;27(9):673–9.
14. Arlettaz A, Portier H, Lecoq AM, et al. Effects of short-term prednisolone intake during submaximal exercise. Med Sci Sports Exerc 2007;39(9):1672–8.
15. Collomp K, Arlettaz A, Portier H, et al. Short-term glucocorticoid intake combined with intense training on performance and hormonal responses. Br J Sports Med 2008;42(12):983–8.
16. Nordsborg N, Ovesen J, Thomassen M, et al. Effect of dexamethasone on skeletal muscle Na+, K+ pump subunit specific expression and K+ homeostasis during exercise in humans. J Physiol 2008;586(5):1447–59.
17. Soetens E, De MK, Hueting JE. No influence of ACTH on maximal performance. Psychopharmacology 1995;118(3):260–6.
18. UNESCO. United Nations Educational, Scientific and Cultural Organization; International convention on the fight against doping, 2005. Available at: http://portal.unesco.org/en/ev.phpURL_ID=31037&URL_DO=DO_TOPIC&URL_SECTION=201.html. Accessed October 19, 2005.
19. Brotman DJ, Girod JP, Garcia MJ, et al. Effects of short-term glucocorticoids on cardiovascular biomarkers. J Clin Endocrinol Metab 2005;90(6):3202–8.
20. Duclos M, Gatti C, Bessiere B, et al. Tonic and phasic effects of corticosterone on food restriction-induced hyperactivity in rats. Psychoneuroendocrinology 2008;34(3):436–45.
21. Roug-Pont F, Deroche V, Le Moal M, et al. Individual differences in stress-induced dopamine release in the nucleus accumbens are influenced by corticosterone. Eur J Neurosci 1998;10:3903–7.
22. Gorostiaga EM, Czerwinski SM, Hickson RC. Acute glucocorticoid effects on glycogen utilization, O2 uptake, and endurance. J Appl Physiol 1988;64(3): 1098–106.
23. Capaccio JA, Galassi TM, Hickson RC. Unaltered aerobic power and endurance following glucocorticoid-induced muscle atrophy. Med Sci Sports Exerc 1985; 17(3):380–4.
24. Lund S, Holman GD, Schmitz O, et al. Contraction stimulates translocation of glucose transporter GLUT4 in skeletal muscle through a mechanism distinct from that of insulin. Proc Natl Acad Sci U S A 1995;92(13):5817–21.
25. Ruzzin J, Jensen J. Contraction activates glucose uptake and glycogen synthase normally in muscles from dexamethasone-treated rats. Am J Physiol Endocrinol Metab 2005;289(2):E241–50.
26. Arlettaz A, Portier H, Lecoq AM, et al. Effects of acute prednisolone intake on substrate utilization during submaximal exercise. Int J Sports Med 2008;29(1): 21–6.
27. Short KR, Nygren J, Bigelow ML, et al. Effect of short-term prednisone use on blood flow, muscle protein metabolism, and function. J Clin Endocrinol Metab 2004;89(12):6198–207.
28. Iuchi T, Akaike M, Mitsui T, et al. Glucocorticoid excess induces superoxide production in vascular endothelial cells and elicits vascular endothelial dysfunction. Circ Res 2003;92(1):81–7.
29. Duclos M, Gouarne C, Martin C, et al. Effects of corticosterone on muscle mitochondria identifying different sensitivity to glucocorticoids in Lewis and Fischer rats. Am J Physiol 2004;286:E159–67.
30. Davis SN, Shavers C, Costa F, et al. Role of cortisol in the pathogenesis of deficient counterregulation after antecedent hypoglycemia in normal humans. J Clin Invest 1996;98(3):680–91.

31. McGregor VP, Banarer S, Cryer PE. Elevated endogenous cortisol reduces autonomic neuroendocrine and symptom responses to subsequent hypoglycemia. Am J Physiol Endocrinol Metab 2002;282(4):E770-7.

32. Guinot M, Duclos M, Idres N, et al. Value of basal serum cortisol to detect corticosteroid-induced adrenal insufficiency in elite cyclists. Eur J Appl Physiol 2007; 99(3):205-16.

33. Henzen C, Suter A, Lerch E, et al. Suppression and recovery of adrenal response after short-term, high-dose glucocorticoid treatment. Lancet 2000;355(9203): 542-5.

34. Broide J, Soferman R, Kivity S, et al. Low-dose adrenocorticotropin test reveals impaired adrenal function in patients taking inhaled corticosteroids. J Clin Endocrinol Metab 1995;80(4):1243-6.

35. Kannisto S, Korpi M, Arikoski P, et al. Biochemical marker of bone metabolism in relation to adrenocortical and growth suppression during the initiation phase of inhaled steroid therapy. Pediatr Res 2002;52:258-62.

36. Todd GR, Acerini CL, Ross-Russell R, et al. Survey of adrenal crisis associated with inhaled corticosteroids in the United Kingdom. Arch Dis Child 2002;87(6): 457-61.

37. Cooper MS, Stewart PM. Corticosteroid insufficiency in acutely ill patients. N Engl J Med 2003;348(8):727-34.

38. Oelkers W. Adrenal insufficiency. N Engl J Med 1996;335(16):1206-12.

Dehydroepiandrosterone to Enhance Physical Performance: Myth and Reality

Stefanie Hahner, MD, Bruno Allolio, MD*

KEYWORDS

- Adrenal insufficiency • DHEA • Androgens
- Doping • Testosterone • Physical performance
- Body composition • Bone

DEHYDROEPIANDROSTERONE AS AN ANDROGENIC PROHORMONE: PHYSIOLOGY

Dehydroepiandrosterone (DHEA) and dehydroepiandrosterone sulfate (DHEAS) are the most abundant steroids in the human circulatory system. They are mainly synthesized in the zona reticularis of the adrenal cortex, whereas the gonads contribute only about 5% to the circulating levels.

Different from cortisol and aldosterone, DHEA secretion follows a characteristic age-related pattern.[1] DHEA is a major secretory product of the fetal adrenal gland, with high circulating concentrations at birth. Serum concentrations then decrease to very low levels until they gradually start to continuously rise again between ages 6 and 10 years.[2] Peak DHEA concentrations are observed in early adulthood and are then followed by a steady decline down to about 20% of maximum levels around age 70 years.[3] This age-associated decrease has been termed adrenopause despite the fact that the activity of cortisol production by the zona fasciculata and aldosterone production by the zona glomerulosa does not change with age. The age-related decline in DHEA levels shows high interindividual variability and may be related to a reduction in size of the zona reticularis.[4] Secretion of DHEA is stimulated by adrenocorticotropic hormone and follows a diurnal rhythm similar to that of cortisol. In contrast, DHEAS, which has a far longer half-life, does not show any diurnal variation.

It had been assumed for a long time that DHEA and DHEAS undergo continuous interconversion, suggesting that most of the circulating DHEA is generated from peripheral DHEAS.[5] However, although a high percentage of circulating DHEAS is generated from DHEA via hepatic DHEA sulfotransferase (SULT2A1) activity, only

Endocrinology and Diabetes Unit, Department of Medicine I, University of Würzburg, Oberdürrbacher Strasse 6, D-97080 Würzburg, Germany
* Corresponding author.
E-mail address: allolio_b@medizin.uni-wuerzburg.de (B. Allolio).

Endocrinol Metab Clin N Am 39 (2010) 127–139
doi:10.1016/j.ecl.2009.10.008
0889-8529/10/$ – see front matter © 2010 Elsevier Inc. All rights reserved.

endo.theclinics.com

minimal amounts of circulating DHEA arise from DHEAS, indicating that peripheral sul-phatase activity does not contribute significantly to circulating DHEA.[6] This observa-tion is of major significance, as often only the level of serum DHEAS is measured, which does not always reflect the level of circulating DHEA adequately.

DHEA has multiple different effects within the organism that are in part not fully understood. Mechanisms of action are categorized as indirect DHEA-mediated and direct DHEA-mediated effects. Indirect actions are mediated by bioconversion to active androgens or estrogens by the adrenal gland or the gonads or as an intracrine effect by local conversion in the peripheral target cell. DHEA itself is often called an adrenal androgen; however, it does not bind to the androgen receptor. The androgenic action of DHEA is mediated by the consecutive conversion to testosterone and dihy-drotestosterone (**Fig. 1**). The necessary enzymes 3β-hydroxysteroid dehydrogenase, 17β-hydroxysteroid dehydrogenase, and 5α-reductase are almost ubiquitously ex-pressed in target tissues.[7] Thus, target cells can produce androgens adapted to their own demand, independent from changes in systemic androgen levels. About 30% to 50% of androgen synthesis in men and 50% to 100% of estrogen synthesis in pre- and postmenopausal women occurs in peripheral target cells.[8]

Administration of DHEA in humans leads to significant increases in circulating sex steroids, whereas conversion to sex steroids shows a sexual dimorphism, with predominant generation of androgens in women and a significant increase of estro-gens in men.[9,10]

DHEA also acts as a neurosteroid. Because of the intracerebral expression of steroidogenic enzymes, it can be synthesized within the human brain.[11,12] DHEA has been shown to directly interact with a variety of neurotransmitter receptors, including *N*-methyl-D-aspartate receptors,[13] gamma-aminobutyric acid receptors, and sigma receptors.[7,14] It may also be converted to other downstream steroids within the brain, modulating neuronal activity.[15,16]

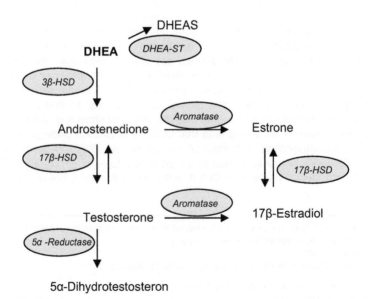

Fig. 1. Conversion of DHEA to active androgens and estrogens.

In addition to its indirect action via conversion to sex steroids and its neurosteroidal activity, there is evidence for a direct action of DHEA via specific membrane receptors. High-affinity binding sites for DHEA have been identified in endothelial cells,[17] and it has been shown that DHEA is able to activate endothelial nitric oxide synthase via a G protein–coupled plasma membrane receptor.[17,18] Furthermore, DHEA affects extracellular signal-regulated kinase I phosphorylation in human muscular smooth muscle cells.[19]

DHEA has also been shown to directly bind to immune cells. It increases interleukin-2 secretion from human T cells in vitro and the activity of natural killer cells.[20] It also inhibits interleukin-6 release by mononuclear cells. Investigations on the effects of DHEA on the immune system in vivo have mainly been performed in patients with systemic lupus erythematosus. It has been demonstrated that DHEA exhibited positive immunomodulatory effects with reduction of disease activity and glucocorticoid dose. However, mostly supraphysiologic doses were administered in these trials.

DHEA EFFECTS IN ADRENAL INSUFFICIENCY (MUSCLE, EXERCISE, BODY COMPOSITION, CARDIOVASCULAR SYSTEM)

Patients with adrenal insufficiency (AI) suffer from severe impairment of DHEA secretion and represent a good model to clarify the physiologic role of DHEA and the effects of DHEA replacement in a clinical setting. Pharmacokinetic studies have demonstrated that oral administration of DHEA, 25 to 50 mg, in patients with AI restores serum DHEA(S) concentrations to the normal range of young adults.[9] Moreover, it has been shown that a single morning dose is sufficient to maintain normal DHEA(S) concentrations throughout the day.[9] All studies in patients with AI have invariably shown that administration of DHEA not only increases circulating DHEA(S) concentrations but also leads to significant increases in circulating sex steroids because of downstream conversion.

Based on the observation of impaired well-being in patients with AI, the effects of DHEA on subjective health status have been most intensively studied in patients with AI. DHEA has beneficial effects on subjective health status, mood, and sexuality, which are often impaired in those patients.[9,21,23–25] These effects could also be demonstrated in men who do not suffer from androgen deficiency owing to the preserved androgen production by their testes, indicating that these effects are in part mediated by neurosteroidal activity.[26,27]

Effects on Insulin-like Growth Factor-1

In the first published DHEA replacement study in AI patients,[9] DHEA led to increased insulin-like growth factor-1 (IGF-1) concentrations. This increase was observed only in women with primary AI, whereas women with secondary AI showed no clear increase in IGF-1, suggesting that DHEA might act via pituitary growth hormone (GH) secretion to influence circulating IGF-1 levels. However, recent studies on GH replacement in patients with hypopituitarism demonstrated that DHEA replacement increased serum IGF-1 concentrations by 18% in female patients, but not in male patients. This indicated that the activity of DHEA is not related to changes in GH secretion. In keeping with this observation, Brooke and colleagues[26] observed that DHEA replacement in patients with hypopituitarism reduced GH dose requirements in female patients on GH replacement. Administration of DHEA led to a 14.6% ± 20% reduction in the dose of GH required to maintain constant serum IGF-1 levels. This effect was maintained for 12 months and was followed by a significant fall in the level of serum IGF-1 2 months after withdrawal of DHEA. No such effect was observed in male patients.

As administration of DHEA increases circulating androgen concentrations in women to the normal range but does little to change the androgen concentrations in men with hypopituitarism receiving androgen replacement, these findings suggest that the increase in the level of IGF-1 is related to androgenic effects of DHEA. However, increases in the level of IGF-1 have not been observed in other studies.[24,28]

Effects on Lipids and Insulin Sensitivity

Dhatariya and colleagues[29] studied 28 hypoadrenal women in a single-center randomized double-blind placebo-controlled crossover study, who received DHEA, 50 mg/d, or placebo for 12 weeks. Fasting insulin and glucagon levels were lower with DHEA, and the average amount of glucose needed to maintain similar blood glucose levels while infusing the same insulin dosages was higher during DHEA administration, whereas endogenous glucose production was unchanged. These findings suggest that DHEA increased insulin sensitivity in hypoadrenal women. However, no effects with DHEA administration on fasting glucose, insulin, or glucose-insulin ratio were observed in other studies.[31,33,34]

Effects on lipids are more consistent. The first study in patients with AI demonstrated a significant decrease of the levels of total cholesterol and high-density lipoprotein (HDL) cholesterol.[9] Similarly, in the study by Dhatariya and colleagues[29] and Srinivasan and colleagues,[35] DHEA reduced not only total cholesterol, low-density lipoprotein cholesterol, and triglycerides but also HDL cholesterol. The mechanisms for the reduction in the levels of HDL and total cholesterol are most likely mediated by the effects of androgens on increasing hepatic lipase activity, thus impairing hepatic cholesterol formation.[36] Further long-term studies are needed to analyze the effect on cardiovascular outcome parameters.

Muscle Function, Body Composition, and Bone

The available data provide no evidence that DHEA improves or changes muscular function in patients with AI.[31]

DHEA, 50 mg, did not change physical performance, body composition, protein metabolism, or muscle mitochondrial biogenesis in 28 women with AI in a prospective, randomized, placebo-controlled, crossover study. However, lowering of messenger ribonucleic acid levels of binding proteins of IGF-1 and myosin heavy chain 1 were reported, suggesting potential effects of longer term treatment.[37]

Similarly, although DHEA binding sites have been detected on endothelial cells, DHEA replacement in 8 patients with adrenal failure had no effect on endothelial function or cardiovascular parameters despite clear changes in androgen status[38]; this has been confirmed in a recent trial in 40 patients with AI who received DHEA, 50 mg, or placebo for 12 weeks in a randomized, double-blind, crossover design. DHEA supplementation did not significantly affect measures of arterial stiffness or endothelial function in those patients.[39]

As the duration of most studies was less than 12 months, changes in bone mineral density (BMD) are difficult to assess. DHEA led to a small decrease in the level of serum osteocalcin in women with AI,[31] whereas bone resorption markers did not change. In one study, an increase in BMD was reported.[23]

In women with systemic lupus erythematosus receiving long-term glucocorticoid therapy, DHEA (200 mg/d) prevented bone loss and significantly increased BMD.[40,41] However, such a dose leads to supraphysiologic concentrations of DHEA(S) and circulating androgens. Longer studies in a sufficient number of patients are needed to clarify the role of DHEA in replacement therapy.

ANABOLIC DHEA EFFECTS IN THE ELDERLY

In aging societies, the quest for measures that delay aging and frailty has become more prevalent. As many hormones, such as DHEA, decline with age, it has been postulated that low hormone levels contribute to age-related phenotypic changes like sexual dysfunction, sarcopenia, osteoporosis, and increased body fat.

Some correlation studies further indicate that DHEA(S) levels are interrelated with functional activities.[42,43] Animal experiments have demonstrated beneficial effects of DHEA on the cardiovascular system and the immune system; furthermore, anti-tumor and antidiabetic effects could be demonstrated. These observations have led to the assumption that DHEA supplementation might stop these aging processes and have resulted in a wide and unreflected use of DHEA as an antiaging hormone. However, as relevant DHEA levels are observed only in higher primates, animal experiments using industrial doses of DHEA have little bearing on human physiology.

Several trials have addressed the effect of DHEA on body composition, metabolic parameters, muscle strength, and bone in elderly subjects. The effect that is most consistently observed is an increase in IGF-I levels comparable with what has been observed in patients with AI (**Table 1**).[44-50]

DHEA replacement has been reported to increase BMD in elderly subjects (see **Table 1**).[45,49-54] Jankowski and colleagues[45] investigated 70 women and 70 men aged 60 to 88 years. They observed an increase in hip bone mass density in both sexes, and in women, additionally, an increase in lumbar spine bone mass density after 1-year treatment with DHEA, 50 mg/d. The changes in BMD were associated with estradiol levels and free estrogen index at 12 months, suggesting that the effects were primarily mediated by increases in serum estradiol.[55] Several other randomized controlled trials reported similar observations with slight increases in bone mass density and changes in markers of bone turnover, mainly in women.[45,49-54] However, the effect is relatively small compared with other treatments established for osteoporosis. Fractures as an outcome have so far not been included.

Effects of DHEA on body composition and physical performance are inconsistent. Morales and colleagues[46] reported an increase in muscle strength in men aged 50 to 60 years after 6 months of treatment with DHEA, 100 mg/d, but not in women. Diamond and colleagues[56] demonstrated that application of a 10% DHEA cream to the skin daily for 12 months led to an increase in femoral muscle area in 15 women aged 60 to 70 years. A decrease in fat mass and an increase in fat-free mass as assessed by dual-energy x-ray absorptiometry measurement was furthermore observed by Villareal and colleagues[54] However, no effect on body composition could be observed in several other large trials (see **Table 1**).[45,49,53,57] As the mild anabolic effects of DHEA might be insufficient to increase muscle mass or strength in sedentary people, the potential of potentiating the response to exercise training has been investigated.

In a randomized, double-blind, placebo-controlled trial, Villareal and Holloszy[58] analyzed the effects of 10 months of administration of DHEA, 50 mg/d, with the addition of weightlifting exercise training during the last 4 months of the study (DHEA exercise group, n = 29; placebo exercise group, n = 27) in 28 women and 28 men aged 65 to 78 years. DHEA alone for 6 months did not significantly increase strength or thigh muscle volume. However, DHEA treatment potentiated the effect of 4 months of weightlifting training on muscle strength and on thigh muscle volume, measured by magnetic resonance imaging. In another study in 31 postmenopausal women, DHEA, 50 mg/d, did not demonstrate additive exercise-related effects on body composition, physical performance, or cardiometabolic risk when administered in

Table 1
DHEA and anabolic effects in elderly people

Authors (Year)	Study Design, Intervention	Subjects, Age Range in y	IGF-I	Muscle Strength	Body Composition	Bone Effects
Weiss[50] (2009)	Randomized placebo-controlled trial in first year, open-label study in second year DHEA, 50 mg	58 f, 55 m 65–75	Increase in serum IGF-I	NA	NA	No change in men, increase in spine BMD
von Mühlen et al[49] (2008)	Randomized, placebo-controlled trial; 12 mo DHEA, 50 mg	115 f, 110 m 55–85	Increase in serum IGF-I only in women	NA	No significant change	BMD increase at lumbar spine only in women
Nair et al[53] (2006)	Randomized double-blind placebo-controlled; 24 mo DHEA, 50 mg po, vs placebo	57 f, 60 m 62–75	NA	No significant change	No significant change	Increase in BMD of ultradistal radius in women, in femoral neck in men
Jankowski et al[45] (2006)	Randomized, double-blinded, controlled trial 12 mo DHEA, 50 mg, vs placebo	70 f, 70 m 60–88	Increase in serum IGF-I	NA	No significant change	Increase in hip BMD in both sexes; in women additionally increase in lumbar spine BMD
Baulieu et al[52] (2000); Percheron et al[57] (2003) (DHEAge study)	Double-blind placebo-controlled; 12 months DHEA, 50 mg po, vs placebo	140 f, 140 m 60–79	No significant change	No change of handgrip or knee muscle strength after 12 mo	No change in muscle or fat cross-sectional area at thigh, no effect on muscular morphologic features	Slight increase in BMD in women, no effect in men

Study	Design/Dose	Subjects				
Kahn et al[30] (2002)	Placebo-controlled, double-blind study; 6 mo DHEA, 90 mg po	43 m 56–80	NA	NA	NA	No significant change in bone turnover parameters in men
Villareal et al[54] (2000)	Open-label, not randomized, no placebo control; 6 mo DHEA, 50 mg po	20 f, 16 m 64–82	Increase in serum IGF-I	NA	Fat mass decreased and fat-free mass increased	BMD of the total body and lumbar spine increased
Flynn et al[22] (1999)	Randomized double-blind, crossover; 9 mo DHEA, 100 mg po	39 m 60–84	NA	NA	No significant change	NA
Morales et al[46] (1998)	Double-blind placebo-controlled, crossover; 6 mo DHEA, 100 mg po	10 f, 9 m 50–65	Increase in serum IGF-I	Knee muscle strength and lumbar back strength increased in men	Fat body mass decreased in men; increase in total body mass in women	NA
Casson et al[44] (1998)	Randomized, placebo-controlled, double-blind trial; 6 mo DHEA, 25 mg	13 f Postmenopausal women	Increase in serum IGF-I	NA	No significant change	No significant change
Labrie et al[32] (1997)	12 months 10% DHEA cream	14 f 60–70	NA	NA	NA	Increase in hip BMD
Diamond et al[56] (1996)	Placebo-controlled, crossover; 12 mo DHEA, 2–5 g/d percutaneous (cream)	15 f 60–70	No significant change	NA	Increase of muscular area, decrease of subcutaneous fat area	NA

Abbreviations: f, female; m, male; NA, not available.

combination with endurance and resistance exercise training, whereas exercising per se significantly increased insulin sensitivity and improved body composition.[59] However, study duration was only 12 weeks.

The DHEAge study included the so far largest group of subjects and addressed the value of reestablishing DHEA levels to levels of young adults in 240 men and women aged 60 to 79 years.[52,57] In women older than 70 years, gains in BMD were detected and libido was increased but no significant changes were observed in men. No influence on well-being or cognition could be demonstrated after 12 months of DHEA treatment.

In the so far longest term randomized, placebo-controlled, double-blind trial, Nair and colleagues[53] investigated the effect of DHEA and testosterone on quality of life, body composition, physical performance, or metabolism in elderly subjects. They found no significant effects of DHEA in these healthy elderly individuals with low baseline DHEA levels. Also, low doses of testosterone led to only a slight increase in fat-free mass and BMD at the femoral neck. No effect of DHEA on quality of life was observed.

A possible explanation for the mild or missing effects of DHEA might be a participation bias due to the preferential recruitment of healthy volunteers. Thus, it is unclear if subjects with further complaints might benefit more from DHEA administration.

DHEA USE IN SPORTS

As DHEA can be converted into the potent endogenous anabolic androgenic steroids testosterone and dihydrotestosterone, it is included in the list of prohibited substances and methods by the World Anti-Doping Agency (WADA) (The 2009 Prohibited List International Standard, 01.01.2009). This inclusion of DHEA has had already major implications. Tyler Hamilton, Olympic gold medalist and professional bicycle racer, recently announced his retirement after testing positive for DHEA. However, there is very limited information on the use of DHEA and other anabolic prohormones in sports. Reeder and colleagues[60] surveyed 475 high school students and reported that 4% of this population of athletes and nonathletes used anabolic precursors within the past year. In addition, the National Collegiate Athletic Association (NCAA) reported in 2001 that 5.3% of their athletes admitted the use of DHEA or androstenedione in the past year.[61] These numbers suggest that a significant percentage of young athletes use prohormones, including DHEA, as ergogenic drugs. However, the true significance of DHEA use in sports remains to be elucidated. According to the WADA rules (WADA technical document—TD2004EAAS), urine samples containing DHEA concentrations greater than 100 ng/mL shall be submitted to isotope ratio mass spectrometry (IRMS) analysis. Recently, Mareck and colleagues[62] reported on the detection of DHEA misuse by means of gas chromatography-combustion-isotope ratio mass spectrometry. In 2006, 11.012 doping control urine samples were analyzed, and 0.9% of these samples yielded concentrations of DHEA greater than 100 ng/mL. However, 99% of the IRMS results did not indicate an administration of exogenous prohormones or testosterone. An IRMS analytical finding was documented in only 1 sample. Again in 2007, 6622 doping control urine samples were analyzed using a DHEA metabolite, which was described as a useful gas chromatography-mass spectrometry marker for screening for DHEA abuse. DHEA concentrations greater than 100 ng/mL were found in 6 urine samples, none of them showing positive IRMS findings.

These observations suggest that the current threshold values for doping controls might need to be reconsidered and also demonstrate a low prevalence of ergogenic DHEA use among athletes.

Scientific evidence for an ergogenic efficacy of DHEA remains virtually nonexistent. Initially, Nestler and colleagues[63] reported a decreased level of body fat in young men aged 20 to 25 years after supplementation with an industrial DHEA dose (1600 mg/d) for 28 days. Although fat mass decreased, overall body mass remained constant, and the investigators concluded that DHEA had led to an increased lean body mass. However, neither muscle performance nor strength was measured. Another study[64] using the same high dose for 4 weeks in healthy males failed to show any change in lean body mass or protein synthesis. Therefore, even these extraordinarily high doses seemed to have no relevant effect on indices of lean body mass, at least in the short term.

Similarly, experienced male weightlifters who received DHEA (100 mg/d) showed no differences in the gains in strength or lean mass.[65] No differences occurred in the gains in strength or lean mass in young, novice weightlifters after injection of DHEA, 150 mg/d, or placebo.[66]

Thus, at least in healthy men and male athletes, it remains to be shown that DHEA possesses ergogenic potential. In fact, based on the above-mentioned conversion of DHEA in males, it is unlikely that even long-term administration of doses up to 100 mg/d have the potential to generate significant anabolic activity in the presence of a background of high endogenous testosterone concentrations. However, comparable studies in female athletes are missing and are more likely to demonstrate an ergogenic potential of DHEA because, unlike in men, DHEA is able to greatly increase circulating testosterone in healthy women in a dose-dependent fashion.[67]

SUMMARY

Multiple studies have convincingly and consistently shown that DHEA is a prohormone that, after exogenous administration, can be converted into potent sex steroids, such as testosterone and estradiol. Accordingly, the WADA has included DHEA in the list of prohibited substances, and first cases of DHEA doping have been reported. However, an ergogenic potential of DHEA has not yet convincingly been demonstrated and remains largely a myth. This is particularly true for male athletes, as extraordinarily high amounts of DHEA are required to demonstrate an increase in circulating testosterone levels against the physiologic background concentration. Whether the pronounced increases in the levels of circulating androgens after ingestion of DHEA may lead to ergogenic activity remains largely unexplored.

The situation might be entirely different in women. Exogenous DHEA administration has been shown to induce an increase in circulating testosterone concentrations in a dose-dependant manner. Thus, very high DHEA doses (eg, 1600 mg/d) have the potential to generate significant anabolic activity. However, no long-term studies in young women or in female athletes have been reported. Concerning the effect of DHEA in women, only the results of studies in women with AI or elderly women are available. As outlined earlier, the published data on the effects of DHEA on muscle mass and strength here are conflicting with most studies that show little or no effect on body composition, muscle mass, or muscle strength. However, in general, replacement doses (eg, 50 mg/d orally) were used in these studies, precluding clear conclusions regarding higher doses of DHEA for longer periods of time in women.

REFERENCES

1. Orentreich N, Brind JL, Rizer RL, et al. Age changes and sex differences in serum dehydroepiandrosterone sulfate concentrations throughout adulthood. J Clin Endocrinol Metab 1984;59:551.

2. Reiter EO, Fuldauer VG, Root AW. Secretion of the adrenal androgen, dehydroepiandrosterone sulfate, during normal infancy, childhood, and adolescence, in sick infants, and in children with endocrinologic abnormalities. J Pediatr 1977; 90:766.
3. Orentreich N, Brind JL, Vogelman JH, et al. Long-term longitudinal measurements of plasma dehydroepiandrosterone sulfate in normal men. J Clin Endocrinol Metab 1992;75:1002.
4. Parker CR Jr, Mixon RL, Brissie RM, et al. Aging alters zonation in the adrenal cortex of men. J Clin Endocrinol Metab 1997;82:3898.
5. Bird CE, Masters V, Clark AF. Dehydroepiandrosterone sulfate: kinetics of metabolism in normal young men and women. Clin Invest Med 1984;7:119.
6. Hammer F, Subtil S, Lux P, et al. No evidence for hepatic conversion of dehydroepiandrosterone (DHEA) sulfate to DHEA: in vivo and in vitro studies. J Clin Endocrinol Metab 2005;90:3600.
7. Martel C, Melner MH, Gagne D, et al. Widespread tissue distribution of steroid sulfatase, 3 beta-hydroxysteroid dehydrogenase/delta 5-delta 4 isomerase (3 beta-HSD), 17 beta-HSD 5 alpha-reductase and aromatase activities in the rhesus monkey. Mol Cell Endocrinol 1994;104:103.
8. Labrie F. Intracrinology. Mol Cell Endocrinol 1991;78:C113.
9. Arlt W, Callies F, van Vlijmen JC, et al. Dehydroepiandrosterone replacement in women with adrenal insufficiency. N Engl J Med 1999;341:1013.
10. Arlt W, Justl HG, Callies F, et al. Oral dehydroepiandrosterone for adrenal androgen replacement: pharmacokinetics and peripheral conversion to androgens and estrogens in young healthy females after dexamethasone suppression. J Clin Endocrinol Metab 1928;83:1998.
11. Compagnone NA, Bulfone A, Rubenstein JL, et al. Steroidogenic enzyme P450c17 is expressed in the embryonic central nervous system. Endocrinology 1995;136:5212.
12. Corpechot C, Robel P, Axelson M, et al. Characterization and measurement of dehydroepiandrosterone sulfate in rat brain. Proc Natl Acad Sci U S A 1981;78: 4704.
13. Bergeron R, de Montigny C, Debonnel G. Potentiation of neuronal NMDA response induced by dehydroepiandrosterone and its suppression by progesterone: effects mediated via sigma receptors. J Neurosci 1996;16:1193.
14. Majewska MD, Demirgoren S, Spivak CE, et al. The neurosteroid dehydroepiandrosterone sulfate is an allosteric antagonist of the GABAA receptor. Brain Res 1990;526:143.
15. Steckelbroeck S, Watzka M, Lutjohann D, et al. Characterization of the dehydroepiandrosterone (DHEA) metabolism via oxysterol 7alpha-hydroxylase and 17-ketosteroid reductase activity in the human brain. J Neurochem 2002;83:713.
16. Zwain IH, Yen SS. Neurosteroidogenesis in astrocytes, oligodendrocytes, and neurons of cerebral cortex of rat brain. Endocrinology 1999;140:3843.
17. Liu D, Dillon JS. Dehydroepiandrosterone activates endothelial cell nitric-oxide synthase by a specific plasma membrane receptor coupled to Galpha(i2,3). J Biol Chem 2002;277:21379.
18. Simoncini T, Mannella P, Fornari L, et al. Dehydroepiandrosterone modulates endothelial nitric oxide synthesis via direct genomic and nongenomic mechanisms. Endocrinology 2003;144:3449.
19. Williams MR, Ling S, Dawood T, et al. Dehydroepiandrosterone inhibits human vascular smooth muscle cell proliferation independent of ARs and ERs. J Clin Endocrinol Metab 2002;87:176.

20. Dillon JS. Dehydroepiandrosterone, dehydroepiandrosterone sulfate and related steroids: their role in inflammatory, allergic and immunological disorders. Curr Drug Targets Inflamm Allergy 2005;4:377.
21. Bilger M, Speraw S, LaFranchi SH, et al. Androgen replacement in adolescents and young women with hypopituitarism. J Pediatr Endocrinol Metab 2005;18:355.
22. Flynn MA, Weaver-Osterholtz D, Sharpe-Timms KL, et al. Dehydroepiandrosterone replacement in aging humans. J Clin Endocrinol Metab 1999;84:1527.
23. Gurnell EM, Hunt PJ, Curran SE, et al. Long-term DHEA replacement in primary adrenal insufficiency: a randomized, controlled trial. J Clin Endocrinol Metab 2008;93:400.
24. Hunt PJ, Gurnell EM, Huppert FA, et al. Improvement in mood and fatigue after dehydroepiandrosterone replacement in Addison's disease in a randomized, double blind trial. J Clin Endocrinol Metab 2000;85:4650.
25. Johannsson G, Burman P, Wiren L, et al. Low dose dehydroepiandrosterone affects behavior in hypopituitary androgen-deficient women: a placebo-controlled trial. J Clin Endocrinol Metab 2002;87:2046.
26. Brooke AM, Kalingag LA, Miraki-Moud F, et al. Dehydroepiandrosterone improves psychological well-being in male and female hypopituitary patients on maintenance growth hormone replacement. J Clin Endocrinol Metab 2006;91:3773.
27. van Thiel SW, Romijn JA, Pereira AM, et al. Effects of dehydroepiandrostenedione, superimposed on growth hormone substitution, on quality of life and insulin-like growth factor I in patients with secondary adrenal insufficiency: a randomized, placebo-controlled, cross-over trial. J Clin Endocrinol Metab 2005;90:3295.
28. Lovas K, Gebre-Medhin G, Trovik TS, et al. Replacement of dehydroepiandrosterone in adrenal failure: no benefit for subjective health status and sexuality in a 9-month, randomized, parallel group clinical trial. J Clin Endocrinol Metab 2003;88:1112.
29. Dhatariya K, Bigelow ML, Nair KS. Effect of dehydroepiandrosterone replacement on insulin sensitivity and lipids in hypoadrenal women. Diabetes 2005;54:765.
30. Kahn AJ, Halloran B, Wolkowitz O, et al. Dehydroepiandrosterone supplementation and bone turnover in middle-aged to elderly men. J Clin Endocrinol Metab 2002;87:1544.
31. Callies F, Fassnacht M, van Vlijmen JC, et al. Dehydroepiandrosterone replacement in women with adrenal insufficiency: effects on body composition, serum leptin, bone turnover, and exercise capacity. J Clin Endocrinol Metab 1968;86:2001.
32. Labrie F, Diamond P, Cusan L, et al. Effect of 12-month dehydroepiandrosterone replacement therapy on bone, vagina, and endometrium in postmenopausal women. J Clin Endocrinol Metab 1997;82:3498.
33. Christiansen JJ, Gravholt CH, Fisker S, et al. Very short term dehydroepiandrosterone treatment in female adrenal failure: impact on carbohydrate, lipid and protein metabolism. Eur J Endocrinol 2005;152:77.
34. Libe R, Barbetta L, Dall'Asta C, et al. Effects of dehydroepiandrosterone (DHEA) supplementation on hormonal, metabolic and behavioral status in patients with hypoadrenalism. J Endocrinol Invest 2004;27:736.
35. Srinivasan M, Irving BA, Dhatariya K, et al. Effect of dehydroepiandrosterone replacement on lipoprotein profile in hypoadrenal women. J Clin Endocrinol Metab 2009;94:761.
36. Tan KC, Shiu SW, Pang RW, et al. Effects of testosterone replacement on HDL subfractions and apolipoprotein A-I containing lipoproteins. Clin Endocrinol (Oxf) 1998;48:187.

37. Dhatariya KK, Greenlund LJ, Bigelow ML, et al. Dehydroepiandrosterone replacement therapy in hypoadrenal women: protein anabolism and skeletal muscle function. Mayo Clin Proc 2008;83:1218.

38. Christiansen JJ, Andersen NH, Sorensen KE, et al. Dehydroepiandrosterone substitution in female adrenal failure: no impact on endothelial function and cardiovascular parameters despite normalization of androgen status. Clin Endocrinol (Oxf) 2007;66:426.

39. Rice SP, Agarwal N, Bolusani H, et al. Effects of dehydroepiandrosterone replacement on vascular function in primary and secondary adrenal insufficiency: a randomized crossover trial. J Clin Endocrinol Metab 1966;94:2009.

40. Mease PJ, Ginzler EM, Gluck OS, et al. Effects of prasterone on bone mineral density in women with systemic lupus erythematosus receiving chronic glucocorticoid therapy. J Rheumatol 2005;32:616.

41. Sanchez-Guerrero J, Fragoso-Loyo HE, Neuwelt CM, et al. Effects of prasterone on bone mineral density in women with active systemic lupus erythematosus receiving chronic glucocorticoid therapy. J Rheumatol 2008;35:1567.

42. Abbasi A, Duthie EH Jr, Sheldahl L, et al. Association of dehydroepiandrosterone sulfate, body composition, and physical fitness in independent community-dwelling older men and women. J Am Geriatr Soc 1998;46:263.

43. Ravaglia G, Forti P, Maioli F, et al. The relationship of dehydroepiandrosterone sulfate (DHEAS) to endocrine-metabolic parameters and functional status in the oldest-old. Results from an Italian study on healthy free-living over-ninety-year-olds. J Clin Endocrinol Metab 1996;81:1173.

44. Casson PR, Santoro N, Elkind-Hirsch K, et al. Postmenopausal dehydroepiandrosterone administration increases free insulin-like growth factor-I and decreases high-density lipoprotein: a six-month trial. Fertil Steril 1998;70:107.

45. Jankowski CM, Gozansky WS, Schwartz RS, et al. Effects of dehydroepiandrosterone replacement therapy on bone mineral density in older adults: a randomized, controlled trial. J Clin Endocrinol Metab 2006;91:2986.

46. Morales AJ, Haubrich RH, Hwang JY, et al. The effect of six months treatment with a 100 mg daily dose of dehydroepiandrosterone (DHEA) on circulating sex steroids, body composition and muscle strength in age-advanced men and women. Clin Endocrinol (Oxf) 1998;49:421.

47. Morales AJ, Nolan JJ, Nelson JC, et al. Effects of replacement dose of dehydroepiandrosterone in men and women of advancing age. J Clin Endocrinol Metab 1994;78:1360.

48. Villareal DT, Holloszy JO. Effect of DHEA on abdominal fat and insulin action in elderly women and men: a randomized controlled trial. JAMA 2004;292:2243.

49. von Muhlen D, Laughlin GA, Kritz-Silverstein D, et al. Effect of dehydroepiandrosterone supplementation on bone mineral density, bone markers, and body composition in older adults: the DAWN trial. Osteoporos Int 2008;19:699.

50. Weiss EP, Shah K, Fontana L, et al. Dehydroepiandrosterone replacement therapy in older adults: 1- and 2-y effects on bone. Am J Clin Nutr 2009;89:1459.

51. Baulieu EE. Dehydroepiandrosterone (DHEA): a fountain of youth? J Clin Endocrinol Metab 1996;81:3147.

52. Baulieu EE, Thomas G, Legrain S, et al. Dehydroepiandrosterone (DHEA), DHEA sulfate, and aging: contribution of the DHEAge Study to a sociobiomedical issue. Proc Natl Acad Sci U S A 2000;97:4279.

53. Nair KS, Rizza RA, O'Brien P, et al. DHEA in elderly women and DHEA or testosterone in elderly men. N Engl J Med 2006;355:1647.

54. Villareal DT, Holloszy JO, Kohrt WM. Effects of DHEA replacement on bone mineral density and body composition in elderly women and men. Clin Endocrinol (Oxf) 2000;53:561.
55. Jankowski CM, Gozansky WS, Kittelson JM, et al. Increases in bone mineral density in response to oral dehydroepiandrosterone replacement in older adults appear to be mediated by serum estrogens. J Clin Endocrinol Metab 2008;93: 4767.
56. Diamond P, Cusan L, Gomez JL, et al. Metabolic effects of 12-month percutaneous dehydroepiandrosterone replacement therapy in postmenopausal women. J Endocrinol 1996;150(Suppl):S43.
57. Percheron G, Hogrel JY, Denot-Ledunois S, et al. Effect of 1-year oral administration of dehydroepiandrosterone to 60- to 80-year-old individuals on muscle function and cross-sectional area: a double-blind placebo-controlled trial. Arch Intern Med 2003;163:720.
58. Villareal DT, Holloszy JO. DHEA enhances effects of weight training on muscle mass and strength in elderly women and men. Am J Physiol Endocrinol Metab 2006;291:E1003.
59. Igwebuike A, Irving BA, Bigelow ML, et al. Lack of dehydroepiandrosterone effect on a combined endurance and resistance exercise program in postmenopausal women. J Clin Endocrinol Metab 2008;93:534.
60. Reeder BM, Rai A, Patel DR, et al. The prevalence of nutritional supplement use among high school students: a pilot study. Med Sci Sports Exerc 2002;34:193.
61. Calfee R, Fadale P. Popular ergogenic drugs and supplements in young athletes. Pediatrics 2006;117:e577.
62. Mareck U, Geyer H, Flenker U, et al. Detection of dehydroepiandrosterone misuse by means of gas chromatography-combustion-isotope ratio mass spectrometry. Eur J Mass Spectrom (Chichester, Eng) 2007;13:419.
63. Nestler JE, Barlascini CO, Clore JN, et al. Dehydroepiandrosterone reduces serum low density lipoprotein levels and body fat but does not alter insulin sensitivity in normal men. J Clin Endocrinol Metab 1988;66:57.
64. Welle S, Jozefowicz R, Statt M. Failure of dehydroepiandrosterone to influence energy and protein metabolism in humans. J Clin Endocrinol Metab 1990;71: 1259.
65. Wallace MB, Lim A, Cutler A, et al. Effects of dehydroepiandrosterone vs androstenedione supplementation in men. Med Sci Sports Exerc 1999;31:1788.
66. Brown GA, Vukovich MD, Sharp RL, et al. Effect of oral DHEA on serum testosterone and adaptations to resistance training in young men. J Appl Phys 1999; 87:2274.
67. Stanczyk FZ, Slater CC, Ramos DE, et al. Pharmacokinetics of dehydroepiandrosterone and its metabolites after long-term oral dehydroepiandrosterone treatment in postmenopausal women. Menopause 2009;16:272.

Procedures for Monitoring Recombinant Erythropoietin and Analogs in Doping

Séverine Lamon, MSc, Neil Robinson, PhD,
Martial Saugy, PhD, PD*

KEYWORDS

- Recombinant erythropoietin • Human EPO • Anti-doping
- Athletic performance

RECOMBINANT ERYTHROPOIETIN

Human erythropoietin (hEPO) was isolated for the first time from a large quantity of urine in 1977,[1] and this was followed by the successful isolation and cloning of the hEPO gene in 1983.[2] Recombinant hEPO (rEPO) became available in the late 1980s as a treatment for acute anemia mainly associated with chronic kidney disease but also with cancer, AIDS, hepatitis C infection, bone marrow transplantation, autoimmune diseases, heart failure, or other chronic infections. The factors causing this so-called anemia of chronic disorders are principally reduced iron availability in the bone marrow, increased hemolysis, and bleeding. rEPO can substitute for endogenous EPO by binding to the EPO receptor and triggering intracellular signaling in a manner identical to that of the native hormone. It raises hemoglobin concentration in a dose-dependant and predictable way. Hemoglobin concentration is one of the principal factors of aerobic power and, consequently, of performance in many types of physical activities. The use of rEPO is, therefore, particularly powerful for improving the physical performances of patients, reducing exertional dyspnea, and, more generally, improving their quality of life. Additionally, it avoids the need for red cells transfusions and abolishes, therefore, the risks of incompatibility reactions, viral infections, and iron overload. rEPO may also slow down the progression of chronic kidney disease. Therapies with rEPO are widely used—this drug is one of the top-selling

Swiss Laboratory for Doping Analyses, University Center of Legal Medicine, West Switzerland, Chemin des Croisettes 22, 1066 Epalinges, Switzerland
* Corresponding author.
E-mail address: martial.saugy@chuv.ch (M. Saugy).

Endocrinol Metab Clin N Am 39 (2010) 141–154
doi:10.1016/j.ecl.2009.10.004
0889-8529/10/$ – see front matter © 2010 Elsevier Inc. All rights reserved.

pharmaceutical products worldwide—and generally well tolerated.[3] Rarely, however, pure red-cell aplasia due to the appearance of neutralizing auto–anti-EPO antibodies is observed after EPO administration.[4] A few articles also report the specific presence of antibodies against rEPO.[5]

The original forms of rEPO, epoetin-α (Eprex) and epoetin-β (Recormon), are engineered in Chinese hamster ovary (CHO) cells transfected with the hEPO gene.[6] Endogenous EPO and rEPO have identical primary and secondary structures, with respect to the peptide backbone of 165 amino acids, the disulfide bonds, and the four glycosylation sites. The molecular composition of the N-linked oligosaccharide side chains of both EPO types presents specific differences, however. The terminal monosaccharide of N-linked side chains is usually a sialic acid residue linked to a galactose residue. The recombinant molecules contain no new structural elements; however, they lack one of the two types of sialic acid–galactose linkage (specifically, the sialic acid 2α→6 galactose linkage) present in the native hormone. It is established that EPO isoforms containing fewer sialic acid residues present a greater affinity for the EPO receptor but a shorter survival in circulation.[7] In addition to endogenous circulating EPO, rEPO has several glycosylation isoforms.

Clinical trials involving a more recent rEPO product, epoetin-ω, were performed in several countries. This rEPO form was produced in baby hamster kidney (BHK) cells and seemed effective for treating anemia. As CHO and BHK cells possess different glycosyltransferase and glycosidase equipments, the glycosylation pattern of rEPO produced in CHO and BHK cells differs slightly. The N-chains of rEPO produced in BHK cells are sulfated to a higher degree. Consequently, their pharmacokinetic properties also differ slightly.[7]

Currently, many forms of other rEPOs are available on the market. Darbepoetin-α, or novel erythropoiesis stimulating protein (NESP), (Aranesp [Amgen AG, Zug, Switzerland]) is a glycoprotein hormone that differs from native hEPO by five amino acids, allowing the attachment of additional oligosaccharide chains. NESP was defined as second-generation EPO. Epoetin-δ (Dynepo [Shire Pharmaceuticals, Basingstoke, UK]) is a more recently engineered rEPO that is produced by gene activation in human fibrosarcoma cells into which a DNA fragment, which activates the EPO promoter, was transfected.[8] Other cell lines were also successfully transfected with the hEPO gene. Pegylated epoetin-β, or continuous erythropoiesis receptor activator (CERA), (Mircera) represents the third generation of erythropoiesis-stimulating agents with respect to the large polyethylene glycol molecule making that CERA has a particularly long half-life compared with other similar drugs.

The patent for epoetin molecules expired in Europe in 2004. From then on, manufacturers have started to bring generic versions of epoetins (so-called biosimilars) to the market.[9] At the time of this writing, two such biosimilar epoetins have been approved by the European Union and others may follow. Many "copy" rEPOs are believed available worldwide, however. Copy EPOs are probably synthesized using similar techniques to the original products, even if their production process is usually not stringent enough to be approved by drug regulatory authorities, such as the Food and Drug Administration in the United States and the European Medicines Agency in Europe. Recently, Macdougall and Ashenden[10] estimated that up to 80 such products may be sold in emergent countries. This fact will strongly influence the future of the fight against rEPO abuse in sport.

ERYTHROPOIETIN ABUSE IN SPORT

rEPO became available in 1990 in Europe, as Eprex (epoetin-α), the first rEPO product, was commercialized. It seemed that this hormone rapidly would be used illicitly in endurance sports. In 1991, Adamson and Vapnek[11] suggested that fact in a correspondence published by the *New England Journal of Medicine* and underlined the potential danger or rEPO abuse for the life and the health of athletes. They also discussed existing speculations that rEPO may have been involved in the deaths of professional cyclists from the Netherlands.

EFFECTS OF RECOMBINANT HUMAN ERYTHROPOIETIN TREATMENT ON PERFORMANCE

It is easily explainable that rEPO has been rapidly abused by athletes looking for an artificial performance enhancer. In humans, maximal aerobic power (Vo_{2max}) is one of the key predictors of race performance in endurance sports.[12,13] In the case of elite athletes, it has been shown that Vo_{2max} is limited more by oxygen delivery than by metabolic capacity.[14] Consequently, as blood O_2 availability increases, Vo_{2max} also increases. At sea level, blood O_2 availability is mainly determined by the hemoglobin concentration. It is well established that hemoglobin concentration, and hematocrit increase significantly after rEPO treatment. For instance, three subcutaneous injections of 20 to 40 IU/kg body mass rEPO per week were shown to induce a haemoglobin concentration increase of more than 15 g/L and a hematocrit increase of more than 5%.[15] Moreover, several studies demonstrated clearly that rEPO administration induced an increase in haemoglobin concentration that was also concomitant in Vo_{2max}.[15–17]

HISTORY OF THE FIGHT AGAINST ERYTHROPOIETIN ABUSE IN SPORT

In 1993, Casoni and colleagues[18] examined 240 elite athletes and a control group that received EPO injections, with the purpose of identifying possible differences in hematologic markers between both groups that would have been useful in identifying EPO use. They proposed a model based on the quantification of a specific red blood cells population, called macrocytic hypochromatic erythrocytes (MacroHypo). These erythrocytes were defined as having a volume above 120 fL and a hemoglobin content below 28 pg. It was observed that all subjects having a MacroHypo level above 0.6% were subjects that had received rEPO. Therefore, this percentage was proposed as a cutoff limit and an athlete presenting a MacroHypo value higher than the limit would have been suspected of EPO misuse. The test was poorly sensitive, however, and 50% of the rEPO containing samples were not detected.

In 1996, Gareau and colleagues[19] suggested, in a correspondence published in *Nature*, that it was possible to diagnose erythropoiesis manipulation by rEPO using erythropoiesis blood parameters, such as soluble transferrin receptor (sTFR) and ferritin. At the same time, many rumors concerning the abuse of rEPO among elite cyclists were circulating. From then on, the Laboratoire suisse d'Analyse du Dopage (LAD), at that time named Unité d'Analyse du Dopage, and the Union Cycliste Internationale decided to perform a study involving blood collection coupled with haematologic and biochemical measurements of athletes taking part in the Tour de Suisse 1996. This project was also aimed at determining if the organization of blood collections during major cycling competitions was applicable in the field.[20]

The samples were collected at the end of a stage of the Tour de Suisse and were immediately analyzed in Lausanne. The obtained results were then compared with blood samples collected from sport students who had performed a controlled endurance effort. Surprisingly, the differences observed between both populations mainly concerned plasma EPO and sTFR concentrations—values were slightly higher in cyclist population than in student population. Both parameters were not significant to demonstrate a general abuse of rEPO by cyclists. It was also observed that the majority of the cyclists had extremely high ferritin concentrations (up to five times the normal expected concentration). At that point, the trend among athletes was to take high quantities of iron (intravenously, preferably), in order (1) to avoid anemia and (2) probably to fulfill the acute iron request linked to EPO stimulation. This observation questioned Gareau's hypothesis, which suggested using the ratio, sTFR/ferritin, as a marker of rEPO intake.[19] These results could reflect two things: that the abuse of rEPO was not generalized in cycling or that the measured secondary parameters were not efficient or selective enough to identify cheating athletes. It was nevertheless established that blood collections "in competition" were realistically feasible.

After this pilot study, the so-called hematocrit program was launched in 1997 by the Union Cycliste Internationale, in collaboration with the LAD. As blood secondary parameters seemed to be not relevant enough to indicate an erythropoiesis manipulation, and as a real antidoping test did not exist at that time, it was decided to establish an empiric hematocrit level that, in case of an athlete, would exceed it and lead to forcing him or her to stop racing for a minimum period of 2 weeks; this suspension is the so-called no-start or competition rule. The establishment of such a cutoff limit aimed at avoiding the expansion of the phenomenon of rEPO abuse to the detriment of equity and health in sport. The chosen hematocrit cutoff was 50%, a value corresponding approximately, in a normal male population, to the mean value plus two SDs. Athletes having a physiologic hematocrit level above this cutoff limit had, on the basis of a regular follow-up of hematologic data, the possibility of obtaining a hematocrit certificate that would specify their individual cutoff limit. Although widely criticized at that time, this limit finally corresponded to the best compromise existing between efficient preventive effect and coherent scientific explanation. At the same time, the International Ski Federation led a similar hemoglobin program that used a cutoff limit of 18.5 g/dL, corresponding to a hematocrit level of approximately 54%. A too elevated limit, however, would have allowed athletes to abuse of rEPO until their hematocrit level reached the cutoff. With time, this hemoglobin limit was effectively considered ineffective to fight against rEPO doping. The hematocrit program of 1997 still constitutes the basis of the biologic follow-up now applied.[20]

Finally, in 2000, shortly before the Sydney Olympic Games, Parisotto proposed a new model taking into account five parameters to demonstrate altered erythropoiesis.[21,22] These indirect markers were hematocrit, reticulocyte hematocrit, percent macrocytes, serum EPO, and sTFR. The ON-model combining these parameters allowed identifying EPO abusers during a period of drug administration, whereas the OFF-model was applicable during the washout period. The International Olympic Committee approved the ON model to be used during the Olympic Games. As a direct detection method was published approximately at the same time,[23] the tests were combined and applied together during the Olympic Games. Apparently, this combination was not effective, as no athlete was proved to have abused rEPO during the competition.

DIRECT DETECTION OF RECOMBINANT HUMAN ERYTHROPOIETIN ABUSE

Taking into consideration the outstanding physiologic effects of rEPO and its (apparently) limited secondary effects short term, this drug soon became one of the athletes' most popular doping agent. Since 1984, all forms of blood doping in sport had been officially banned. In 1990, the International Olympic Committee medical commission, which was in charge of the antidoping regulations at that time, added rEPO to the list of prohibited drugs in sports, even if a direct test allowing detection of the molecule would become available after only a decade.

In addition to the indirect approach, scientists were working on the direct detection of rEPO in blood and urine. A direct detection method would have the undeniable advantage of identifying the drug itself (or its metabolites), even if it would probably be unable to detect an EPO intake dating from more than a few days previously.

The most powerful way to discriminate between endogenous EPO and rEPO is probably based on the glycosylation differences existing between both types of molecules. Glycosylation of epoetins-α and -β takes place in CHO cells rather than in human cells.[24] As a result, recombinant molecules exhibit fewer sialic acid residues on their surface. Recombinant molecules are, therefore, less negative than endogenous ones. The consequent differences of charge carried by the different sugar structures allows discriminating between endogenous and exogenous EPO isoforms.[25] In 1995, Wide and colleagues proposed a method able to separate both types of molecules in blood and urine.[26] The median charge of EPO was determined, in blood or in urine concentrates, thanks to an electrophoresis in a 0.10% agarose suspension at pH 8.6. It was then expressed in terms of electrophoretic mobility. This technique was reliable, as it allowed clearly identifying the presence of rEPO in urine and blood. Although the proposed method was powerful as long as the biologic samples were collected within 24 hours after the last rEPO injection, it seemed far less sensitive in samples that were collected later after injection. After 3 days after the last rEPO injection, more than half of the subjects could not be declared positive. Furthermore, all samples did not present any traces of rEPO after 7 days. Nevertheless, this study showed for the first time that administered rEPO could be detected in urine. Compared to the blood parameters philosophy, this method allowed detecting directly the presence of rEPO in biologic fluids. It seemed, however, to be time consuming and expensive. Moreover, this technique could not be reproduced in another laboratory and, therefore, was never applied in an antidoping context. At that time, a detection method based on electrophoresis represented a completely new trend for the antidoping world. The current trend was instead orientated toward complex analytic mass spectrometry tools targeting anabolic steroids and biochemical methods, such as electrophoresis, were not familiar to the antidoping authorities.

THE ISOELECTRIC FOCUSING TEST

In June 2000, a few weeks before the Sydney Olympic games, Lasne and de Ceaurriz[23] proposed, in *Nature*, an innovative test based on the isoelectric separation of the urinary EPO isoforms on a polyacrylamide gel followed by a double-blotting process.[27,28] The principle of this method was again based on the charge differences existing between the endogenous and the recombinant hormone. The isoelectric focusing allows the separation of proteins regarding their individual isoelectric points. The isoforms of epoetins-α and -β were demonstrated as less acidic than the endogenous isoforms of hEPO.[29] Therefore, a particular isoelectric pattern could be defined for each EPO form.[30]

In spite of the fact that the isoelectric focusing test (IEF) was as expensive and time consuming as the method proposed by Wide, it seemed to be reproducible and reliable and, therefore, worthwhile in the antidoping context. Breidbach and colleagues[31] rapidly assessed the sensitivity of the method. In 2003, they observed that all the subjects who received nine injections of 50 IU/kg epoetin-α were tested positive 3 days after the last EPO injection. Moreover, on the seventh day after the last rEPO dose, approximately half of the subjects were still detectable. In spite of difficult beginnings, due to the unsuccessful campaign led against rEPO doping during the Sydney Olympic games, IEF finally was imposed as the official test recommended by the World Anti-Doping Agency (WADA) for the screening of rEPO abuse in athletes. In 2001, the LAD reported the first positive rEPO doping case, which incriminated the Danish cyclist, Bo Hamburger. This case was brought in front of the court (Court of Arbitration for Sport [CAS], Lausanne). At that time, discrepancies still existed between the laboratories of Lausanne and Paris concerning the criteria that must be fulfilled to declare a case positive. Lausanne requested that 80% of the EPO bands had to be located in the basic area of the gel, whereas Paris set this limit at 85%. This inconsistency resulted in the loss of the case and underlined the fact that positivity criteria had to be harmonized between laboratories. A few years later, Hamburger openly admitted to having abused rEPO.

Initially, the test was designed to separate the classic first-generation EPOs (epoetins-α, -β, and -ω) from endogenous EPO in urine. With time, it has been adapted to other rEPO forms, such as darbepoetin-α (NESP)—the first NESP-positive cases were reported in cross-country skiers[32] (Larissa Lazutina and Johann Muelleg) during the Salt Lake City Olympic Games; epoetin-δ (Dynepo); and, more recently, generic (biosimilar) and copy EPOs. The rapid and incessant evolution of the antidoping problem continually forces the test to develop. Among other actual evolutions, the sample preparation technique, which basically consisted of several concentration and ultrafiltration steps allowing concentrating 20 mL of urine to 20 to 40 μL of an urinary extract called retentate, will undergo significant changes. Improvement of the quality and the purity of EPO extracts and extraction of EPO from the blood matrix constitute the main challenges. Immunoaffinity-based techniques, such as the ones recently proposed by Lasne and colleagues[33] and Lönnberg and colleagues,[34] probably are the most promising tool for reaching these goals (**Fig. 1**). One of the main

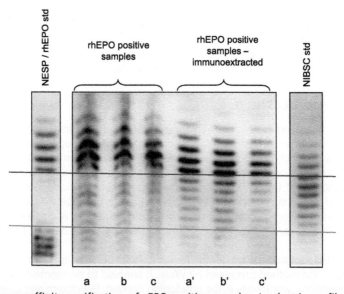

Fig. 1. Immunoaffinity purification of rEPO-positive samples. Isoelectric profiles of three rEPO-positive samples prepared with the classic retentate method (a–c) and with immunoaffinity purification (a'–c'). Immunopurification is an efficient tool to clean up the urine extract and obtain better images. In addition, a potential cross-reactivity of the anti-EPO antibody is excluded. (*From* Reichel C. Identification of zinc alpha-2-glycoprotein binding to clone AE7A5 antihuman EPO antibody by means of nano-HPLC and high-resolution high-mass accuracy ESI-MS/MS. J Mass Spectrom 2008;43(7):916–23; with permission.)

advantages of combining immunoaffinity-based and IEF resides in the use of two distinct anti-EPO antibodies in the same procedure, which is of major importance for excluding all types of cross-reactions with other antigens.

QUESTIONING THE ISOELECTRIC FOCUSING TEST

IEF is currently the only official accredited EPO screening method used on a routine basis in the antidoping laboratories of the world. Since the publication of the test in 2000, however, it has been continuously challenged. During the past 9 years, many articles have been published by different groups, attacking various aspects of the method. This constitutes the background of a continual ideologic war matching the defenders of the IEF method against its detractors. In 2006, Franke and Heid[35] challenged no fewer than six scientific parameters of the method aimed at proving that IEF was not suitable for antidoping purposes. Principally, and like other investigators,[36–38] they questioned the specificity of the anti-EPO antibody—the AE7A5 clone, a monoclonal mouse antibody manufactured by R & D Systems, recommended by the WADA for IEF. Proposing a new 2-D gel-based separation method, Khan and colleagues[38] claimed the existence several urinary proteins cross-reacting with the AE7A5 clone and suggested the return of false-positive results in the past. IEF experts responded by mentioning the poor quality of the presented 2-D gels and the total absence of any bands in the window used for interpretation of the isoelectric profiles in the case of samples devoid of EPO deposited on an IEF gel.[39] Nevertheless, in 2008, Reichel[40] proved the existence of a nonspecifically interacting protein, identified as zinc $\alpha 2$-glycoprotein, using a shotgun proteomics approach, including nano-HPLC peptide separation, and high-resolution, high-mass accuracy, electrospray ionization–tandem mass spectrometry peptide sequencing. This binding occurred, however, outside the used pH range for evaluating EPO profiles.

Another key element frequently subject to controversy concerns the claimed occurrence of false-positive results due to the atypical EPO patterns generated by strenuous efforts (**Fig. 2**).[36] It is true that, in early uses of this method, some false-positive results were reported by antidoping laboratories on the basis of atypical basic profiles, which seemed to illustrate the recently described phenomenon of effort urines.[41] The case involving the athlete Rutger Beke was resolved after the fact in front of a panel of experts.

After the Bernard Lagat incident in 2003, an additional parameter was considered in order to avoid, with the greatest possible degree of certainty, the occurrence of false-positive cases. The A sample (screening and confirmation analyses) of this athlete presented an atypical, extremely basic EPO profile that was suggested as due to a bacterial degradation of the urine. Lagat's B sample (counter-analysis performed in presence of the athlete), however, tested negative. The conservation and transport conditions of the samples were nevertheless questioned. Consequently, an additional assay, called a stability test, was added to the WADA requirements for rEPO screening. The stability test aims at demonstrating that no bacterial activity occurred in the urine. Therefore, rEPO and NESP are added to the sample before one night's incubation at 37°C. The sample is then deposited on a gel and, in the case of the bands position of both EPO forms, is not altered when compared with the corresponding controls; any bacterial activity can be excluded (see **Fig. 2**). Currently, no first-generation EPO-positive result can be returned without performing a stability test.

ESTABLISHMENT OF THE ACTUAL POSITIVITY CRITERIA

Despite the negative image of the test they conveyed, these incidents created a basis for refining the positivity criteria. The percentage of basic bands (the so-called 80%

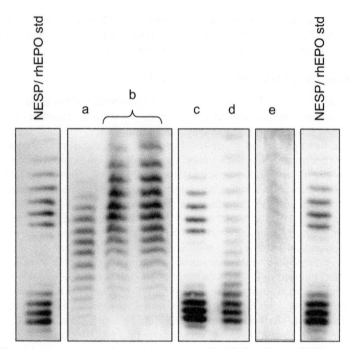

Fig. 2. Effort urine and active urine. (a) EPO isoform distribution of a negative urine sample collected before a strenuous physical effort. (b) EPO isoform distribution of negative urine samples of the same individual collected after a strenuous physical effort. (c) EPO isoform distribution of a negative urine sample spiked with epoetin-β and NESP. (d) EPO isoform distribution of an active urine sample spiked with epoetin-β and NESP. (e) EPO isoform distribution of an active urine sample.

rule) was gradually replaced by new, more discriminating criteria focusing on similarity in terms of band position, distribution, and intensities between the sample and a reference preparation corresponding to rEPO. Currently, these criteria are summarized in a WADA EPO technical document, which is regularly updated.[42] They rely on the definition of a basic area on a gel, going from the cathode edge up to and including band 1 of Biologic Reference Preparation, a 50:50 (weight/weight) blending of two erythropoietin preparations currently available on the European market, namely, epoetin-α and epoetin-β), and of an acidic area, going from the anode edge up to and including band A of Aranesp. By exclusion, an endogenous area is defined between the basic and the acidic area (**Fig. 3**).

The identification criteria define the requisites that the image has to fulfill to consider that an adverse analytic finding corresponding to the presence of rEPO or NESP has occurred. For rEPO, the actual identification criteria are as follows:

1. In the basic area (as defined in **Fig. 4**), there must be at least three acceptable, consecutive bands assigned as 1, 2, and 3 in the corresponding reference preparation.
2. The two most intense bands measured by densitometry in the basic area must be consecutive and must be bands 1, 2, or 3.
3. Each of the two most intense bands in the basic area must be more intense (approximately twice or more) than any band in the endogenous area, as measured by densitometry.

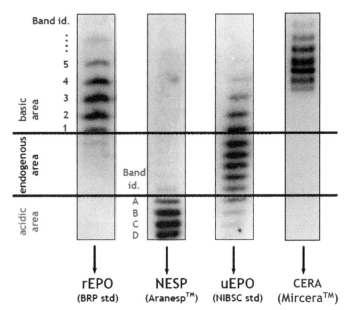

Fig. 3. Image of the identification window of lanes corresponding to the analysis of rEPO, CERA, NESP, and urinary EPO (uEPO). Basic and acidic areas are defined, as described, by the position of the bands corresponding to the rEPO Biologic Reference Preparation (BRP) of the European Pharmacopeias (equimolar mixture of epoetin-α and -β), NESP (Aranesp, Amgen), and, by exclusion, the endogenous area is defined in-between (uEPO). The bands in the basic, endogenous and acidic areas are identified by numbers and letters as shown. CERA shows a different pattern with some bands approximately colocalized with those defined by rEPO and others bisecting rEPO bands (particularly in the region between band 4 and 6). Those bands are intense and specifically identify CERA. (*Adapted from* http://www.wada-ama.org; with permission.)

Similar criteria exist for NESP and CERA. To apply these criteria, the gel must, however, previously fulfill acceptance criteria, ensuring that spots, smears, and areas of excessive background significantly interfering with the application of the identification criteria are not present and that comparison to reference samples allow assignment of band numbers in an athlete's sample. Application of the stability test allowing exclusion of the presence of active urines is the third requirement for the evaluation of an EPO IEF gel. In addition, the technical document mentions that a second opinion is mandatory in case of adverse analytic finding (positive sample).

Laboratories usually report urinary EPO analyses as follows:

- Negative: EPO bands distribution and intensity correspond to those of urinary NIBSC standard.
- Positive: EPO bands distribution and intensity correspond to those of rEPO, NESP, or CERA standards and fulfill the corresponding positivity criteria.
- Undetectable: it has not been possible to detect any traces of EPOs in this sample.
- Atypical: EPO bands distribution and intensity do not correspond to NIBSC standard or to any documented rEPO.

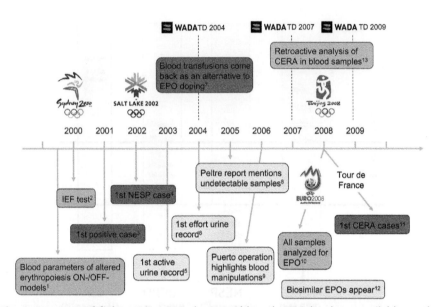

Fig. 4. Ten years of fight against EPO doping. Although rEPO has been available on the market for a decade, a direct detection test (IEF), replacing the secondary parameters models that were used until there, was proposed just before the Sydney Olympic Games. This test allowed finding the first rEPO-positive case in 2001, followed by the first NESP-positive case 1 year later. The subsequent period probably corresponded to the comeback of blood transfusions as an undetectable alternative to EPO doping, a fact supported by the results of the Puerto operation in 2006. Despite the specificity of the new test, the laboratories observed atypical EPO patterns, identified as active urines and effort urines. An official report auditing the IEF test also mentioned the common occurrence of undetectable EPO profiles. During the subsequent years and thanks to blood indicators, the fight against EPO doping was improved, particularly through large campaigns targeting many athletes in a more precise way. From 2007, biosimilar EPOs and CERA have become available and positive cases were immediately reported. The positivity criteria, which were harmonized for the first time in 2004 (WADA technical document [TD] 2004), evolved over the years to improve the sensitivity of the method and to adapt to the new molecules. (*Data from* Refs.[3,8,11,12,15–18,31,36,42–44])

- Suspect: the result for rEPOs is considered as suspect for one of the following reasons: (1) the isoelectric pattern of the sample does not meet all the positivity criteria or (2) all the acceptability criteria of the technique are not entirely fulfilled

Active urines and effort urines are usually reported as negative, as far as supporting evidence allows ensuring their origin (stability test or urinary excretion marker). These comments are usually included in the analytic reports so that the federations have an additional tool for targeting suspect athletes.

ALTERNATIVES TO THE ISOELECTRIC FOCUSING TEST

Since 2000 and the publication of the IEF test, this test has been subject to serious controversies. These incessant challenges are an advantage, however, in that the method has been incessantly questioned and several groups have worked simultaneously at improving its sensitivity and specificity. New EPOs with variable IEF profiles and active urines and effort urines have made additional strategies necessary. Active defenders of IEF recently revealed that the test still allowed athletes using rEPO microdoses to evade doping controls,[43] thus highlighting the necessity to continuously update the method and the corresponding positivity criteria. Alternative methods were also developed. In 2003, it was suggested that epoetin-α and -β and darbepoietin-α could be separated by means of 2-D electrophoresis.[44] The main advantage of 2-D–based methods resides in the separation of the molecules by their isoelectric point and molecular mass. The sensitivity of the proposed technique, however, was too low to consider its application for antidoping purposes. Two years later, Khan and colleagues' group,[38] one of the most virulent IEF detractors, described a more sensitive 2-D gel electrophoresis method and suggested replacing IEF with 2-D. The technique was, however, subject to controversy.[39]

During the past 10 years, the research of an IEF-orthogonal method, which could be used as a screening or a confirmation method, has occupied many scientists in the antidoping field. A few of them developed the idea that hEPO and rEPO molecules have a slightly different apparent molecular mass and proposed a sodium dodecyl sulfate polyacrylamide gel electrophoresis (SDS-PAGE) variant as a complementary method to IEF.[45] Endogenous and exogenous EPOs are discriminated in terms of relative electrophoretic mobility on a denaturant gel, the molecular masses of rEPOs being typically higher than that of hEPO. Although epoetins-α and -β showed subtle differences in electrophoretic mobility when compared with hEPO, this method seemed beneficial in relation to active and effort urines. Moreover, epoetin-δ (Dynepo) presents a characteristic and clearly identifiable pattern, as do darbepoietin-α (NESP) and other heavy pegylated EPOs, such as CERA. This may not be the case for some biosimilar EPOs, however, that could not be differentiated from hEPO using this method.

One of the most promising approaches for rEPO screening in urine is the membrane-assisted isoform immunoassay (MAIIA).[46] This new technology, recently developed by a Swedish group, is able to distinguish minor differences in protein carbohydrate structure, requiring a small amount of each isoform. MAIIA chips are microimmunoaffinity columns composed of a separation zone, containing anion exchange groups or ligands, such as lectins, and a capturing zone with immobilized specific antibodies. In the case of EPO isoforms detection, the separation zone contains wheat germ agglutinin groups, where isoforms interacting with the ligands are retarded. After having passed the separation zone, the weak binding isoforms are captured and detected in the antibody zone. This completely innovative technology is still being developed. Nevertheless, it may represent a powerful alternative to IEF in a few years.

Currently, complex analytic approaches based on mass spectrometry tools are the technique of choice for the screening many abused molecules in urine. Although mass spectrometry has demonstrated its utility for peptide and proteins on various occasions in the past, no conclusive approach has been established for EPO. In 2005, epoetin-α and -β and NESP could be differentiated by matrix-assisted laser desorption/ionization mass spectrometry applying a high-resolution time of flight. The discrimination of the three molecules was based on the identification of distinct molecular substructures at the protein level triggered by specific enzymatic reactions.[47] In 2008, a method allowing the differentiation and identification of rEPO and NESP in equine plasma by liquid chromatography coupled to tandem mass spectrometry was published by Guan and colleagues.[48] Recently, the same group proposed an extension of the proposed method in human plasma.[49] Although this method is powerful for the identification of NESP in human plasma, it is not applicable to rEPO because it cannot differentiate the recombinant from the endogenous molecule. In summary, the main obstacles encountered seem to be the low amounts of EPO available in urine specimens and the heterogeneity of endogenously produced EPO and rEPO molecules. In addition, the extensive characterization that was achieved for rEPO was never performed on human endogenous EPO because its standard is not available in sufficient quantity.[50]

REFERENCES

1. Miyake T, Kung CK, Goldwasser E. Purification of human erythropoietin. J Biol Chem 1977;252(15):5558–64.
2. Lin FK, Suggs S, Lin CH, et al. Cloning and expression of the human erythropoietin gene. Proc Natl Acad Sci U S A 1985;82(22):7580–4.
3. Cea Bauer. Erythropoietin: molecular physiology and clinical application. New York: M. Dekker; 1993.
4. Schonholzer C, Keusch G, Nigg L, et al. High prevalence in Switzerland of pure red-cell aplasia due to anti-erythropoietin antibodies in chronic dialysis patients: report of five cases. Nephrol Dial Transplant 2004;19(8):2121–5.
5. Peces R, de la Torre M, Alcazar R, et al. Antibodies against recombinant human erythropoietin in a patient with erythropoietin-resistant anemia. N Engl J Med 1996;335(7):523–4.
6. Davis JM, Arakawa T, Strickland TW, et al. Characterization of recombinant human erythropoietin produced in Chinese hamster ovary cells. Biochemistry 1987;26(9):2633–8.
7. Jelkmann W. The enigma of the metabolic fate of circulating erythropoietin (Epo) in view of the pharmacokinetics of the recombinant drugs rhEpo and NESP. Eur J Haematol 2002;69(5–6):265–74.
8. Barbone FP, Johnson DL, Farrell FX, et al. New epoetin molecules and novel therapeutic approaches. Nephrol Dial Transplant 1999;14(Suppl 2):80–4.
9. Schellekens H. The first biosimilar epoetin: but how similar is it? Clin J Am Soc Nephrol 2008;3(1):174–8.
10. Macdougall IC, Ashenden M. Current and upcoming erythropoiesis-stimulating agents, iron products, and other novel anemia medications. Adv Chronic Kidney Dis 2009;16(2):117–30.
11. Adamson JW, Vapnek D. Recombinant erythropoietin to improve athletic performance. N Engl J Med 1991;324(10):698–9.
12. Bulbulian R, Wilcox AR, Darabos BL. Anaerobic contribution to distance running performance of trained cross-country athletes. Med Sci Sports Exerc 1986;18(1):107–13.
13. Craig NP, Norton KI, Bourdon PC, et al. Aerobic and anaerobic indices contributing to track endurance cycling performance. Eur J Appl Physiol Occup Physiol 1993;67(2):150–8.
14. Wagner PD. New ideas on limitations to VO2max. Exerc Sport Sci Rev 2000;28(1):10–4.
15. Berglund B, Ekblom B. Effect of recombinant human erythropoietin treatment on blood pressure and some haematological parameters in healthy men. J Intern Med 1991;229(2):125–30.
16. Audran M, Gareau R, Matecki S, et al. Effects of erythropoietin administration in training athletes and possible indirect detection in doping control. Med Sci Sports Exerc 1999;31(5):639–45.

17. Ekblom B, Berglund B. Effect of erythropoietin administration on mammal aerobic power. Scand J Med Sci Sports 1991;1(2):88–92.
18. Casoni I, Ricci G, Ballarin E, et al. Hematological indices of erythropoietin administration in athletes. Int J Sports Med 1993;14(6):307–11.
19. Gareau R, Audran M, Baynes RD, et al. Erythropoietin abuse in athletes. Nature 1996;380(6570):113.
20. Robinson N, Mangin P, Schattenberg L, et al. Origine du suivi hématologique: les contrôles hématocrites dans le cyclisme. (février 2003). Revue Française des Laboratoires 2003;350:53–9 [in French].
21. Parisotto R, Gore CJ, Emslie KR, et al. A novel method utilising markers of altered erythropoiesis for the detection of recombinant human erythropoietin abuse in athletes. Haematologica 2000;85(6):564–72.
22. Parisotto R, Wu M, Ashenden MJ, et al. Detection of recombinant human erythropoietin abuse in athletes utilizing markers of altered erythropoiesis. Haematologica 2001;86(2):128–37.
23. Lasne F, de Ceaurriz J. Recombinant erythropoietin in urine. Nature 2000; 405(6787):635.
24. Wang MD, Yang M, Huzel N, et al. Erythropoietin production from CHO cells grown by continuous culture in a fluidized-bed bioreactor. Biotechnol Bioeng 2002;77(2):194–203.
25. Choi D, Kim M, Park J. Erythropoietin: physico- and biochemical analysis. J Chromatogr B Biomed Appl 1996;687(1):189–99.
26. Wide L, Bengtsson C, Berglund B, et al. Detection in blood and urine of recombinant erythropoietin administered to healthy men. Med Sci Sports Exerc 1995; 27(11):1569–76.
27. Lasne F. Double-blotting: a solution to the problem of nonspecific binding of secondary antibodies in immunoblotting procedures. J Immunol Methods 2003; 276(1–2):223–6.
28. Lasne F, Martin L, Crepin N, et al. Detection of isoelectric profiles of erythropoietin in urine: differentiation of natural and administered recombinant hormones. Anal Biochem 2002;311(2):119–26.
29. Wide L, Bengtsson C. Molecular charge heterogeneity of human serum erythropoietin. Br J Haematol 1990;76(1):121–7.
30. Catlin DH, Breidbach A, Elliott S, et al. Comparison of the isoelectric focusing patterns of darbepoetin alfa, recombinant human erythropoietin, and endogenous erythropoietin from human urine. Clin Chem 2002;48(11):2057–9.
31. Breidbach A, Catlin DH, Green GA, et al. Detection of recombinant human erythropoietin in urine by isoelectric focusing. Clin Chem 2003;49(6 Pt 1): 901–7.
32. Wide L, Wikstrom B, Eriksson K. A new principle suggested for detection of darbepoetin-alpha (NESP) doping. Ups J Med Sci 2003;108(3):229–38.
33. Lasne F, Martin L, Martin JA, et al. Isoelectric profiles of human erythropoietin are different in serum and urine. Int J Biol Macromol 2007;41(3):354–7.
34. Lönnberg M, Drevin M, Carlsson J. Ultra-sensitive immunochromatographic assay for quantitative determination of erythropoietin. J Immunol Methods 2008;339(2):236–44.
35. Franke WW, Heid H. Pitfalls, errors and risks of false-positive results in urinary EPO drug tests. Clin Chim Acta 2006;373(1–2):189–90.
36. Beullens M, Delanghe JR, Bollen M. False-positive detection of recombinant human erythropoietin in urine following strenuous physical exercise. Blood 2006;107(12):4711–3.

37. Kahn A, Baker M. Non-specific binding of monoclonal human erythropoietin antibody AE7A5 to *Escherichia coli* and *Saccharomyces cerevisiae* proteins. Clin Chim Acta 2006;379:173–5.
38. Khan A, Grinyer J, Truong ST, et al. New urinary EPO drug testing method using two-dimensional gel electrophoresis. Clin Chim Acta 2005;358(1–2):119–30.
39. Rabin OP, Lasne F, Pascual JA, et al. New urinary EPO drug testing method using two-dimensional gel electrophoresis. Clin Chim Acta 2006;373(1–2):186–7.
40. Reichel C. Identification of zinc-alpha-2-glycoprotein binding to clone AE7A5 antihuman EPO antibody by means of nano-HPLC and high-resolution high-mass accuracy ESI-MS/MS. J Mass Spectrom 2008;43(7):916–23.
41. Lamon S, Martin L, Robinson N, et al. Effects of exercise on the isoelectric patterns of erythropoietin. Clin J Sport Med 2009;19:311–5.
42. WADA. Technical document TD2009 EPO. Available at: http://www.wada-ama.org. Accessed 2009.
43. Ashenden M, Varlet-Marie E, Lasne F, et al. The effects of microdose recombinant human erythropoietin regimens in athletes. Haematologica 2006;91(8):1143–4.
44. Caldini A, Moneti G, Fanelli A, et al. Epoetin alpha, epoetin beta and darbepoetin alfa: two-dimensional gel electrophoresis isoforms characterization and mass spectrometry analysis. Proteomics 2003;3(6):937–41.
45. Reichel C, Kulovics R, Jordan V, et al. SDS-PAGE of recombinant and endogenous erythropoietins: benefits and limitations of the method for application in doping control. Drug Test Anal 2009;1:43–50.
46. Lonnberg M, Carlsson J. Lab-on-a-chip technology for determination of protein isoform profiles. J Chromatogr A 2006;1127(1–2):175–82.
47. Stubiger G, Marchetti M, Nagano M, et al. Characterisation of intact recombinant human erythropoietins applied in doping by means of planar gel electrophoretic techniques and matrix-assisted laser desorption/ionisation linear time-of-flight mass spectrometry. Rapid Commun Mass Spectrom 2005;19(5):728–42.
48. Guan F, Uboh CE, Soma LR, et al. Differentiation and identification of recombinant human erythropoietin and darbepoetin Alfa in equine plasma by LC-MS/MS for doping control. Anal Chem 2008;80(10):3811–7.
49. Guan F, Uboh CE, Soma LR, et al. Identification of darbepoetin alfa in human plasma by liquid chromatography coupled to mass spectrometry for doping control. Int J Sports Med 2009;30(2):80–6.
50. Groleau PE, Desharnais P, Cote L, et al. Low LC-MS/MS detection of glycopeptides released from pmol levels of recombinant erythropoietin using nanoflow HPLC-chip electrospray ionization. J Mass Spectrom 2008;43(7):924–35.

Anorexia, Bulimia, and the Female Athlete Triad: Evaluation and Management

Felicia A. Mendelsohn, MD[a],*, Michelle P. Warren, MD[b]

KEYWORDS

• Anorexia • Bulimia • Athlete • Amenorrhea

ANOREXIA AND BULIMIA
Definitions and Epidemiology

Anorexia nervosa is characterized by a triad of amenorrhea, weight loss, and psychiatric disturbance. According to the definition in the *Diagnostic and Statistical Manual of Mental Disorders*, fourth edition (DSM-IV), the diagnosis of anorexia nervosa requires 4 criteria: refusal to maintain weight within a normal range for height and age (more than 15% below ideal body weight), intense fear of gaining weight or getting fat, severe body image disturbance or denial of the seriousness of the current low body weight, and absence of the menstrual cycle for greater than 3 cycles in postmenarchal females.[1] Anorexia is then divided into 2 subtypes: restricting and binge eating/purging. Patients with the restricting subtype primarily use restriction of food intake to reduce their weight, whereas those suffering with the binging/purging subtype tend to use vomiting, laxatives, or diuretics to control their weight. Either subtype may also engage in compulsive exercise as a means to reduce weight.

The criteria for the diagnosis of bulimia nervosa listed by the DSM-IV include: recurrent episodes of binge eating with a sense of lack of control; recurrent inappropriate compensatory behavior to prevent weight gain (such as self-induced vomiting, laxatives, diuretics, or excessive exercise); the binge eating and compensatory behavior to occur at least twice per week for 3 months; and self-evaluation unduly influenced by body shape and weight. These disturbances must not occur exclusively during

[a] Department of Obstetrics and Gynecology, Columbia College of Physicians and Surgeons, 4 Dearfield Drive, Suite 102, Greenwich, CT 06831, USA
[b] Department of Obstetrics and Gynecology and Medicine, Columbia College of Physicians and Surgeons, 622 West 168th Street, PH 16-127, New York, NY 10032, USA
* Corresponding author.
E-mail address: mendelsohn@hotmail.com (F.A. Mendelsohn).

Endocrinol Metab Clin N Am 39 (2010) 155–167
doi:10.1016/j.ecl.2009.11.002
0889-8529/10/$ – see front matter © 2010 Elsevier Inc. All rights reserved.

episodes of anorexia nervosa. Bulimia is further divided into purging and nonpurging subtypes.[1] Weight may fluctuate, generally not to dangerously low levels, but many metabolic problems cause serious health issues. Bulimia is often associated with impulsive behavior, alcohol or drug use, promiscuity, and stealing or shoplifting.[2,3]

The prevalence of these disorders has been increasing, with the lifetime prevalence of anorexia nervosa in women at 0.3% to 1.0% and prevalence rates of 1% to 1.5% for bulimia. Many more (3%–5%) have disordered eating but do not fulfill strict criteria for anorexia nervosa or bulimia nervosa, instead meeting criteria for an eating disorder not otherwise specified (NOS). All conditions are much more common in women, with a ratio favoring females of 10:1 for anorexia. The physical consequences of these disorders can include hypothalamic amenorrhea, low peak bone mass, stress fractures, and infertility.[2–4]

Clinical Features

Common physical symptoms associated with anorexia include constipation, intolerance to cold, dry skin, and hair loss. Lanugo type hair may be present on the body. Hypercarotenemia may give a yellowish tinge to the skin. Petechiae, pedal edema, and acrocyanosis can occur. Bradycardia is common, as well as hypotension and hypothermia. Laboratory tests may be normal but also may show leukopenia with a relative lymphocytosis, azotemia due to dehydration, and electrolyte abnormalities such as hyponatremia, hypokalemia, hypophosphatemia, and hypoglycemia. Additional features that should be looked for specifically with bulimia include parotid gland enlargement from vomiting, erosion of the enamel on the anterior surface of teeth because of chronic acid exposure, and Russell's sign, which signifies skin lesions on the fingers used to induce vomiting. The incidence of menstrual irregularity with bulimia is highly variable. Patients with bulimia may have anovulation with normal estrogen secretion.

Hormonal Abnormalities

Anorexia nervosa is associated with multiple hormonal abnormalities, and has been more extensively studied than bulimia. There are data suggesting that patients with bulimia may have an increased accumulation of visceral fat.[5] Regarding bone mineral density (BMD), low bone mass in persons with bulimia is usually associated with preceding anorexia.[6] Functional hypothalamic amenorrhea is now a required element in the diagnosis of anorexia. The underlying pathophysiology in hypothalamic amenorrhea is a suppression of gonadotropin secretion due to a decrease in pulse amplitude or frequency of gonadotropin releasing hormone (GnRH) from the medial central area of the hypothalamus. As GnRH pulses decline, luteinizing hormone (LH) and follicle-stimulating hormone (FSH) pulses decrease in number (**Fig. 1**). Without ovarian stimulation by the gonadotropins LH and FSH every 60 to 90 minutes, estrogen levels decrease. Any restraining metabolic signal, including inadequate nutritional intake, abnormal eating behavior, excessive exercise, and weight loss, can suppress normal GnRH pulsatility and prevent the resumption of menses. A reduction in a woman's percentage of body fat can lead to a reduction in the production of adipokines, particularly leptin.[7] In one study, the administration of recombinant methionyl human leptin restored an ovulatory menstrual cycle in 3 of 8 subjects with functional hypothalamic amenorrhea, suggesting that this hormone can potentially reverse the suppression caused by energy deficiency.[8] Even though leptin seems to be critical for menstrual cyclicity, this hormone alone is insufficient for normal cyclicity and likely must interact with other signals that indicate adequate nutritional intake. Another hormone that also affects GnRH pulsatility is ghrelin. Ghrelin is an orexigenic peptide

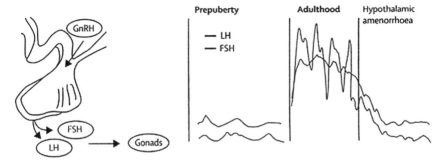

Fig. 1. Luteinizing hormone (LH) and follicle-stimulating hormone (FSH) pulsatility in hypothalamic amenorrhea. (*From* Chan J, Mantzoros C. Role of leptin in energy-deprivation states: normal human physiology and clinical implications for hypothalamic amenorrhoea and anorexia nervosa. Lancet 2005;366:74–5; with permission.)

secreted by the oxyntic cells of the stomach, and is thought to be both a short-term regulator of food intake and a regulator of long-term energy balance.[9] Ghrelin is likely an important component of the restraining metabolic signal in functional hypothalamic amenorrhea, and may help to explain why women who have regained normal weight or who have ceased to exercise, but still show distorted eating patterns, can have prolongation of amenorrhea.[10,11] Peptide YY (PYY) is an anorexigenic peptide derived from the gut that is secreted in response to caloric intake.[7] Patients with anorexia nervosa have been found to have elevated levels of PYY. It has been hypothesized that these elevated levels may predispose a person to anorexia and the associated reduced food intakes. Elevated PYY levels also correlate with changes in bone markers signifying decreased turnover of bone, and may contribute to bone loss.[12]

Anorexia can result in a delayed age of menarche in some girls, and thus a common presenting feature may be primary amenorrhea. The adolescent years are a period of crucial bone development, and girls with amenorrhea may not achieve optimal bone mass because of this.[13,14] Failure to reach an optimal peak bone mass will put these women at greater risk of fracture even later in life, particularly when they are postmenopausal.

Another hormonal abnormality seen in patients with anorexia nervosa is androgen deficiency, demonstrated by low free testosterone levels and low levels of dehydroepiandrosterone sulfate (DHEA-S) in certain studies.[15] These androgen deficiencies may contribute to bone loss as well as some of the psychiatric comorbidities associated with anorexia, such as anxiety and depression.[16] One study examined 61 adolescent girls with anorexia and found an inverse correlation between serum DHEA-S and urinary cross-linked N-telopeptides (NTx).[17] Patients with lower serum DHEA-S levels had higher urinary NTx levels, implying higher amounts of bone resorption. A study randomized 33 women with anorexia nervosa and relative testosterone deficiency to different doses of transdermal testosterone or placebo for 3 weeks.[18] Markers of depression and spatial cognition improved, and some but not all markers of bone formation improved.

Abnormalities of the hypothalamic-pituitary-adrenal axis are seen in anorexia nervosa as well. Elevated levels of cortisol are found in the serum, urine, and saliva of anorexic patients compared with healthy controls.[19,20] A study of adolescents revealed that the raised urine and serum cortisol levels in these patients could be explained by increases in the pulse frequency of cortisol secretion.[19] There is also some evidence for neuroendocrine dysregulation of the hypothalamic-pituitary-adrenal axis in patients with bulimia nervosa.[21]

Another hormonal characteristic of anorexia nervosa is an acquired resistance to growth hormone (GH), manifested by elevated GH levels and low insulinlike growth factor (IGF)-1 levels.[22,23] A study also demonstrated that the bioactivity of IGF-1 in serum of patients at different stages of anorexia is significantly reduced.[24] Of importance is that abnormalities in this GH-IGF-1 axis have been shown to reverse with refeeding.[25] The excess of GH is shown to be a sequela of both increased basal secretory rates and an increased frequency of secretory bursts.[22,23] A possible explanation attributes the GH excess to a lack of IGF-1 mediated negative feedback because of the block in IGF-1 secretion by the liver in starvation states.[7] GH acts directly on bone and indirectly through IGF-1 with anabolic effects. One study examined the effects of recombinant human IGF-1 (rhIGF-1) and oral contraceptives on BMD in 60 osteopenic women.[26] Women treated with rhIGF-1 for 9 months had small beneficial changes in their bone density, particularly when combined with oral contraceptives. Treatment with oral contraceptives alone did not improve bone density in malnourished patients. However, treatment with rhIGF-1 has not been approved for this indication.

Nutritional deficiencies alone can lead to bone loss, and reversing this caloric restriction can lead to large increases in bone density.[27,28] One study found that the recovery of bone metabolism may be a biphasic process.[29] This study showed that an improvement in bone formation is directly related to refeeding. Bone resorption remains elevated, however, until the return of menses and a restoration of endogenous estrogen production. It is possible that the restoration of menses is associated with improvement in the secretion of other important neuropeptides that may positively affect bone mass. The importance of nutrition and weight gain is also demonstrated in a study of women with anorexia who underwent an intensive 3-month nutritional rehabilitation program.[30] Significant weight gain resulted in an increase in BMD at both the spine and hip, and this correlated with appropriate improvements in both bone formation and bone resorption markers. If the weight is maintained, the bone density can improve by almost 1 standard deviation within 1 year. Another study examined women with anorexia and found that their low body weight was associated with a hypoestrogenic state.[31] These women demonstrated elevated levels of bone resorption markers and low levels of bone formation markers. This imbalance was reversed with weight gain, and BMD similarly improved.

The malnutrition associated with anorexia can also lead to the typical changes seen with sick euthyroid syndrome.[7] T3 levels are usually low, with elevated reverse T3 concentrations and T4 to T3 ratios.[32,33] T4 levels can also be decreased in some patients with anorexia.[32] Serum thyroid-stimulating hormone (TSH) levels may be within the normal range or mildly reduced.[34] These changes in thyroid hormone levels are thought to be normal physiologic adaptations to malnutrition, and patients should not be treated with thyroid hormone replacement based merely on these numbers.[7]

THE FEMALE ATHLETE TRIAD
Definition

In June of 1992, the American College of Sports Medicine identified and defined a triad of disorders observed in adolescent and young adult female athletes, now commonly known as the female athlete triad.[35,36] This triad of disorders includes disordered eating, amenorrhea, and osteoporosis. The triad is particularly common in athletic sports that emphasize a lean body build or subjective scoring of performance.

Epidemiology and Pathophysiology

Two large studies examined the prevalence of clinical eating disorders based on appropriate definitions by the DSM-IV. The first study examined 263 Australian male and female elite athletes and the same number of nonathletes to determine the prevalence of eating disorders.[37] Eating disorders were revealed in 31% of the female athletes in "thin-build" sports compared with 5.5% of the control population. Another study examined 1620 male and female Norwegian elite athletes and a similarly sized group of controls, evaluating them for the presence of eating disorders, including anorexia nervosa, bulimia nervosa, and eating disorders NOS.[38] The study found that 25% of female athletes competing in endurance sports, aesthetic sports, and weight-class sports had clinical eating disorders compared with 9% of the general control population. A recent cross-sectional study from Brazil evaluated 78 female elite swimmers.[39] The researchers found that 44.9% of the athletes met the criteria for disordered eating, 19.2% for menstrual irregularity, and 15.4% for low bone mass. Only 35.9% of the women did not meet the criteria for any of the end points assessed.

The presence of primary amenorrhea is found in less than 1% of the general population, but has been demonstrated in more than 22% of college girls competing in cheerleading, diving, and gymnastics.[40] Secondary amenorrhea has been shown in 2% to 5% of the general population, versus up to 69% of ballet dancers[41] and 65% of long-distance runners.[42] Menarche has also been shown to be significantly delayed in athletes who start physical activities before the onset of menstruation.[42] Subclinical menstrual disorders can also be found in eumenorrheic athletes. Luteal phase deficiency or anovulation was demonstrated in 78% of eumenorrheic recreational runners in at least 1 out of every 3 menstrual cycles.[43]

Low BMD has been associated with disordered eating in eumenorrheic athletes, but has been shown to be even lower in amenorrheic athletes.[36] A systematic review was conducted of studies that used World Health Organization (WHO) T-scores for diagnosis of osteopenia and osteoporosis. The investigators found a prevalence in female athletes of osteopenia from 22% to 50% and a prevalence of osteoporosis between 0% and 13%, compared with only 12% and 2.3% respectively in a normal population.[44]

A significant number of female athletes suffer from one of the components of the female athlete triad, but a few actually suffer from all 3 components of the triad. A study examined the prevalence of disordered eating, menstrual dysfunction, and low BMD among 112 United States college athletes in 7 different sports including diving, swimming, cross-country, track, tennis, field hockey, and softball.[45] Twenty-five percent (28/112) of athletes met the criteria for disordered eating, and 26% (29/112) met the criteria for menstrual dysfunction. Two athletes had a low BMD with a Z-score below −2.0. In total, 10 athletes met the criteria for a combination of 2 disorders, whereas only 1 athlete met the criteria for all 3 disorders. However, if a Z-score below −1.0 is considered significant, then an additional 2 athletes met the criteria for all 3 components of the triad. Another study examined 170 female high school athletes from 8 different sports.[46] In total, 18.2% of the athletes met the criteria for disordered eating, 23.5% had menstrual irregularity, and 21.8% had low BMD with Z-scores below −1.0. Ten girls (5.9%) met criteria for 2 components of the triad, and 2 girls (1.2%) met criteria for all 3 components of the triad. Amenorrhea and low bone density are more common in sports for which a low weight is desirable.[47]

The current description of the female athlete triad focuses on low energy availability as the key disorder underlying all the components of the triad.[48] Energy availability or energy drain refers to the amount of dietary energy still present to be used for other bodily functions after exercise is completed. This energy availability or energy drain thus takes into account the total intake of energy from diet minus the amount of energy expended with exercise.[36] When the total net energy availability is not sufficient, to promote survival natural physiologic mechanisms will reduce the amount of energy used for growth and reproduction. Sufficient energy is necessary to maintain eumenorrhea and adequate estrogen production and thus sustain good bone health. Unhealthy athletes may have reduced energy availability because they are restricting their diet and energy intake, because they are suffering from an actual clinical eating disorder, or because of prolonged periods of increasing energy expenditure through exercise without increasing dietary energy intake. Low energy availability can affect hypothalamic function and result in depression of gonadotropin secretion, resulting in amenorrhea and low estrogen levels. One study looked at 15 ballet dancers aged 13 to 15 years who maintained a high level of physical activity.[49] Menarche occurred at a mean age of 15.4 years in this group, which was significantly delayed compared with the average age of 12.5 years in normal controls and 12.6 years in normal music students. Sexual development progressed and menarche occurred in 10 girls after a decrease in exercise or an injury causing forced rest of at least a 2-month duration, despite only minimal or no weight gain during this period. The study concluded that energy drain may play an important modulatory effect on the hypothalamic pituitary set point at puberty and may induce amenorrhea, prolonging the prepubertal state. Suppression of bone formation and an increase in bone resorption is most likely due to nutritional factors, as the lack of estrogen causes an increase in both formation and resorption. Young women runners with amenorrhea for greater than 4 years have been shown to have a reduction in bone turnover, but in particular a reduction in bone formation.[28] It is possible that it is actually an energy deficit that is predominantly affecting bone metabolism in these women.

Bone strength and the risk for fracture depends on multiple variables, including BMD, the internal structure of the bone mineral, and the quality of the bone protein (**Box 1**).[50] Current tools for screening and diagnosis of osteoporosis are based solely on BMD. Osteoporosis can be caused by accelerated bone mineral loss in adulthood

---

Box 1
Clinical determinants of low bone mass in anorexia nervosa

Presentation at younger age particularly before menarche or before 18 years

Duration of anorexia

Duration of amenorrhea

Duration of postmenarchal menses before amenorrhea

Estrogen deprivation exposure time

Low body mass index (BMI), weight, and lean body mass

BMI at follow up

Subtype of anorexia (binge-eating purging subtypes more at risk than restrictive)

Frequency of vomiting

Depression

Data from Jayasinghe Y, Grover SR, Zacharin M. Current concepts in bone and reproductive health in adolescents with anorexia nervosa. BJOG 2008;115:304–15.

or by not accumulating enough optimal BMD during childhood and adolescence. The WHO uses criteria to diagnose osteopenia and osteoporosis in postmenopausal women based on T-scores that compare individuals to average peak adult BMD. However, the International Society for Clinical Densitometry (ISCD) recommends that BMD in premenopausal women and children be expressed instead as Z-scores to compare these individuals to age- and sex-matched controls.[51] The ISCD suggests that Z-scores below −2.0 be termed "low bone density below the expected range for age" in premenopausal women and as "low bone density for chronological age" in children. The ISCD also recommends that the term osteopenia not be used in this population, and that the diagnosis of osteoporosis should only be given in this population when low BMD is present along with secondary risk factors that suggest an increased short-term risk of bone mineral loss and fracture. Secondary risk factors include chronic malnutrition, eating disorders, hypogonadism, glucocorticoid exposure, and previous fractures. The American College of Sports Medicine (ACSM) defines "low bone mineral density" as a history of nutritional deficiencies, hypoestrogenism, stress fractures, or other secondary clinical risk factors for fracture, together with a BMD Z-score between −1.0 and −2.0.[36] Further, ACSM defines "osteoporosis" as secondary clinical risk factors for fracture with BMD Z-scores less than or equal to −2.0.

A female athlete's bone mineral density is a manifestation of multiple factors including nutrition as reflected in her cumulative history of energy availability, her menstrual status, her innate genetics, and her experience with other nutritional and behavioral factors (**Table 1**).[36] Thus, when evaluating a female athlete it is important to know her current BMD and to also take into consideration in what direction her BMD is currently moving. It is important to remember that the onset of amenorrhea will not immediately affect her BMD. Stress fractures have been shown to occur more often in physically active women with irregular menstrual cycles or low BMD. In one study, the relative risk of stress fracture was demonstrated to be 2 to 4 times greater in amenorrheic than eumenorrheic athletes.[52]

Screening

The optimal timing of screening for the female athlete triad should occur at the physical examination before participating in a sport, or at annual health checkups.[36] Other opportunities that present itself include visits for related problems such as amenorrhea or stress fractures. If a female athlete is found to have one component of the triad, she should be evaluated for the other components of the triad as well. Regarding the patient's history, important information including energy intake, dietary practices, weight fluctuations, and exercise energy expenditure needs to be ascertained. Other important components of the history include menstrual history and current menstrual status, and factors associated with low BMD including prior stress fractures. Height, weight, and vital signs should be recorded during the physical examination. Important signs to look for on examination include bradycardia, orthostatic hypotension, cold hands and feet, hypercarotenemia (most easily seen as orange discoloration of the palms), lanugo hair, and parotid gland enlargement.[53] Pelvic examination may reveal vaginal atrophy if hypoestrogenism is present. For patients with disordered eating, initial laboratory assessment should include a chemistry profile with electrolytes, a complete blood count, thyroid function tests, and urinalysis. Laboratory tests in the workup of secondary amenorrhea should include a pregnancy test, LH, FSH, estradiol, prolactin, and TSH. If signs of androgen excess are present on physical examination, then testosterone and dehydroepiandrosterone sulfate levels should also be checked.[36] BMD should be assessed with dual-energy x-ray absorptiometry (DXA) after a stress fracture or fracture from minimal trauma, or after amenorrhea,

Table 1
Causes of low bone mass in anorexia nervosa

Factor	Proposed Effect
Estrogen deficiency	Increased bone resorption. Possibly decreased bone formation, as shown to correlate with low osteocalcin
IGF-1 deficiency, GH resistance	Low IGF-1 levels are resistant to the bone anabolic effects of GH. Strong association between low IGF-1 and low osteocalcin synthesis
Low DHEA-S	Possible loss of anabolic and antiosteolytic properties, mediated by low IGF-1
Low free testosterone	Correlates with bone resorption and bone formation markers in AN
Hypercortisolemia	Strong inverse correlation with bone formation markers, but not resorption markers. Possibly decreases bone formation
Ghrelin resistance	Perhaps mediated by high cortisol and GH resistance, and lack of response to the signal to increase nutritional intake in anorexia
Increased osteoprogerin	Decreases bone resorption. Increased levels indicate a compensatory (yet suboptimal) bone remodeling process
Reduced leptin	May possibly have role in the central and peripheral regulation of bone formation but relationship has not been established. Administration of recombinant leptin has increased bone formation markers
Undernutrition	Seems to be an independent contributor to BMD, in adolescents. In adults with AN, GH and catecholamines function as intermediates of undernutrition and bone resorption. Relationship of calcium and vitamin D intake on BMD in AN unclear
Exercise	Moderate exercise (<3 h/wk) is a significant predictor of BMD
PYY	Inversely associated with bone turnover markers. Increased PYY may possibly cause reduction of osteoblastic activity via its receptor (Y2)
Low T3	Perhaps because of low osteocalcin expression and low IGF-1 release from osteoblasts
Adrenergic regulation	Adrenaline, noradrenaline associated with increased bone resorption in AN

Abbreviations: AN, anorexia nervosa; BMD, bone mineral density; DHEA-S, dehydroepiandrosterone sulfate; GH, growth hormone; IGF, insulinlike growth factor; PYY, peptide YY.
Data from Jayasinghe Y, Grover SR, Zacharin M. Current concepts in bone and reproductive health in adolescents with anorexia nervosa. BJOG 2008;115:304–15.

oligomenorrhea, or disordered eating have been present for 6 months.[54] DXA should be repeated after 12 months in those patients who have persistent disorders of the female athlete triad at that time. Serial DXA studies should ideally be performed on the same machine for more accurate comparisons. Both the posterior-anterior (PA) spine and the hip (femoral neck or total hip) should be measured, and the diagnosis of low BMD is based on the lowest Z-score of either of these sites.[55]

Treatment

Prevention and treatment of the female athlete triad should involve multiple specialists acting as a team, including a physician, a registered dietician, and a mental health practitioner if evidence of an eating disorder is present.[36] Other valuable assistance may come from a certified athletic trainer, an exercise physiologist, an athlete's coach, and parents. The primary emphasis should be on education for prevention, and optimizing energy availability. Athletes should be counseled on nutritional recommendations including adequate calcium and vitamin D intake.

One of the strongest contributors to exercise-induced amenorrhea is a chronic energy deficit. Therefore, the first goal of therapy to restore normal menstrual cycles should be to modify diet and exercise behaviors to increase energy availability.[56] Increases in BMD can accompany regain of weight and menstrual function. A study of a cohort of athletes over a 15.5-month period compared amenorrheic athletes who regained menses, those who remained amenorrheic, and athletes with regular cycles. Initially, amenorrheic athletes who regained menses had an increase in bone density in the vertebral spine of 6.3% compared with a 3.4% continued loss of bone in the 2 athletes who remained amenorrheic during the study period.[57] A positive correlation was shown between BMI, serum levels of bone formation markers, and serum estradiol.[58] Another study examined 7 female runners with exercise-induced amenorrhea and decreased BMD, and reexamined them 15 months later. During this time period, 4 runners reduced their weekly running distance by 43% and took supplemental calcium. These athletes had an average body weight increase of 5% and regained menses. These women also increased their bone mineral content from 1.003 ± 0.097 g/cm^2 to 1.070 ± 0.089 g/cm^2. The other 3 runners took supplemental calcium as well, but did not reduce their running distance. Body weight did not change significantly, and they did not have regain of menses. These athletes had no significant change in bone mineral content.[59]

Athletes with disordered eating should be referred for nutrition counseling. Adequate amounts of vitamins including calcium (1000–1300 mg/day) and vitamin D (800 IU/day) should be consumed through a combination of healthy diet and supplements if needed. Athletes with eating disorders who do not comply with treatment may need to be restricted from training or competition.[36]

Pharmacologic interventions with hormone replacement therapy or oral contraceptives will not completely reverse the underlying mechanisms causing impairment of bone formation, and thus such treatment alone will not fully restore BMD. A study conducted at the authors' institution examined 55 ballet dancers, including 24 who were amenorrheic.[60] Amenorrheics were randomized to receive placebo or conjugated estrogens (Premarin), 0.625 mg for 25 days monthly, with medroxyprogesterone (Provera), 10 mg for 10 of these 25 days, for 2 years. These women were compared with normally menstruating controls. The study participants also received 1250 mg calcium per day. BMD was measured at the foot, wrist, and lumbar spine. Results showed no significant difference in bone density between the placebo and treated groups after 2 years. Five patients (all of whom were receiving placebo) did resume menses during the study period and did show an increase in BMD, but did not normalize their BMD. These findings suggest that other factors aside from hypoestrogenism, possibly related to nutrition, may be involved and necessary for the normalization of bone density.

Bisphosphonates are approved for the treatment of postmenopausal osteoporosis; however, they should not be used in young women. First, the use of these medications in this population has not been well studied and thus potential risks and long-term effects are not known.[61] Also, bisphosphonates have been shown to cross the placenta in animal studies, and it is known that bisphosphonates may reside in bone for several years, thus are potentially able to cause harm to the developing fetus of a woman of childbearing age.[62]

SUMMARY

The female athlete triad is an increasingly prevalent condition involving disordered eating, amenorrhea, and osteoporosis. An athlete can suffer from all 3 components of the triad, or just 1 or 2 of the individual conditions. The main element underlying all the aspects of the triad is low energy availability. Sufficient energy is required to maintain eumenorrhea and, thus, adequate estrogen production and good bone health. Good nutrition is also arguably the most important determinant of return of menses and improvement in bone density. Screening for these disorders should be an important component of an athlete's care. Prevention and treatment should involve a team approach, including a physician, a nutritionist, and a mental health provider.

REFERENCES

1. American Psychiatric Association. Diagnostic and statistical manual of mental disorders. 4th edition. Washington, DC: American Psychiatric Association; 1994.
2. Warren MP, Dominguez JE. Eating disorders and the reproductive axis. Encyclopedia of Endocrine Diseases. 2004;2:1–5.
3. Warren MP, Locke RJ. Anorexia nervosa and other eating disorders. In: KL B, editor. Principles and practice of endocrinology and metabolism. 3rd edition. Philadelphia: JB Lippincott Co; 2001. p. 1251–6.
4. Miller KK, Grinspoon SK, Ciampa J, et al. Medical findings in outpatients with anorexia nervosa. Arch Intern Med 2005;165(5):561–6.
5. Ludescher B, Leitlein G, Schaefer JE, et al. Changes of body composition in bulimia nervosa: increased visceral fat and adrenal gland size. Psychosom Med 2009;71(1):93–7.
6. Naessen S, Carlstrom K, Glant R, et al. Bone mineral density in bulimic women—influence of endocrine factors and previous anorexia. Eur J Endocrinol 2006; 155(2):245–51.
7. Lawson EA, Klibanski A. Endocrine abnormalities in anorexia nervosa. Not Found In Database 2008;4(7):407–14.
8. Welt CK, Chan JL, Bullen J, et al. Recombinant human leptin in women with hypothalamic amenorrhea. N Engl J Med 2004;351(10):987–97.
9. Wynne K, Stanley S, Bloom S. The gut and regulation of body weight. J Clin Endocrinol Metab 2004;89(6):2576–82.
10. Warren MP, Voussoughian F, Geer EB, et al. Functional hypothalamic amenorrhea: hypoleptinemia and disordered eating. J Clin Endocrinol Metab 1999; 84(3):873–7.
11. Schneider LF, Warren MP. Functional hypothalamic amenorrhea is associated with elevated ghrelin and disordered eating. Fertil Steril 2006;86(6):1744–9.

12. Misra M, Miller KK, Tsai P, et al. Elevated peptide YY levels in adolescent girls with anorexia nervosa. J Clin Endocrinol Metab 2006;91(3):1027–33.
13. Misra M, Aggarwal A, Miller KK, et al. Effects of anorexia nervosa on clinical, hematologic, biochemical, and bone density parameters in community-dwelling adolescent girls. Pediatrics 2004;114(6):1574–83.
14. Grinspoon S, Miller K, Coyle C, et al. Severity of osteopenia in estrogen-deficient women with anorexia nervosa and hypothalamic amenorrhea. J Clin Endocrinol Metab 1999;84(6):2049–55.
15. Miller KK, Lawson EA, Mathur V, et al. Androgens in women with anorexia nervosa and normal-weight women with hypothalamic amenorrhea. J Clin Endocrinol Metab 2007;92(4):1334–9.
16. Miller KK, Wexler TL, Zha AM, et al. Androgen deficiency: association with increased anxiety and depression symptom severity in anorexia nervosa. J Clin Psychiatry 2007;68(6):959–65.
17. Gordon CM, Goodman E, Emans SJ, et al. Physiologic regulators of bone turnover in young women with anorexia nervosa. J Pediatr 2002;141(1):64–70.
18. Miller KK, Grieco KA, Klibanski A. Testosterone administration in women with anorexia nervosa. J Clin Endocrinol Metab 2005;90(3):1428–33.
19. Misra M, Miller KK, Almazan C, et al. Alterations in cortisol secretory dynamics in adolescent girls with anorexia nervosa and effects on bone metabolism. J Clin Endocrinol Metab 2004;89(10):4972–80.
20. Putignano P, Dubini A, Toja P, et al. Salivary cortisol measurement in normal-weight, obese and anorexic women: comparison with plasma cortisol. Eur J Endocrinol 2001;145(2):165–71.
21. Birketvedt GS, Drivenes E, Agledahl I, et al. Bulimia nervosa—a primary defect in the hypothalamic-pituitary-adrenal axis? Appetite 2006;46(2):164–7.
22. Stoving RK, Veldhuis JD, Flyvbjerg A, et al. Jointly amplified basal and pulsatile growth hormone (GH) secretion and increased process irregularity in women with anorexia nervosa: indirect evidence for disruption of feedback regulation within the GH-insulin-like growth factor I axis. J Clin Endocrinol Metab 1999;84(6):2056–63.
23. Misra M, Miller KK, Bjornson J, et al. Alterations in growth hormone secretory dynamics in adolescent girls with anorexia nervosa and effects on bone metabolism. J Clin Endocrinol Metab 2003;88(12):5615–23.
24. Stoving RK, Chen JW, Glintborg D, et al. Bioactive insulin-like growth factor (IGF) I and IGF-binding protein-1 in anorexia nervosa. J Clin Endocrinol Metab 2007;92(6):2323–9.
25. Golden NH, Kreitzer P, Jacobson MS, et al. Disturbances in growth hormone secretion and action in adolescents with anorexia nervosa. J Pediatr 1994;125(4):655–60.
26. Grinspoon S, Thomas L, Miller K, et al. Effects of recombinant human IGF-I and oral contraceptive administration on bone density in anorexia nervosa. J Clin Endocrinol Metab 2002;87(6):2883–91.
27. Zanker CL. Bone metabolism in exercise associated amenorrhoea: the importance of nutrition. Br J Sports Med 1999;33(4):228–9.
28. Zanker CL, Swaine IL. Bone turnover in amenorrhoeic and eumenorrhoeic women distance runners. Scand J Med Sci Sports 1998;8(1):20–6.
29. Dominguez J, Goodman L, Sen Gupta S, et al. Treatment of anorexia nervosa is associated with increases in bone mineral density, and recovery is a biphasic process involving both nutrition and return of menses. Am J Clin Nutr 2007;86(1):92–9.

30. Viapiana O, Gatti D, Dalle Grave R, et al. Marked increases in bone mineral density and biochemical markers of bone turnover in patients with anorexia nervosa gaining weight. Bone 2007;40(4):1073–7.
31. Bolton JG, Patel S, Lacey JH, et al. A prospective study of changes in bone turnover and bone density associated with regaining weight in women with anorexia nervosa. Osteoporos Int 2005;16(12):1955–62.
32. Croxson MS, Ibbertson HK. Low serum triiodothyronine (T3) and hypothyroidism in anorexia nervosa. J Clin Endocrinol Metab 1977;44(1):167–74.
33. Leslie RD, Isaacs AJ, Gomez J, et al. Hypothalamo-pituitary-thyroid function in anorexia nervosa: influence of weight gain. Br Med J 1978;2(6136):526–8.
34. Kiyohara K, Tamai H, Takaichi Y, et al. Decreased thyroidal triiodothyronine secretion in patients with anorexia nervosa: influence of weight recovery. Am J Clin Nutr 1989;50(4):767–72.
35. Yeager KK, Agostini R, Nattiv A, et al. The female athlete triad: disordered eating, amenorrhea, osteoporosis. Med Sci Sports Exerc 1993;25(7):775–7.
36. Nattiv A, Loucks AB, Manore MM, et al. American College of Sports Medicine position stand. The female athlete triad. Med Sci Sports Exerc 2007;39(10): 1867–82.
37. Byrne S, McLean N. Elite athletes: effects of the pressure to be thin. J Sci Med Sport 2002;5(2):80–94.
38. Sundgot-Borgen J, Torstveit MK. Prevalence of eating disorders in elite athletes is higher than in the general population. Clin J Sport Med 2004;14(1):25–32.
39. Schtscherbyna A, Soares EA, de Oliveira FP, et al. Female athlete triad in elite swimmers of the city of Rio de Janeiro, Brazil. Nutrition 2009;25(6):634–9.
40. Beals KA, Manore MM. Disorders of the female athlete triad among collegiate athletes. Int J Sport Nutr Exerc Metab 2002;12(3):281–93.
41. Abraham SF, Beumont PJ, Fraser IS, et al. Body weight, exercise and menstrual status among ballet dancers in training. Br J Obstet Gynaecol 1982;89(7): 507–10.
42. Dusek T. Influence of high intensity training on menstrual cycle disorders in athletes. Croat Med J 2001;42(1):79–82.
43. De Souza MJ, Miller BE, Loucks AB, et al. High frequency of luteal phase deficiency and anovulation in recreational women runners: blunted elevation in follicle-stimulating hormone observed during luteal-follicular transition. J Clin Endocrinol Metab 1998;83(12):4220–32.
44. Khan KM, Liu-Ambrose T, Sran MM, et al. New criteria for female athlete triad syndrome? As osteoporosis is rare, should osteopenia be among the criteria for defining the female athlete triad syndrome? Br J Sports Med 2002;36(1):10–3.
45. Beals KA, Hill AK. The prevalence of disordered eating, menstrual dysfunction, and low bone mineral density among US collegiate athletes. Int J Sport Nutr Exerc Metab 2006;16(1):1–23.
46. Nichols JF, Rauh MJ, Lawson MJ, et al. Prevalence of the female athlete triad syndrome among high school athletes. Arch Pediatr Adolesc Med 2006;160(2): 137–42.
47. Fenichel RM, Warren MP. Anorexia, bulimia, and the athletic triad: evaluation and management. Curr Osteoporos Rep 2007;5(4):160–4.
48. Bonci CM, Bonci LJ, Granger LR, et al. National athletic trainers' association position statement: preventing, detecting, and managing disordered eating in athletes. J Athl Train 2008;43(1):80–108.
49. Warren MP. The effects of exercise on pubertal progression and reproductive function in girls. J Clin Endocrinol Metab 1980;51(5):1150–7.

50. National Institutes of Health Consensus Development Panel. Osteoporosis prevention, diagnosis, and therapy. JAMA 2001;285:785–95.
51. Writing Group for the ISCD Position Development Conference. Diagnosis of osteoporosis in men, premenopausal women, and children. J Clin Densitom 2004;7(1):17–26.
52. Bennell K, Matheson G, Meeuwisse W, et al. Risk factors for stress fractures. Sports Med 1999;28(2):91–122.
53. Becker AE, Grinspoon SK, Klibanski A, et al. Eating disorders. N Engl J Med 1999;340(14):1092–8.
54. Khan AA, Hanley DA, Bilezikian JP, et al. Standards for performing DXA in individuals with secondary causes of osteoporosis. J Clin Densitom 2006;9(1):47–57.
55. Hans D, Downs RW Jr, Duboeuf F, et al. Skeletal sites for osteoporosis diagnosis: the 2005 ISCD official positions. J Clin Densitom 2006;9(1):15–21.
56. Kopp-Woodroffe SA, Manore MM, Dueck CA, et al. Energy and nutrient status of amenorrheic athletes participating in a diet and exercise training intervention program. Int J Sport Nutr 1999;9(1):70–88.
57. Drinkwater BL, Nilson K, Ott S, et al. Bone mineral density after resumption of menses in amenorrheic athletes. JAMA 1986;256(3):380–2.
58. Zanker CL, Swaine IL. Relation between bone turnover, oestradiol, and energy balance in women distance runners. Br J Sports Med 1998;32(2):167–71.
59. Lindberg JS, Powell MR, Hunt MM, et al. Increased vertebral bone mineral in response to reduced exercise in amenorrheic runners. West J Med 1987;146(1):39–42.
60. Warren MP, Brooks-Gunn J, Fox RP, et al. Persistent osteopenia in ballet dancers with amenorrhea and delayed menarche despite hormone therapy: a longitudinal study. Fertil Steril 2003;80(2):398–404.
61. Miller KK, Klibanski A. Clinical review 106: amenorrheic bone loss. J Clin Endocrinol Metab 1999;84(6):1775–83.
62. Patlas N, Golomb G, Yaffe P, et al. Transplacental effects of bisphosphonates on fetal skeletal ossification and mineralization in rats. Teratology 1999;60(2):68–73.

Growth Factors, Muscle Function, and Doping

Geoffrey Goldspink, PhD, ScD, FRCS[a,b,*], Barbara Wessner, PhD[c], Harald Tschan, PhD[c], Norbert Bachl, MD[c]

KEYWORDS

• Growth factors • Muscle function • Doping • Olympic Games

The Olympic Games, in addition to being known for which city they were held in, have also cynically been named after the prevalent type of doping that has been used. For example, there are the β-agonist games, the erythropoietin games, the steroid games, and so forth. Based on current interest, the new games may retrospectively be called the growth factor games. The realization that there are systemic and local growth factors dates back to early studies of pituitary function and the role of growth hormone (GH) in inducing the liver to produce insulinlike growth factor 1 (IGF-1), which was originally called somatomedin C. This anabolic factor influences the growth of tissues, including the promotion of muscle mass skeletal muscle during postnatal growth. It is now apparent, however, that the enhancement of muscle development in young adults has to be viewed separately from control of muscle growth during puberty and the point at which the epiphyses close because muscles respond to traction associated with longitudinal bone growth. Rennie[1] has pointed out that it is not sensible to extrapolate the actions of GH in adults to that of prepubescent growth and use for doping aimed at increasing muscle mass. Some of these situations are complex, however, and GH does strengthen connective tissue; therefore, athletes are able to engage in a higher level of resistance training. With techniques in molecular and cell biology and the considerable recent intensive interest shown by the big pharmaceutical companies in developing a treatment of muscle cachexia and sarcopenia, the potential for increasing muscle mass and strength has attracted considerably interest for nonmedical uses. Although efforts to develop treatment of conditions, such as

[a] Department of Surgery, University College Medical School, University of London, Rowland Hill Street, London NW3 2PF, England, UK
[b] Department of Anatomy and Developmental Biology, University College Medical School, University of London, Rowland Hill Street, London NW3 2PF, England, UK
[c] Department of Sports and Exercise Physiology, Centre for Sports Sciences and University Sports, University of Vienna, Auf der Schmelz 6, A-1150 Vienna, Austria
* Corresponding author. Department of Surgery, University College Medical School, University of London, Rowland Hill Street, London NW3 2PF, England, UK.
E-mail address: gb.goldspink@btinternet.com (G. Goldspink).

Endocrinol Metab Clin N Am 39 (2010) 169–181
doi:10.1016/j.ecl.2009.11.001
0889-8529/10/$ – see front matter © 2010 Published by Elsevier Inc.

muscular dystrophy, or to prevent age-related sarcopenia are laudable, the same therapeutic methods of increasing muscle strength and endurance inevitably may be used by athletes. Attempts at keeping events, such as the Olympic Games, "clean" are thwarted by the increased availability of performance-enhancing agents, including growth factors, undermining the concept of open and fair competition. It has to be pointed out, however, that those methods not only are used at the level of competitive athletics at the highest sports levels but also by an increasing percentage of leisure-time sportspeople purchasing drugs from the black market. In addition, it can be speculated that different methodologies for gene transfer to enhance the biologic activity of growth factors may be misused to increase endurance capacity or muscle mass, thus strength, in different disciplines in sport.[2] Athletes in the power events and participants in sports, such as American football, rugby, handball, and soccer, today seem so well muscled compared with those seen in photographs of approximately 30 years ago that many people find it difficult to believe that in all cases this is due to improvements in training methods, although these clearly have contributed. Because growth factors are available over the Internet, it is also difficult to believe that taking these are not part of the training regime of many international-level athletes and body builders. Therefore, it is necessary to increase knowledge about the mode of action of growth factors concerning muscle growth, in particular, the associated dangers to long-term health, and to develop methodologies to counteract their misuse during training and competitions. Hence, a brief description of the development of methods of detection of growth factor doping is included.

THE GROWTH HORMONE/INSULINLIKE GROWTH FACTOR 1 AXIS AND MUSCLE HYPERTROPHY

Other contributors to this issue of *Endocrinology and Metabolism Clinics of North America* discuss aspects of GH and mature IGF-1 as a doping agent. In this article, GH is discussed in relation to its control of the levels of other growth factors. The liver is the main source of circulating IGF-1, and GH up-regulates not only the synthesis of IGF-1 but also the insulinlike growth factor–binding proteins. It became clear, however, that when the IGF-1 receptor was deleted from skeletal muscles,[3] a functional insulinlike growth factor receptor was found not necessary for load-induced skeletal muscle hypertrophy. Therefore, previous claims that IGF-1 initiates muscle hypertrophy have not been substantiated and, as its distribution is ubiquitous in all tissues, including muscle, those claims that it initiates the hypertrophy process do not make physiologic sense. The IGF-1 receptor knockout experiments require a new way of thinking about the GH/IGF-1 axis, also emphasizing the importance of the direct effect of GH on tissues and the role of autocrine/paracrine IGF-1 derived by alternate splicing of the IGF-1 gene, in particular the mechano growth factor (MGF) splice variant, which has been shown to be produced in response to mechanical strain and muscle cell damage. The C-terminal peptide of this IGF-1 isoform has been shown to have a specific actions that are not mediated via the IGF-1 receptor.[4,5] In younger individuals, there is also the situation in which bone lengthening imposes mechanical stress on the musculature. Levels of GH and IGF-1 reach their peak levels during adolescence and thereafter, there is a marked decline in the circulating levels of GH and a somewhat smaller decline in circulating IGF-1. From clinical practice, in young adults who are GH deficient, the administration of recombinant human GH (rhGH) has positive effects on muscle mass function and decreased body fat. These findings indicate that older individuals with decreased levels of circulating GH and IGF-1 may benefit from GH therapy, which probably encourages the illicit use of GH among athletes, even those competing. Young athletic individuals post puberty, however, are not GH deficient, and recent experiments[6] in which human GH (hGH) was administered to physical education students, who were in regular training but not in competitive sports, showed no increase in maximum strength although their circulating IGF-1 levels were markedly increased. To evaluate the effects of using hGH for enhancing performance, a randomized double-blind trial with a crossover design was funded by the World Anti-Doping Agency (WADA). Seven young fit subjects were randomly assigned to a group receiving daily injections of a clinically permitted recombinant hGH or placebo for a 2-week period. After a 1-month washout, the groups were reversed. It was found that rhGH increased circulating IGF-1 markedly from 31.8 to 109 nmol/L ($P<.05$). There was no increase in maximum strength or in muscle-specific IGF-1Ea and IGF-1Ec (MGF) RNA transcript expression, however. Unlike in the liver, the muscle class 1 and class 2 IGF-1 expression did not change significantly in these young athletes after administration of rhGH. The findings contrast with those of a previous study in GH-deficient elderly men that resulted in higher muscle IGF-1Ea after rhGH administration When this was combined with resistance training there was also a marked increase in MGF (human IGF-1Ec) and in muscle cross-sectional area.[7] This is in accord with the conclusion drawn by Rennie[1] for healthy young individuals who are post puberty; there seems to be no point in using hGH to enhance performance. There are a few acromegalic individuals who continue to show a marked improvement in performance into their early 20s but it can be argued that in these cases this aspect of puberty is not complete. Therefore, in these somewhat unusual individuals, extra hGH production of an episodic nature cannot be ruled out as a means of performance enhancement. hGH is available over the Internet and is still used by many individuals, including film stars, in the hope that it will build up and maintain their muscles, but as far as athletes are concerned, extraneous GH is detectable, as naturally produced hGH exists as a major and a minor isoform for which antibodies are available. The ratio of these isoforms in plasma provides a means of detecting its misuse although there was a rumor that hGH was being extracted using the original method of using pituitaries of corpses. In this way the ratio of the major and minor isoforms would be the same. The use of hGH for doping cannot be dismissed as it has several functions, one of which is to increase the level of IGF-1 in blood and other tissues. As discussed previously, in acromegaly, which is associated with high hGH levels and, hence, high serum levels of IGF-1 due to an active pituitary, this is associated with a higher propensity to develop cancer. This alone should deter individuals from using high dosages of hGH for purposes of body building and enhancing performance in sporting events.

INSULINLIKE GROWTH FACTOR 1 (MATURE INSULINLIKE GROWTH FACTOR 1)

The GH/IGF-1 axis is involved directly or indirectly in muscle growth, particularly up to adolescence. Thereafter, it is uncertain just what role GH plays, as Goldberg in 1967[7] showed that in hypophysectomized rats muscle hypertrophy could be induced by overload. This also applies to the liver type of IGF-1 (mature IGF-1 from IGF-1Ea). More recently, load-induced muscle growth was shown to still occur in transgenic animals in with the IGF-1 receptor was ablated.[3] A survey of the literature shows that the conclusions concerning IGF-1's autocrine role were almost exclusively drawn from transgenic studies in which exogenous IGF-1 was overexpressed and that did not take account of the physiologic role of mechanical loading on muscle tissue. Several groups have published data that indicate serum and muscle IGF-1 levels increase as a result of resistance exercise in animal models, thus presumably explaining why it has been tried as an enhancing substance and why it is on the banned list. Pharmaceutical and biotech companies have made versions of the IGF-1 protein but earlier studies in relation to muscle development used antibody detection,[8] which recognized the main spherical part domains A to D that all the isoforms of the IGF-1 possess. This was a problem as these manufactured versions are related to IGF-1 and did not include any C-terminal side chains encoded in the IGF-1 gene, which are different in the three main types of IGF-1 isoforms and are responsible for some of their unique properties. Several articles on IGF-1 complementary DNA (cDNA) transfer using viral vectors started at the University of Pennsylvania[9–11] and more recently some of these publications are aimed at reconciling their results.[12,13] These involved viral vectors and included a muscle-specific expression element and the IGF-1 cDNA, designated mIGF-1. These have shown as beneficial for slowing the progress of muscular dystrophy and amyotrophic lateral sclerosis (ALS) in animal models of these diseases and are claimed to be safe, as the IGF-1 is expressed only in muscle fibers. Understandably, there is concern that methods of gene transfer will be used for gene doping particularly if they include IGF-1 splice variants. This subject has previously been reviewed by several investigators,[2,14] and there was a WADA-sponsored conference in Helsinki at which this subject was discussed. At this stage it seems dangerous for anyone to use this approach for introducing exogenous IGF-1, as even by incorporating a muscle-specific expression element into the viral vector, the chances are that the carcinogenic IGF-1 product may not completely stay in the muscle cells. It is not known how much IGF-1 would be produced in other cell types by leaky expression, particularly in liver tissue, where viral genes tend to accumulate. Also, there are concerns that the introduction of anabolic IGF-1, which is hyperglycemic and carcinogenic, cannot be reversed. Last but not least, it would be difficult to adjust the free mature IGF-1 levels, which are particularly important for IGF-1, because of the role of their binding proteins in prereceptor regulation. Another group at the University of Pennsylvania, working on hemophilia, using a similar viral vector with the coding sequence of factor nine together with muscle response elements. These trials were stopped after the death of the patient, however, which was related to accumulation of the gene constructs in the liver, one patient being treated with a similar viral construct. Plasmid vectors that do not integrate with the chromosomes are probably safer, as plasmids are known to exist in most cells, and when they contain a muscle-specific regulatory element, they can deliver growth factors. These affect only the injected tissue, but systemic delivery of plasmid vectors to defined organ systems is being attempted in animals using pressure, although this requires sophisticated equipment and is unlikely to be used by athletes. In spite of the several reviews that have been published on gene doping, it is probable that gene transfer technology will take several years to perfect until it is regarded as reasonably safe. Also, the use of recombinant mature IGF-1 or IGF-1Ea protein is potentially dangerous as it disturbs glucose homeostasis and has carcinogenic properties. Also, there is no direct evidence that serum IGF-1 induces muscle hypertrophy or acts as more than a general anabolic agent.

DIFFERENT GROWTH FACTORS DERIVED FROM THE INSULINLIKE GROWTH FACTOR 1 GENE

It is now appreciated that in human muscle the IGF-1 gene can be spliced to produce at least three types of insulinlike growth factors[15,16] but the number is double as these may be class 1 or class 2. Exons 1 and 2 that give rise to these are shown in **Fig. 1** and are different start sequences that precede the exons that code for the different

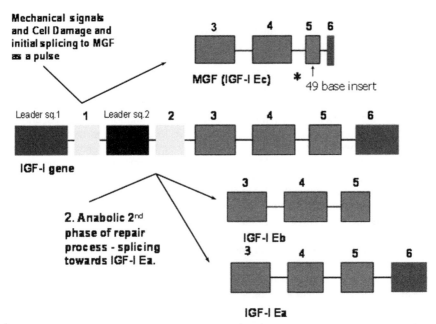

Fig. 1. Illustration of the way the IGF-1 gene is spliced in response to resistance exercise or tissue damage: first to MGF (IGF-1Ea in the human), which involves a reading frame shift that results in a unique C-terminal peptide, and later to the IGF-1Ea, which is the liver type of IGF-1 in rodents and in humans.

domains the three main splice variants. All of these main types have the same tertiary structure with a spherical body, the configuration of which is maintained by three S-S bonds, but there is a side chain that differs for the IGF-1s A, B, and C and which is encoded by different E domains. The main spherical body of the molecule is encoded by A to D domains of the IGF-1 gene is sometimes referred to mature IGF-1 and is responsible for the anabolic properties of all the splice variants of IGF-1. This main body of IGF-1Ea is responsible for this form of IGF-1 binding to at least eight different binding proteins and has the IGF-1 receptor recognition site, which presumably is exposed when it is in nonbound form. In IGF-1Ea the side chain is glycosylated and large but this is probably cleaved off when it released in what may be a time-release manner, and for this reason serum levels of IGF-1 do not reflect the marked diurnal of hGH production by the liver and other tissues. Commercially produced versions of IGF-1 have altered amino acid (aa) sequences to reduce peptidase activity and in some cases to prevent this form of mature IGF-1 from binding to its binding proteins. These are available for research purposes but are unlikely to be used for doping. Recombinant mature IGF-1, which is produced in a way similar to human insulin and is much less expensive, is likely to be misused; some individuals have been using human insulin even against strong medical advice.

MECHANO GROWTH FACTOR, A SPLICE VARIANT OF THE INSULINLIKE GROWTH FACTOR 1 GENE IN RESPONSE TO MECHANICAL STRESS

The MGF splice variant of IGF-1, equivalent to human IGF-1Ec (IGF-1Eb), is expressed in response to mechanical stimulation[17,18] and peaks earlier than IGF-1Ea mRNA.[19,20]

It is a potent growth factor for increasing muscle strength by its role in activating muscle satellite (stem) cell proliferation after muscle damage.[21] A single injection of a MGF-cDNA–containing plasmid vector resulted in a 25% increase in the fiber cross-sectional area of the injected normal muscle and a 30% increase in dystrophic mouse muscle within 3 weeks[22] compared with IGF-1Ea viral vector transfection, which lasted more than 4 months and developed a minor result. Although these experiments are not strictly comparable, it seems that MGF is more potent in activating muscle hypertrophy, probably due to its dual effect on satellite cell proliferation and anabolic properties, and the effect may be different at different ages.[23] Serum GH levels decrease markedly during aging and it has been found that its administration combined with resistance exercise considerably improved MGF mRNA levels in the thigh muscles of elderly men relative to either treatment alone, although IGF-1Ea levels were not up-regulated by resistance training in these elderly subjects.[15,24] In all cases, mechanical signals (muscle contraction and stretch) generated during resistance exercise cause splicing toward MGF. Therefore, it is not surprising that the first hits received when entering MGF into a Google search lead to sport and bodybuilding forums. So, the use of this growth factor probably is not restricted to clinical studies anymore. It also has been detected in other tissues, such as tendons (after mechanical stress), the myocardium (in which it prevents cell death),[25,26] and the central nervous system (n which it was also shown to promote the retention of motor units in ALS).[27] This suggests that MGF that is produced by natural exercise helps protect the myocardium, the central nervous system, and musculoskeletal tissues. Recombinant MGF has been produced in China[28] and Russia[29] but this is presumably the full MGF molecule of 70 plus amino acids with the mature IGF-1 part and a side chain (E domain), which itself has several of the unique growth properties. In addition to having different expression kinetics to IGF-1Ea, MGF has a unique C-terminal peptide that activates the expansion of the muscle stem cell pool. Using *quantitative reverse transcription* (qRT)–polymerase chain reaction (PCR) with primers to this unique E domain sequence, it was found that MGF expression peaks earlier than that of total IGF-1 mRNA and that after muscle damage, MGF is produced as a pulse lasting only approximately a day.[19] It was also found that the role of the terminal 24 amino acids of E domain peptide is to activate the muscle satellite (progenitor) cells to proliferate[21] and also prevents them entering the myogenic pathway. These mononucleated muscle stem cells are usually positioned just beneath the basal lamina but outside the membrane of the myofiber, and by activating them, this small unique sequence of MGF kick starts the hypertrophy process. In muscle that is a postmitotic tissue, these cells provide the extra nuclei for postnatal growth and repair after local injury of muscle fibers. Ates and colleagues[5] using defined muscle stem (progenitor) cells from human muscle biopsies, confirmed that initially with mouse muscle cell-line cultures.[4] These findings are in accord with work published by Jacqueimin and colleagues,[30] who showed that although IGF-1 does not initiate the replication of satellite cells, it is involved in the second stage by causing them to fuse and enter the myogenic pathway once they are in the muscle fiber. The expression of MGF in response to resistance exercise provides the rationale for treating age-related sarcopenia, particularly in the frail elderly. Using the 24 aa peptide of the MGF E domain on human on stem muscle cells, it was encouraging to find that even in conditions, such as muscular dystrophy and ALS, and in normal muscle, these progenitor cells could be activated to multiply. Thus, it may not be necessary to transplant muscle stem cells if the progenitor cell pool can be replenished by administration of MGF provided as the peptide or by gene therapy. In addition to activating the muscle stem cells, the C-terminal peptide was found to be protective against cellular damage in several tissues. For example, using isolated brain slices treated with free radical generator compounds, when the MGF C-terminal peptide was applied, free radical damage and cell death was considerably reduced.[31] This helps explain why regular exercise is beneficial not only for the musculature but also for the maintenance of other tissues.

As far as doping is concerned, MGF is a prime candidate, although it was described in body builder blogs as effective in enhancing muscle hypertrophy but expensive (which is the case for the synthetic 24 aa peptide). Soon this will no longer be the case because it can now be produced by recombinant methods in yeast and *Escherichia coli*. As a consequence, in the next few years its increasing availability will no doubt increase it use for doping.

MYOSTATIN INHIBITORS

In recent years, a negative muscle regulatory factor, myostatin, has been discovered, which, as its name implies, reduces muscle growth. A defect in the myostatin gene was first studied with respect to double muscling in Belgian Blue cattle[32] and in recent years a double-allele knockout was found in one individual[33] whose mother was an athlete with just one silenced allele. Myostatin retards muscle development, which led to the idea that knocking out or knocking down myostatin at the protein or gene level offered potential for increasing muscle mass and strength. Although this led to an increase in muscle mass, the increase in strength was not commensurate and specific strength is actually decreased. As this negative regulator pushes satellite cells into the quiescent state, the muscle satellite (stem) cell does not expand.[34] As these are the source of the extra myonuclei of this postmitotic tissue in which mitotic divisions of nuclei cease after embryologic formation, this does not result in normal muscle growth, as presumably the extra nuclei are required particularly for massive increase in contractile protein.[35] The tissues in mice that are myostatin knockout or knockdown animals is abnormal and give rise to a greater number of muscle fibers, whereas adults develop larger and more muscle fibers. After myostatin knockdown, however, the most relevant point from a doping standpoint is that muscle size and muscle strength do not develop proportionally and the specific muscle strength is actually less.[36] In transgenic mice in which both alleles are silenced, the hypertrophic muscles show reduced capillarization and impaired force generation, possibly due to overdevelopment of sarcoplasmic reticulum coupled with a deficiency in mitochondria.[37] Nevertheless, research on blocking myostatin is developing and commercial products are offered over the Internet. The scientific evidence showed that targeted postnatal inactivation of the myostatin gene that resulted in a myostatin nul mouse had a decreased number of active satellite cells, helping to explain the imbalance between functional and nonfunctional protein that results in decreased muscle-specific contractile force and decreased oxidative capacity of the muscles in addition to impaired respiratory and cardiovascular function. This would handicap rather than provide an advantage in most athletic events the exception of those that require gross strength, such as the top body weight groups. Somewhat more promising results for treating genetic muscle disorders come from groups[38] who are using an alternatively spliced cDNA of follistatin, which is an inhibitor of myostatin. The results showed increased muscle size and strength in species ranging from mice to monkeys. Antimyostatin antibodies are being evaluated in phase I/II trials, but phase III trials and approvals for human clinical use are not yet foreseen. Sadly, sports history is replete with examples of athletes willing to risk severe side effects, long-term damage, or even death in the pursuit of victory, and the possibility exists that athletes might try to obtain untested or prototype therapeutics. Considering the requests and offers in Internet forums of nonprofessional athletes, it cannot be excluded that some kind of antimyostatin treatment is already being used in humans. The only extant antimyostatin treatment is a herbal supplement of questionable efficacy.

OTHER GROWTH FACTORS INVOLVED IN SKELETAL MUSCLE ADAPTATION AND REPAIR

There is a realization that the signaling involved in muscle hypertrophy and increase in fatigue resistance involves a matrix of signaling cascades and several growth factors. Intervention in these processes might be upstream or downstream for the purposes of therapeutic and doping methods. The misuse of other growth factors that influence muscle adaptation and repair seems less imminent compared with that of the GH/IGF-1 axis but complementary administration for increased blood flow to the target tissues will no doubt be on the agenda of some professional coaches who have a strong science background to produce medal winners to secure their positions. Angiogenesis is a common adaptive response that improves the duration of training, which is mediated through the upregulation of angiogenic factors, such as vascular endothelial growth factor (VEGF) and basic fibroblast growth factor (bFGF or FGF2). The underlying natural mechanism of this response is not clear, but the reduced oxygen tension or related metabolic alterations in the skeletal muscle might act as possible stimuli. Therefore, training at high altitude, which induces these growth factors, is considered a legitimate means of increasing these angiogenic factors. Many preclinical and some clinical experiences in trials of peripheral artery diseases indicate that the administration of bFGF probably enhances neovascularization of musculoskeletal tissues. Nakamura and colleagues[39] induced neovascularization in a mural model using a controlled release of biologically active bFGF molecules from a self-produced carrier, which was injected directly into the back of mice. Efthimiadou and colleagues[40,41] administered bFGF after tenotomy of the rat gastrocnemius muscle and achieved a significant prevention of atrophy-induced decrease of blood vessels. Many studies concerning angiogenesis have addressed with the therapeutic effect of VEGF, a highly specific mitogen for vascular endothelial cells with very short half-life in circulation and an essential coordinator of chondrocyte death, chondroclast function, extracellular matrix remodelling, angiogenesis, and bone formation in the growth plate. This article, however, is concerned only with doping post puberty. Today, more than 30 animal studies report evidence the usefulness of VEGF in angiogenesis therapy, which has already entered the phase of clinical trials. Baumgartner and colleagues[42] successfully performed a phase 1 clinical trial in nine patients with critical limb ischemia by intramuscular injection of a VEGF-plasmid followed by improved collateral flow and an amelioration of clinical status. Similar positive results were obtained by Kim and colleagues[43] by gene transfer in patients using a naked plasmid with the cDNA of VEGF. In mouse models of differently induced muscular damage, the delivery of VEGF-165 using an adeno-associated virus vector markedly improved muscle fiber reconstitution, angiogenesis, and regeneration.[44] Hence, VEGF causes new blood vessels to grow, which in theory could move more oxygen and nutrients between muscles, lungs, and the heart and more effort could be expended on athletic performance. Unregulated VEGF-induced vessel growth also seems to promote tumor growth and metastasis, which is a serious risk for enhancing athletes performance.

MANIPULATION OF PROTEIN SYNTHESIS AND BREAKDOWN

The size of tissues in the body is determined mainly by a balance between the rate at which proteins are synthesized and the rate they are broken down. Every few days, approximately half the enzyme molecules within the body break down and are replaced. The turnover of the contractile proteins of muscle, such as actin and myosin, takes a little longer with half of them replaced every approximately 2 weeks. This higher turnover of muscle protein is part of the tissue adaptation that is taking place during early postnatal growth and development.[45] Using nonradioactive isotope methods, it was found that with age, muscle proteins are degraded and rebuilt at less frequent intervals but the process is still dynamic. Protein degradation requires energy as does the synthesis of muscle proteins and it seems that the balance is more toward decreased protein synthesis, except in some disease states, for example, endotoxin poisoning, in which muscle protein breakdown can be rapid at all ages. Pharmaceutical companies have shown an interest not only in increasing synthesis using growth factors but also in reducing the rate of their degradation. Proposals[46] for increasing muscle mass by slowing down the degradation process during healthy aging, however, would seem physiologically undesirable as continual replacement of proteins is important in tissues, in particular mechanical tissues, as this is a way of ensuring there is no build up of nonfunctional proteins and a reduction in specific strength. At present there seems to be a consensus of opinion that exercise training should be performed a couple of hours after the main high protein meal, which has a good proportion of the essential amino acids. This used to be the case when most people were engaged in manual work but in most countries this is no longer true, as the main meal with the highest quality protein is taken in the evening before retiring to their bed. This, therefore, offers a simple and legitimate method of improving training.

NEW APPROACHES TO THE DETECTION OF DOPING FOR ENHANCED PERFORMANCE

In addition to an initial method for screening large numbers of sports people, it is necessary to have at least one confirmatory test that will stand up in a court of law, as it is necessary to convince a judge that a substance had been taken to alter an individual's physiology advantageously. Developments in mass spectrometry combined with robotics and analyzed by powerful computer programs, such as neural networks, allow hundreds of blood and urine samples to be analyzed within a few days and a change in the metabolic profile can be detected. To establish the methods, collaborative work was performed with analytical chemists at Nottingham Trent University and the racehorse testing laboratories at Horseracing Forensic Laboratory Fordham (Cambridgeshire, United Kingdom), which have expertise in mass spectrometry using blood samples. In these particular examples, blood was used from samples from mice[47] and from human volunteers[47] who had been doped using hGH. The principle is shown in **Fig. 2**, in which red bars indicate use of an illicit substance and blue the normal controls.

Although the initial experiments were set up to detect abnormal IGF-1 levels, other biomarkers, such as leucine-rich glycoprotein, have proved to be good indicators of this type of doping. This automated mass spectrometry approach is developing rapidly into a new branch of biochemistry, named metabolomics. Therefore, the use of advanced automated proteomic equipment and powerful computer programs are not restricted to detecting individuals who have probably taken a banned substance and who should be can subjected to further tests; rather, the whole of this science is becoming more sophisticated and powerful.

For the confirmatory test, human white blood cells were maintained in culture and the changes in the MGF mRNA, as determined by the sensitive quantitative qRT-PCR method, were measured after the human white cells were exposed to one small

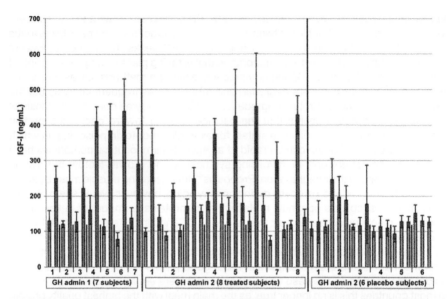

Fig. 2. The principle of the use of automated mass spectrometry for detecting abnormal profile of metabolites in an experiment that involved doping young fit male volunteers with hGH. The dark gray bars show abnormal serum IGF-1 metabolites after hGH doping. (*From* Kay RG, Barton C, Velloso CP, et al. High-throughput ultra-high-performance liquid Chromatography/tandem mass spectrometry quantitation of insulin-like growth factor–I and leucine-rich alpha-2-glycoprotein in serum as biomarkers of recombinant human growth hormone administration. Rapid Commun Mass Spectrom 2009;23:1–10.)

drop of blood from mice or human volunteers that had received. It was found that after hGH administration to mice this confirmatory test also worked well on C2C12 cells.[48] The objective was to illustrate how this generation of molecular biology and advanced analytical chemistry tests without giving sensitive data it is important to protect the Olympic Games and other sporting events **Fig. 3.**

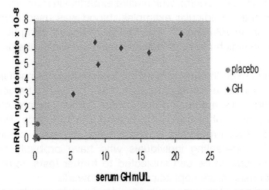

Fig. 3. An example of a test that may be used for confirmation of hGH doping, based on adding one drop of serum from a doping suspect onto normal human white blood cells in culture medium.

SUMMARY

Improved understanding of the local control of muscle mass and strength and the role of growth factors in muscle protection and repair offers the possibility of treating a range of diseases, particularly by using MGF, a splice variant of the IGF-1 gene. The genuine medical use of treating muscle cachexia associated with many diseases also presents a major problem for misuse in athletic events that require power, however, as there is a selection of substances already available over the Internet. For young athletes and their parents, it is important to know that excelling in sports can be achieved without resorting to using drugs. Also, for the major sporting events, for example the Olympic Games, to continue to flourish and maintain the attention of millions of spectators, it is important that sport is kept clean.

ACKNOWLEDGMENTS

Professor Geoffrey Goldspink was a visiting professor at the University of Vienna. Previous funding for the MGF work was from the Wellcome Trust, WADA, and a European Union Framework 5 PENAM Grant. The experiments on administration of hGH to young fit volunteers were funded by a grant from the WADA to Professor Goldspink at University College, London (United Kingdom).

REFERENCES

1. Rennie MJ. Caims for the anabolic effects of growth hormone; a case of the emperor's new clothes? Br J Sports Med 2003;37(2):100–5.
2. Sweeney HL. Gene Doping. Sci Am 2004;291:62–9.
3. Spangenburg EE, Le Roith D, Ward CW, et al. A functional insulin-like growth factor receptor is not necessary for load-induced skeletal muscle hypertrophy. J Physiol 2008;586(1):283–91.
4. Yang SY, Goldspink G. Different roles of the IGF-I Ec peptide (MGF) and mature IGF-I in myoblast proliferation and differentiation. FEBS Lett 2002; 522:156–60.
5. Ates K, Yang SY, Orrell RW, et al. IGF-I splice variant (MGF) increases progenitor cells in ALS, dystrophic and normal muscle. FEBS lett 2007;581: 2727–32.
6. Aperghis M, Velloso CP, Hameed M, et al. Serum IGF-I levels and IGF-I splicing in healthy young males receiving hGH. Growth Horm IGF Res 2009;19(1):61–7.
7. Goldberg AL. Work-induced growth of skeletal muscle in normal and hypophysectomized rats. Am J Phys 1967;213(5):1193–8.
8. Zhan Y, Biggs RB, Booth FW. Insulin like growth factor immunoreactivity increases in muscle after acute eccentric contractions. J Appl Phys 1993;74(I):410–4.
9. Barton-Davies E, Shoturma DI, Musaro A, et al. Viral mediated expression of insulin-like growth factor I blocks the aging-related loss of skeletal muscle function. Proc Natl Acad Sci U S A 1998;95:15603–7.
10. Musaro A, McCullagh K, Paul A, et al. Localized Igf-1 transgene expression sustains hypertrophy and regeneration in senescent skeletal muscle. Nat Genet 2001;27:195–200.
11. Shavlakadze T, Davies M, White JD, et al. Early regeneration of whole skeletal muscle grafts is unaffected by overexpression of IGF-1 in MLC/mIGF-1 transgenic mice. J Histochem Cytochem 2004;52(7):873–83.
12. Barton ER. The ABCs of IGF-I isoforms: impact on muscle hypertrophy and implications for repair. Appl Physiol Nutr Metab 2006;31(6):791–7.

13. Shavlakadze T, Winn N, Rosenthal N, et al. Reconciling data from transgenic mice that overexpress IGF-I specifically in skeletal muscle. Growth Horm IGF Res 2005;15(7):4–18.
14. Goldspink G, Wessner B, Bachl N. Growth factors muscle function and doping. Curr Opin Pharmacol 2008;8(3):352–7.
15. Hameed M, Lange KH, Andersen JL, et al. The effect of recombinant human growth hormone and resistance training on IGF-I mRNA expression in the muscles of elderly men. J Physiol 2004;555(1):231–40.
16. McKay BR, O'Reilly CE, Philips SM, et al. Coexpression of the IGF-I family members with myogenic regulatory factors following acute damaging muscle lengthening contractions in humans. J Physiol 2008;586(22): 5549–60.
17. Yang S, Alnaqeeb M, Simpson H, et al. Cloning and characterization of an IGF-1 isoform expressed in skeletal muscle subjected to stretch. J Muscle Res Cell Motil 1996;17:487–95.
18. Goldspink G, Yang SY. The splicing of the IGF-I gene to yield different muscle growth factors. Adv Genet 2004;52:23–49.
19. Hill M, Goldspink G. Expression and splicing of the insulin-like growth factor gene in rodent muscle is associated with muscle satellite (stem) cell activation following local tissue damage. J Physiol 2003;549(Pt2):409–18.
20. Haddad F, Adams GR. Selected contribution: acute cellular and molecular responses to resistance exercise. J Appl Phys 2002;93:394–403.
21. Hill M, Wernig A, Goldspink G. Muscle satellite (stem) cell activation during local tissue injury and repair. J Anat 2003;203(1):89–99.
22. Goldspink G, Goldspink PH, Yang SY. US patent MGF E peptides, published 2006.
23. Barton ER. Viral expression of insulin-like growth factor-1 isoforms promotes different responses in skeletal muscle. J Appl Phys 2006;100:1778–84.
24. Hameed M, Orrell RW, Cobbold M, et al. Expression of IGF-I splice variants in young and old human skeletal muscle after high resistance exercise. J Physiol 2003;547:247–54.
25. Carpenter V, Matthews K, Devlin G, et al. Mechano-growth factor reduces loss of cardiac function in acute myocardial infarction. Heart Lung Circ 2008;17: 33–9.
26. Shioura KM, Los T, Greenen DI, et al. The unique E-domain of an IGF-I isoform expressed in muscle preserves cardiac function and prevents apopotosis following cardiac infarction [meeting abstracts]. Circulation 2006;114:232–3.
27. Riddoch-Contreras J, Yang SY, Dick JR, et al. Mecahno growth factor, an IGF-I splice variant rescues motoneurons and improves muscle function in SOD 1 mice. Exp Neurol 2009;215(2):281–9.
28. Zhang B, Jiang P, Xian C, et al (2008). Sheng Wu Gong Cheng Xue Bao 1180–85 [in Chinese].
29. Kuznetsova TV, Schulga AA, Wulfson AN, et al. Producing human mechano growth factor (MGF) in E coli. Protein Expr Purif 2008;58(1):70–7.
30. Jacqueimin V, Furling D, Biogot A, et al. IGF-I induces human myotube hypertrophy by increasing cell replacement. Exp Cell Res 2004;299:148–58.
31. Dluzniewska J, Sarnowska A, Beresewicz M, et al. A strong neuroprotective effect of the autonomous C-terminal peptide of IGF-I Ec (MGF) in brain ischemia. FASEB J 2005;19:1896–904.
32. Arthur PF. Double muscling in cattle. Aust J Agric Res 1999;46:1493–515.

33. Schuelke M, Wagner KR, Stolz LE, et al. Myostatin mutation associated with gross muscle hypertrophy in a child. N Engl J Med 2004;350:2682–8.
34. McMahon CD, Popovic L, Oldham JM, et al. Myostatin-deficient mice lose more skeletal muscle mass than wild type controls during hind limb suspension. Am J Physiol Endocrinol Metab 2003;285:E82–7.
35. Amthor H, Macharia R, Navarrete R, et al. Lack of myostatin results in excessive muscle growth but impaired force generation. Proc Natl Acad Sci U S A 2007; 104:1835–40.
36. McCroskery S, Maxwell TM, Sharme M, et al. Myostatin negatively regulate satellite cell activation and self renewal. J Cell Biol 2003;162:1135–47.
37. Grobet L, Pirottin D, Farnir F, et al. Modulating skeletal muscle mass by postnatal, muscle specific inactivation of the myostatin gene. Genesis 2003;35: 227–38.
38. Gilson H, Schakman O, Kallista S, et al. Follistatin induces muscle hypertrophy through satellite cell proliferation and inhibiton of myostain and activin. Am J Physiol Endocrinol Metab 2009;297:E157–64.
39. Nakamura N, Shino K, Natsuume T, et al. Early biological effect of in vivo gene transfer of platelet-derived growth factor (PDGF)-B into healing patellar ligament. Gene Ther 1998;5(9):1165–70.
40. Efthimiadou A, Asimakopoulos B, Nikolettos N, et al. Angiogenic effect of intramuscular administration of basic and acidic fibroblast growth factor on skeletal muscles and influence of exercise on muscle angiogenesis. Br J Sports Med 2006;40(1):35–9.
41. Efthimiadou A, Nikolettos NK, Lambropoulou M, et al. Angiogenic effect of intramuscular administration of basic fibroblast growth factor in atrophied muscles: an experimental study in the rat. Br J Sports Med 2006;40(4):355–8.
42. Baumgartner I, Pieczek A, Manor O, et al. Constitutive expression of phVEGF165 after intramuscular gene transfer promotes collateral vessel development in patients with critical limb ischemia. Circulation 1998;97(12):1114–23.
43. Kim HJ, Jang SY, Park JI, et al. Vascular endothelial growth factor-induced angiogenic gene therapy in patients with peripheral artery disease. Exp Mol Med 2004; 36(4):336–44.
44. Arsic N, Zacchigna S, Zentilin L, et al. Vascular endothelial growth factor stimulates skeletal muscle regeneration in vivo. Mol Ther 2004;10(5):844–54.
45. Goldspink DF, Goldspink G. Age-related changes in protein turnover and ribonucleic acid of the diaphragm muscle of normal and a dystrophic hamsters. Biochem J 1977;162:191–4.
46. Sacheck JM, Ohtsuka A, McLary SC, et al. IGF-I stimulates muscle growth by suppressing protein breakdown and expression of atrophy-related ubiquitin ligases, atrogin-1 and MuRF1. Am J Physiol Endocrinol Metab 2004;287: E591–601.
47. Kay RG, Barton C, Velloso CP, et al. High-throughput ultra-high-performance liquid chromatography/tandem mass spectrometry quantitation of insulin-like growth factor-I and leucine-rich alpha-2-glycoprotein in serum as biomarkers of recombinant human growth hormone administration. Rapid Commun Mass Spectrom 2009;23:1–10.
48. Velloso CP, Harridge SDR, Bouloux P, et al. Cultured muscle cells as a system for analysis of IGF-I splicing regulation by factors present in the circulation [abstract from Nottingham meeting of the British Physiological Society]. J Physiol 2004; 558:C5.

Training Modalities: Impact on Endurance Capacity

Martin Flueck, PhD*, Wouter Eilers, MSc

KEYWORDS

- Exercise • Muscle • Mitochondria • Efficiency
- Economy • Gene

Endurance athletes are characterized by a high economy of power output during muscle work. This functional capacity is conditioned by high volumes of exercises that are graded with regard to seasonal planning in different intensity zones. This article addresses the basic biologic principles underlying adjustments of aerobic power output to commonly used training schemes and modes of action of complementary training. A special focus is laid on the implication of genomic mechanisms in the to nature and nurture of the metabolic trait of endurance performance.

BIOENERGETICS OF MUSCLE ACTION

Exercise duration is critically limited by the intensity required to perform a motor task. High power output (>400 W), which is sufficient to accelerate body weight maximally during a sprint, can only be maintained for a few seconds (**Fig. 1**).[1] Continuing exercise beyond a minute is typically accompanied by an approximately 6-fold reduction of power output.

The decline in maximal muscle power with increasing duration of exercise reflects flux rates and delayed activation of the metabolic pathways that fuel muscle contraction (**Fig. 2A**). Maximal muscle activity can only be maintained for a few seconds because the internal energy stores of creatine phosphate are depleted. This high-energy phosphate constitutes the main energy source for the conformation change of myosin molecules that drives the power stroke that shortens muscle fibers on

This work was supported by a start-up grant from Manchester Metropolitan University.
Disclaimer: The presented concepts may not necessarily reflect the consensus in the field and may be limited by the general lack of knowledge on the adaptive mechanism in the professional athlete. Due to restrictions in space, not all relevant literature can be addressed in the context of the article.
Institute for Biomedical Research into Human Movement and Health, Manchester Metropolitan University, Oxford Road, Manchester M1 5GD, UK
* Corresponding author.
E-mail address: m.flueck@mmu.ac.uk (M. Flueck).

Endocrinol Metab Clin N Am 39 (2010) 183–200
doi:10.1016/j.ecl.2009.10.002
0889-8529/10/$ – see front matter © 2010 Elsevier Inc. All rights reserved.

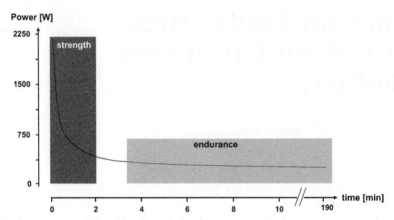

Fig. 1. Bioenergetic relationship. The relation between maximal power output and sustainable time. The highlighted zones reflect those typically assigned to strength and endurance sports. The hyperbolic fit is based on the equation Power $= E + A/t - E \times T [exp - (t/T)]$.

neuronal activation. This high-energy phosphate must be recharged through the synthesis of adenosine triphosphate (ATP) to cover the metabolic cost of the processes associated with fiber contraction and to allow muscle action to continue.[2]

The energy for this recharging is provided by the induced production of ATP through the conversion of the organic substrates glucose and lipids and derived free fatty acids stores.[3] An aerobic and anaerobic biochemical pathway of energy provision can be distinguished with regard to their efficiency and economy of ATP synthesis. Shortly after onset of contraction, the anaerobic conversion of glucose in the sarcoplasma covers most energy demands. This mode of ATP production by glycolytic conversion of glucose into pyruvate is very powerful but is limited by substrate supply and can only produce a limited number of ATPs per split glucose molecule (ie, 2 ATPs per glucose). This energy deficit is compensated by an increase in the abundance of myocellular glucose through contraction-induced elevations of blood flow and substrate import and the delayed elevation of mitochondrial respiration in contracting muscle fibers.[2,4] This latter process enables the oxidative conversion of pyruvate-derived acetyl coenzyme A in mitochondria, which increases the number of ATP molecules being produced per converted glucose to 36.[5] Mitochondrial oxidation of glucose alone, however, cannot cover the energy demands when exercise is continued beyond a few minutes. Concurrently the more economical but slower conversion of imported fatty acid via beta oxidation and the Krebs cycle in mitochondria comes into play. This mode of combustion delivers a considerably larger amount of ATP per fatty acid molecule (ie, 131 ATPs per palmitate; see **Fig. 2**A). Henceforth, the oxidation of pyruvate and fatty acids is the preferred metabolic pathway for exercise activities for which economic energy production becomes a priority because mechanical output needs to be maintained for a prolonged period of time (see **Fig. 2**B).[1,6]

Fatty acid combustion, however, does not occur at a very high rate and is limited by oxygen diffusion at high metabolic demand. Therefore, when oxygen tension is reduced at high intensity of exercise, the conversion of glucose-derived pyruvate in mitochondria is circumvented via sarcoplasmic fermentation to produce 2 additional ATP molecules and the byproduct lactate, with a debated inhibitory role in muscle contraction.[7] Full capacity of these energy pathways relies on the cardiovascular system and is driven by oxygen uptake via lung ventilation.[5] With prolonged duration

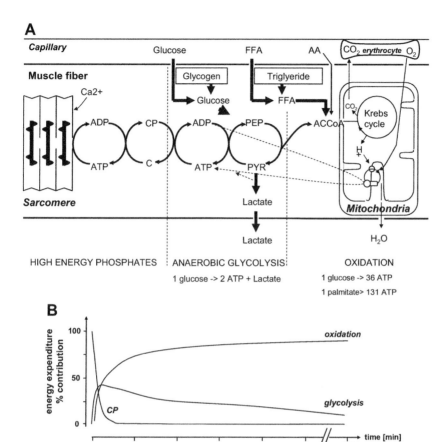

Fig. 2. Metabolic pathways of muscle work. (*A*) Main metabolic pathways that fuel muscle contraction by the conversion of organic substrates. (*B*) Quantitative contribution of aerobic and anaerobic metabolic pathways to time-dependent maximal power output based on previous modeling. AA, amino acid; ADP, adenosine diphosphate; C, creatine; CP, creatine phosphate; FFA, free fatty acid; PEP, phosphoenolpyruvate; PYR, pyruvate. (*Data from* Beneke R, Boning D. The limits of human performance. Essays Biochem 2008;44:11.)

of muscle work, an increasing role is assigned to the buffering and elimination of wasteful metabolic products and substrate supply from intramuscular, hepatic, and adipose stores to prevent fatigue.[1,3,5,8–10]

DESIGN OF THE ENDURANCE ATHLETE

The bioenergetic relationships between muscle power and time set the maxima in muscle-dependent exercise performance (**Fig. 3**). In this complex equation, a high aerobic power output and a large capacity for the containment of waste products are the main variables that characterize exceptional endurance. This is largely explained by an elevated capacity of the shared components of the aerobic pathway of energy provision in mitochondria as it is measurable through maximal oxygen uptake, Vo_2max.[11] The high oxygen/substrate transport capacity is primarily driven via the cardiovascular system and a high capillary and mitochondrial density in

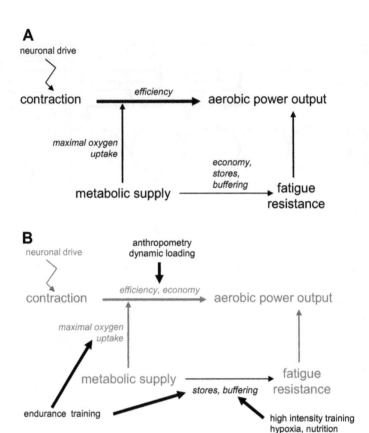

Fig. 3. Principal factors of endurance capacity. (*A*) Main factors that determine endurance performance. (*B*) Points of influence of training interventions for the tuning of endurance performance.

locomotor muscle.[12] Muscle makeup reflects these relationships. Whereas the typical muscle fiber of endurance athletes is surrounded by up to 2.7 capillaries per muscle and contains 11% of mitochondria and 2% of lipid stores, these percentages are significantly lower in untrained populations, which demonstrate larger volumes of fat outside muscle fibers.[13,14]

A main consideration regarding energy expenditure during exercise is that the metabolic cost of muscle work is 3 to 5 times larger than the actual external work being performed. Improvements in the biomechanical efficiency of locomotion are thus of prime importance for the endurance athlete. This view is supported by the measures of power output or velocity of locomotion for a given metabolic cost. Elevations of both parameters of biomechanical efficiency essentially contribute to the superior endurance performance of champions.[7,15] Biochemical efficiency shows a strong association with distance running performance[16] and relates to the content of slow muscle fiber types,[17] which contract more economically than fast-twitch fibers during the normal frequencies of movement.[18] In addition, architectural factors of muscle fibers and the muscle-tendon complex determine muscle force and power.[19] This is indicated by the association of short moment arms of the Achilles tendon and the economy of running in elite endurance athletes.[20] This highlights the fact that the optimization of endurance performance reflects the integrated amelioration of the economy of the power stroke and the efficiency of its conversion into propulsion.

This specialization of economic pathways in endurance athletes is different from the differentiation of muscular features associated with a strength phenotype. This difference is illustrated in decathletes who excel in speed and throwing or endurance disciplines but not both.[21] The allocation trade-offs in the optimization of endurance and force can be explained by the fact that these 2 properties show an inverse relationship with regard to body mass. Endurance capacity is reduced with increasing body mass because of the elevated metabolic cost of moving larger masses. By contrast, strength increases with elevated muscle mass because it is proportional to the cross-sectional area of muscle. This relationship has its foundation in the construction plan of muscle fibers, in which the contractile motor (the sarcomere) and the main cellular powerhouse (mitochondria) are all contained within the same fiber (see **Fig. 2**A). Consequently, mitochondrial content that sets oxygen uptake and sarcomere number that determines muscle force cannot be jointly improved in muscle without affecting body mass. This is a disadvantage for running events over longer distances, owing to elevated overall metabolic cost with the augmented body weight. This is also reflected in the observation that the size of muscle fibers is reduced in marathon runners concomitantly with an increase in specific power.[22]

CONDITIONING OF ENDURANCE PERFORMANCE

Exercise performance is not fixed but specifically tailored by functional demand.[23] This is illustrated by the sizable improvements of aerobic capacity and power output in previously untrained subjects[12,24] after a training program that lasts for only a few weeks. The adaptations, which amount in the order of 40%, involve the remodeling in skeletal muscle and the cardiovascular system.

This plasticity involves increases in the capacity of the biochemical pathways underlying aerobic energy production (see **Fig. 3**). This includes elevations of the volume percentage of mitochondria and capillarity. These adjustments optimize diffusion distances and capacities for oxidative conversion of blood-derived substrates and elimination of waste products, which becomes increasingly important when exercising for extended duration.[10] The maximal achievement in aerobic capacity is strongly reliant on the lung because this respiratory organ limits oxygenation of red blood cells but shows no apparent plasticity.[11]

At the cardiovascular level, advancement in performance with exercise involves modified hemodynamics via elevated stroke volume and improved perfusion through an increased surface of the vascular tree and the antihypertensive effect of exercise.[25,26] Thus the metabolic adjustments to endurance training reflect an integrated compensatory response of the elements that set aerobic capacity. These adjustments are graded with respect to the repetition number (volume) of contractions and distinguish to the effects of mechanical loading.[23,27] Highly repetitive, low-load forms of training (typical 500–10,000 contractions at 200–300 W in endurance events) mainly increase the capacity of metabolic pathways.[28] By contrast, high-load, less-repetitive type of contractions (typically 5–10 contractions at 800–2000 W) elevate muscle power by promoting muscle fiber growth via sarcomere addition.[23] Consequently, opposing biologic strategies explain the conditioning of muscles working at the opposite extremes of the power continuum during short-term strength or endurance type of exercise.

The nurture-dependent specialization of (aerobic) muscle function is rapidly reversed when training is stopped. The activity of several mitochondrial proteins in muscle is halved when training is discontinued for 2 weeks.[25,29] This is accompanied by a decline in stroke volume and Vo_2max.[30] By contrast, muscle capillarization and sarcomere content are stable for up to 4 weeks of detraining before they start to deteriorate. Consequently, Vo_2max declines and becomes manifest as an important reduction in aerobic performance in the endurance athlete.[31] However, Vo_2max remains higher compared with untrained subjects even after 84 days of detraining. Thus the relationships between the occupational stimulus of exercise and muscle oxidative capacity set the window under which endurance performance is maintained in a steady state during periods of rest.

FINE-TUNING FATIGUE RESISTANCE

Training adaptations are driven by cycles of fatigue and recovery after exercise (**Fig. 4**). Accordingly, the elevated amounts and activity of metabolic proteins and organelles are the results of an increase in protein production during the recovery phase from each bout of exercise.[32,33] The accumulation of the surplus with repetition of exercise would explain the improved myocellular capacity for aerobic metabolism in a training steady state.[34]

The recommended training volume to achieve a physiologic effect in the healthy is at least 30 min/d, 3 to 5 d/wk for 4 to 8 weeks.[35] Such endurance work for just thirty 30-minute sessions at high intensity (65% of peak aerobic power output or 85% of maximal heart rate) on a bicycle ergometer improves system parameters of aerobic capacity in previously untrained subjects (Vo_2max approximately 40 mL O_2/min/kg). This concerns a 14% elevation of Vo_2max and an increase in maximal maintained power by 33%, which relates to a relatively larger increase in the volume density of total mitochondria (+40%).[12,28] The induced mitochondrial biogenesis raises the volume percentage of mitochondria in muscle fibers of recruited muscle groups to 4% to 6% in proportion with gains in aerobic performance.[34,36]

The sites of aerobic metabolism that show plasticity to exercise are, however, not confined to muscle alone. The site of adaptation depends on whether muscular (local) or cardiovascular (central) factors constitute 'bottlenecks' of performance.[37] Remodeling can thus concern any step upstream of mitochondria and downstream to the lung that may represent a bottleneck for maximal oxygen uptake.[38]

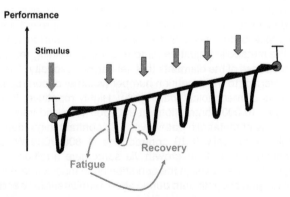

Fig. 4. Exercise-induced microadaptations explain training effect. Cycles of fatigue and recovery after an exercise stimulus drive improvement of aerobic performance with repetition of exercise during training.

The local adjustments of oxidative capacity are graded with regard to exercise intensity, whereby training at lower intensity induces more moderate adjustments.[36] The synopsis of training effects implies that the pace of adaptation in bulk mitochondrial protein is highest in the recently trained and amounts to approximately 1% per session. Higher volumetric increases of the myocellular powerhouse have been seen in endurance athletes after years of training, taking volume density to an incredible 11%.[13]

Consequently, the processes involved in the production of aerobic power output improve best with intense exercise.[7] Typically these adaptations are noted when training intensity or volume is sizably increased. Examples for fine-tuning include elevations of capillary density/capillary-to-fiber ratio and running economy.[7,39,40] Extra adjustment of aerobic metabolism is supported by the decoupled increases in maximal oxygen uptake and fatigue resistance with exercise regimes that enhance metabolic stress during exercise because of reduction of inspired oxygen.[41] Thus endurance performance may be enhanced by targeting the training interventions to those elements of metabolic flux and biomechanics that limit aerobic power output in a particular subject.

The physiologic parameters setting endurance capacity also come into play, to a varying degree, in different sports disciplines. For instance, in marathon runners who perform at a lower percentage of $V_{O_2}max$ (85%) than 1.5- to 10-km runners (95%–100%), exceptional lung function is not possibly the main variable for high capacity.[7] Rather, improvements in metabolic enzymes and elimination of waste products via capillary become increasingly important.[5,10] In addition, modified biomechanical efficiency and the economy of movement may essentially contribute to the capacity to excel in competition, as shown in the case of the current female world record holder in marathon.[7] This possibly reflects the increased capacity of storage and release of elastic energy by increasing the stiffness of the muscles and tendons with running and more efficient mechanics leading to less energy wasted on braking forces and excessive vertical oscillation.[16] The destruction or transfer of energy toward the ground during this form of exercise puts higher mechanical stress on the musculoskeletal system than bicycling exercise, which is the common reference for studying endurance-type exercise.

TUNING OF ENDURANCE PERFORMANCE

The adaptive capacity of human performance is exploited by athletes and their coaches in specific training cycles that meet discipline-specific requirements. The training protocols used by athletes who have achieved their maxima after years of training are pronouncedly different from those of beginners who have elevated their endurance performance with a few weeks of training.[24] The well-trained population is used to working out at higher loads and volumes and prioritizes the training plan because of imposed periods of competition. Because adaptation to exercise fades as a result of the repetition effect, it is also important for the athlete to maximize the adaptive stimulus and compensation phase to maintain and optimize performance.

The commonly used training interventions can be grouped with regard to their effects on the main components of endurance sports: aerobic capacity, resistance to fatigue, biomechanical efficiency, and economy (**Table 1**). Aerobic capacity is mainly improved by endurance exercise at moderate-to-high intensity for 30 minutes and more. This is mediated by targeting aerobic metabolism comprised by mitochondrial biogenesis, fat oxidation, and angiogenesis. Resistance to fatigue is typically addressed with extensive exercise for durations between 1 and 3 hours. Interventions

Table 1
Training schemes of endurance athletes

Complement of Endurance Exercise	Training Intensity	Training Duration	Features	Specificity of Improvement	References
Moderate intensity training	60%–70% peak power output	5 × 30 min/wk for 6 wk	Aerobic metabolism Performance enhancement		12,36,42
Polarized training (extended low intensity zone)	Ventilatory threshold, running	5 mo	Performance enhancement		43
High intensity training	≥80% peak power output, 150% leg Vo_2max	4 wk	Performance enhancement Blood flow capacity Peak oxygen uptake	Vascular tree	39,44,45
Hypoxia during exercise Living low-training high	Anaerobic threshold "High intensity"	6 wk	Anaerobic enzymes, myoglobin Performance enhancement	Muscle	46
Hypoxia during exercise Living high-training low	Anaerobic threshold "High intensity"	4 wk	Hematocrit Performance enhancement	Erythrocyte	47
Strength training	Supramaximal	9 wk	Power output, efficiency	Neuromuscular?	48
Eccentric contractions	54%–65% peak heart rate	8 wk	Power output damage protection	Muscle	49
Plyometric training	Supramaximal	3 × 30 min/wk for 9 wk	Efficiency	Muscle, tendon?	50
Passive intervention					
Fasting before exercise			Lipolysis	Muscle	51

Studies with well-trained participants were included in the table.
Training intensities are described from the perspective of aerobic power production.

that improve biomechanical efficiency and economy are constantly sought after by athletes, coaches, and sport scientists. High-intensity training (HIT) over periods of weeks is believed to be important for the improvement of biomechanical efficiency.[7,15] A training modality that is known to specifically improve this aspect in already highly trained athletes is HIT/supramaximal intermittent exercise.[24,52] This intervention comprises short bouts of exercise at high intensity, that is, typically 4- to 5-minute sessions at 80% to 85% of peak aerobic power output. Six HIT sessions may be suffi-cient to increase peak work rate and exercise speed in competitive cyclists.[35] Alterna-tively, when the amount of training is significantly reduced, HIT may allow the maintenance of muscle oxidative capacity in already trained individuals.[53]

Simultaneous explosive-strength and endurance training is another complement that has been shown to improve the running time in well-trained endurance athletes through elevations in running economy.[48] This observation contrasts with the general belief that the incorporation of a high-strength component has to reflect sport-specific muscle coordination to allow a positive transfer into propulsion.[54]

Because maximal performance cannot be maintained over a full season, the training protocols of the endurance athlete involve macro- and microcycles of preparation that are targeted to ameliorate the various aspects that govern sport-specific maximal velocity for competition. This comprises high-intensity or high-volume training to build up specific performance in the preparative macrocycles before discipline-specific endurance capacity is acquired, and training volume is cut to maximize the body's physical and mental constitution before competition (**Fig. 5**).

The optimal reduction or taper in intense training to recover from exhaustive exercise before a competition is poorly understood. Progressive rather than abrupt reduction of training volume during taper was shown to elevate endurance performance in competition.[24] Several studies document the effectiveness of including an exercise protocol with highly intense activity at reduced volumes in the taper phase.[24,55] This is pointed out by small but significant gains in performance during the pre-event taper across a number of sports.[24] The ameliorations are associated with integrated responses of the cardiorespiratory, metabolic, hormonal, neuromuscular, and psychological systems that restore previously impaired physiologic capacities and the capacity to tolerate training.

A related aspect in training protocols is the polarization of the stimulus and recovery phases.[43] For instance, the increase of the percentage of training in low-intensity

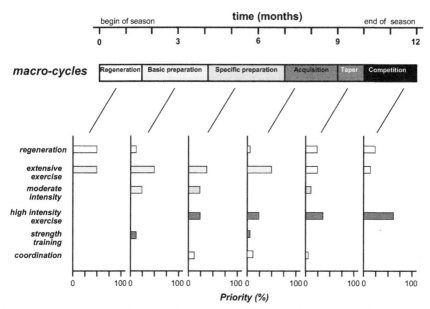

Fig. 5. Staging of training protocols during seasonal macrocycles. An example of periodizing an endurance training program. The whole training effort during multiple macrocycles is directed toward achieving maximum performance during a competition phase at the end of season. (*Bottom*) Bar graphs visualizing the priorities put on the conditioning of the features of the endurance phenotype during each macrocycle.

zones with maintained high-intensity phases can improve performance more than when maintaining a higher percentage of moderate-intensity exercise. Probably this is effective by optimizing the recovery from intense exercise, which is believed to be the key to supercompensation. Equally, regenerative measures such as massages or sauna are an essential part of the successful recovery from high loads of intense exercise activities.

Within the past decade, several physical and nutritional complements that enhance the exercise stimulus to skeletal muscle have been developed, but these are probably not major part of current training schemes of the athlete. One intervention that was shown to improve endurance capacity involves the reduction in the oxygen content of inspired air (hypoxia). Two protocols that distinguish whether hypoxia is added at rest or during exercise are in use. The passive exposure to hypoxia while continuing training at lower altitude levels (living high-training low) for several weeks elevates maximal oxygen uptake via increasing erythrocyte mass.[56] By contrast, living low-training high can improve fatigue resistance in well-trained endurance athletes at high altitude and variably at sea level.[42,46] This is related to the tighter coupling of creatine phosphate replenishment[57] and elevated buffer capacity.[58] Such tuning of the metabolic machinery is the possible consequence of compensation forced by the elevated metabolic stress with increased muscle deoxygenation during exercise. Thus the living high-training low and living low-training high approaches offer complementary ways to improve metabolic flux during endurance exercise by modifying the compartment that demonstrates plasticity.

Because effects are not always observed after training high-living low in the highly trained,[47,59] an important role of the training circumstances is indicated. Accordingly, the lack of effect in some studies may be related to the integration of a hypoxia protocol at the end of a season when the regenerative potential is exhausted or to not cutting the overall training load, as was the case in successful protocols.[41] The consequently reduced absolute intensity (velocity) of exercise under reduced oxygenation may not have been sufficiently high to maintain biochemical economy.

PASSIVE AFFECTION OF ENDURANCE PERFORMANCE

Apart from physical interventions, nutritional interventions are the best-understood passive manipulations of endurance capacity. Their effect is mediated by affecting fuel supply via the alteration of substrate concentration in intramuscular, hepatic, and adipose stores. The use of dietary supplements is based on the early work showing supercompensation of muscular glycogen stores by the combination of carbohydrate diet and exercise.[60] Less common are new applications that support the benefits of a fat-rich diet for ultra endurance events, for which moderately intense exercise is the norm.[61] This is mediated via an increased capacity for the amount of fat oxidation during exercise despite concomitantly reduced glucose oxidation.[62] The role of nutrition as a possible modulator of aerobic metabolism in muscle is highlighted by the changes in substrate use induced by fasting.[51] This includes the upregulation of negative regulators of mitochondrial oxidation of pyruvate, with a concomitant elevation of fatty acid conversion in mitochondria. This raises the possibility that training in the fasting state (in contrast to the earlier belief) can promote the capacity for fatty acid consumption, which is a key determinant in ultra endurance events.

The reduced pace in world record accretion with increased antidoping controls implies that the excellence in human exercise performance cannot solely be explained by training.[63] This is supported by the increasing medical surveys and public exposure of certain athletes as doping victims.[64] The implication of pharmaceutical complements in the exceptional endurance performance of modern times is illustrated by published doping practices.[65] These comment on the hazardous combination of stimulants in some elite cyclists. The list includes hormones with well-known effects on red blood cell count (Epo[66]), lipolysis (human growth hormone[67]), general arousal (cortisol), and muscle anabolism (testosterone). These agents influence the hormonal axes, which are restored with taper.[24,55] This observation supports the fact that the efficiency of doping practices lies in the circumvention of biologic mechanisms that reduce stamina to protect against the consequences of heavy exercise loads. Because the doping agents mentioned earlier are consumed without altering the co-variables of exercise-induced stress, serious health risks are to be expected from turning off these physiologic safety mechanisms.[68]

EXPOSING THE MECHANISM OF ENDURANCE TRAINING

Most training protocols used by athletes reflect heuristic approaches without in-depth knowledge of the underlying physiologic mechanisms. Although numerous reference points are applied for selecting the intensities of training sessions (Umberg R, personal communication, 2004), the optimal dosage to promote performance is not known before long training intervals have elapsed. Even then, the improvements in perfor-mance after months of training are in the order of a small percentage[35] and therefore hard to quantify in field test. Best preparation becomes, however, increasingly critical to excel at the highest level. This is particularly indicated considering that there is a plateau in world record performance in endurance sports.[63]

A clear understanding of the adaptive process to a training stimulus would allow the tailoring of exercise regimes for individual sports persons. Data gleaned through the recent introduction of biochemical and molecular biologic technology into sports biology indicate that the orchestration of muscle remodeling by exercise can be exposed by molecular diagnostics of muscle biopsies. This view is based on the acti-vation of the building plan for mitochondrial biogenesis after the repeated impact of exercise. This mechanism involves the retrieval (expression) of genomic information via the production of diffusible gene messengers (transcripts) and their translation into protein on physiologic stimulation (**Fig. 6**A).

The implication of gene expression in feed-forward control of aerobic muscle perfor-mance is visualized by the augmentation of the template (transcript) levels and synthesis rates of several mitochondrial proteins during the first 24 hours of recovery from an endurance workout.[28,32] These concomitant changes indicate that control of mitochondrial biogenesis after exercise is coordinated by the simultaneous control at the levels of both gene transcription and translation.[32,33] The microadaptation of mito-chondrial proteins to consecutive bouts of exercise results in a gradual accumulation of mitochondrial content per volume of muscle fiber.[34] Therefore, feed-forward control of muscle performance through exercise-induced biogenesis of the mitochondrial organelle is reflected at the level of gene expression.

The recent characterization of all expressed muscle transcripts (ie, the muscle tran-scriptome) with high-throughput technology demonstrates that several metabolic pathways are regulated by single and repeated endurance exercise.[28,69,70] The broad response involves elements of those metabolic pathways that maximize oxidative metabolism (see **Fig. 2**A). This includes increased levels of transcripts of dozens of factors involved in aerobic metabolization of glucose-derived pyruvate and fatty acids in mitochondria.[69,71] This regulation reflects that biochemical pathways represent the functional interaction of multiple proteins in complexes and cell organelles. Regulation of metabolic pathways is also specific as shown by the marginal effect of endurance

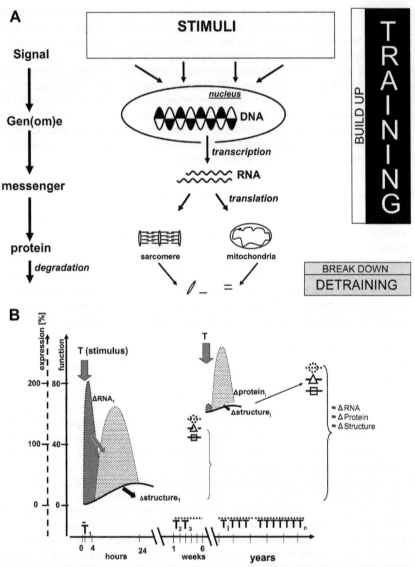

Fig. 6. Expression reprogramming reflects exercise-induced muscle remodeling. (*A*) Paradigm of gene expression. Connected steps of gene expression underlying the buildup of muscle organelles with the impact of the physiologic stimulus of training and their breakdown during detraining. (*B*) The implication of gene expression in control of local oxidative capacity. Transient upregulation of gene transcripts and translation on exercise increases mitochondrial content (structure) by instructing mitochondrial biogenesis during recovery from exercise. The enhancement of local oxidative capacity in a training steady state is evident through corresponding elevations of transcripts, protein, and structure of mitochondria. The implication of mitochondrial transcript expression (but not protein translation) in exercise-induced mitochondrial turnover is reduced in a training state.

exercise on protein synthesis for myofibrillar factors.[28,32] Thus the increased aerobic capacity of muscle with endurance training has its foundation in the concerted regulation of multiple pathways during the recovery phase from exercise.

The genome-dependent response to exercise also provides a rationale for the attenuation of the adaptive scope with increased muscle performance.[12,72] This is indicated through the blunting of the transcript response in vastus lateralis muscle to intense exercise after endurance training[28] but when mitochondrial protein synthesis is still increased[32] (**Fig. 6**B). This implies that posttranslational regulation of this trait of aerobic performance becomes increasingly important in a trained state.

This dampened exercise responsiveness by training relates to the observation that the levels of templates for multiple enzymes of the pathways fueling aerobic substrate conversion in mitochondria are elevated in an endurance-trained state. This concerns transcript levels of the factors involved in mobilization of free fatty acids, pyruvate import, beta oxidation, Krebs cycle, and oxidative phosphorylation, the basal augmentation of which corresponds in skeletal muscle to structural correlates of aerobic metabolism.[28,34,69,71] This suggests that the pronounced role of protein translation after the repetition of an exercise stimulus reflects the new steady state between transcript decay and synthesis rates.

The desensitization of transcript expression to exercise in a trained state is related to the lowered response of oxidative metabolism with training.[34] For instance, mitochondrial density is considerably elevated by just 30 exercise sessions of endurance training in the previously untrained (from 4% to 6%) but years of training are necessary to induce another such increase to 8%.[59,60] This becomes apparent through the comparison of the increases in steady-state transcript levels for oxidative metabolism between recently trained subjects and athletes who continued training for years.[69,71] This comparison reveals that the upregulation of the transcripts of aerobic metabolism in the untrained after 6 weeks of endurance training is virtually identical to the permanent transcript upregulation after years of training (ie, mean increase of 128% vs 80%).[28,69] This view is supported by the observation that the inclusion of 6 weeks of intermittent type of high-intensity endurance training provokes little changes in transcript levels of the vastus lateralis muscle of well-trained runners.[42] The dampened responsiveness possibly reflects increased turnover in athletic individuals because these have arrived at the maxima of possible structural malleability of fuel supply in muscle after years of hard training and competition.

Accordingly, the measure of gene expression allows conclusions on the pace and mode of adaptation of metabolic pathways to single exercise and its repetition in training. The further improvement in endurance performance with continuation of intense training must, therefore, be related to remodeling of auxiliary components of endurance phenotype associated with biomechanical efficiency and fatigue resistance.

Molecular biologic diagnostics also bolsters the specificity/effectiveness of recently introduced training complements. For instance, transcript measures demonstrate that expression reprogramming of glucose import, mitochondrial hydration of carbon dioxide, and lactate elimination correlates with improvements in time to exhaustion in a treadmill test under the training high-living low protocol.[42,73] These adjustments are possibly related to the gain in importance of glycolysis and waste elimination with prolonged work under reduced arterial oxygenation.

FACTORS CONTRIBUTING TO WORLD EXCELLENCE

The modeling of world records illustrates that both endurance- and strength-type disciplines have improved in a piecewise manner over the 111 years since the reintroduction of the Olympic games.[63] Historical events, together with improved preparation and training methods, may have worked synergistically to shape the pattern of human performance improvement.

There is increasing evidence that the athletic excellence of champions is mediated by a unique combination of nature and nurture of the power lines of muscle work.[74] Natural (ie, intrinsic and possible genetic) factors are now known to contribute to the exceptional achievements of both endurance and strength performances of Olympic athletes.[74–77] This is exposed through the association of genetic modifications of a few master regulators of oxidative metabolism with the exceptional phenotype of Olympic athletes. For instance, functionally important mutations in the receptor for the blood hormone erythropoietin, which enhances oxidative capacity by elevating hematocrit, were identified as a key factor of the exceptional stamina of a triple Olympic champion.[78] Also, distinct mitochondrial haplotypes influence the elite endurance status in Kenyan athletes.[77] Finally, it was recently demonstrated that an elevated proportion of gene mutations in transcriptional regulators of oxidative metabolism and slow muscle fiber type is associated with endurance status in Russian athletes compared with control populations.[75] These correspondences support the fact that permanent modification of single master steps of the biomechanical economy of movement contributes importantly to the shaping of the endurance phenotype.

SUMMARY

The exceptional performance of endurance athletes is under feed-forward control by use-related stimuli through the interaction of the environment with genomic mechanisms. Athletes boost their performance by forcing compensation of the power lines of muscle work with various forms of training. The adaptive mechanism distinguishes the training response between untrained and trained populations. The data support the view that untrained individuals gain endurance mainly by building up local and cardiovascular capacity for oxidative metabolism. Competitive athletes refine these adjustments of mitochondrial pathways in muscle through hard work and show critical improvements in the efficiency of prolonged muscle work through understudied metabolic and biomechanical processes. New observations imply that the incorporation of exercise complements in training macrocycles offers means to overcome specific bottlenecks in traits of muscle performance. Functional relationships between muscle performance and gene expression subsequent to exercise indicate the feasibility of using expression profiling to tailor training paradigms to the individual endurance athlete.

REFERENCES

1. Beneke R, Boning D. The limits of human performance. Essays Biochem 2008;44:11.
2. Greenhaff PL, Timmons JA. Pyruvate dehydrogenase complex activation status and acetyl group availability as a site of interchange between anaerobic and oxidative metabolism during intense exercise. Adv Exp Med Biol 1998;441:287.
3. Jeukendrup AE. Modulation of carbohydrate and fat utilization by diet, exercise and environment. Biochem Soc Trans 2003;31:1270.
4. Clifford PS, Hellsten Y. Vasodilatory mechanisms in contracting skeletal muscle. J Appl Phys 2004;97:393.
5. Weibel ER. Powerlines for muscle work: functional limits and structural design in the oxygen and fuel pathways. Med Sci Sports Exerc 2002;34:136.

6. Romijn JA, Coyle EF, Sidossis LS, et al. Regulation of endogenous fat and carbo-hydrate metabolism in relation to exercise intensity and duration. Am J Phys 1993;265:E380.
7. Joyner MJ, Coyle EF. Endurance exercise performance: the physiology of champions. J Physiol 2008;586:35.
8. Oberholzer F, Claassen H, Moesch H, et al. [Ultrastructural, biochemical and energy analysis of extreme duration performance (100km run)]. Schweiz Z Sportmed 1976; 24:71 [in German].
9. Sherman WM, Costill DL. The marathon: dietary manipulation to optimize performance. Am J Sports Med 1984;12:44.
10. Sjogaard G. Muscle morphology and metabolic potential in elite road cyclists during a season. Int J Sports Med 1984;5:250.
11. di Prampero PE. Factors limiting maximal performance in humans. Eur J Appl Physiol 2003;90:420.
12. Hoppeler H, Howald H, Conley K, et al. Endurance training in humans: aerobic capacity and structure of skeletal muscle. J Appl Phys 1985;59:320.
13. Hoppeler H. Exercise-induced ultrastructural changes in skeletal muscle. Int J Sports Med 1986;7:187.
14. Kayar SR, Hoppeler H, Howald H, et al. Acute effects of endurance exercise on mitochondrial distribution and skeletal muscle morphology. Eur J Appl Physiol Occup Physiol 1986;54:578.
15. Cavanagh PR, Kram R. Mechanical and muscular factors affecting the efficiency of human movement. Med Sci Sports Exerc 1985;17:326.
16. Saunders PU, Pyne DB, Telford RD, et al. Factors affecting running economy in trained distance runners. Sports Med 2004;34:465.
17. Coyle EF, Sidossis LS, Horowitz JF, et al. Cycling efficiency is related to the percentage of type I muscle fibers. Med Sci Sports Exerc 1992;24:782.
18. Fitts RH, Widrick JJ. Muscle mechanics: adaptations with exercise-training. Exerc Sport Sci Rev 1996;24:427.
19. Fitts RH, McDonald KS, Schluter JM. The determinants of skeletal muscle force and power: their adaptability with changes in activity pattern. J Biomech 1991; 24(Suppl 1):111.
20. Scholz M, Bobbert MF, van Soest AJ, et al. Running biomechanics: shorter heels, better economy. J Exp Biol 2008;211:6.
21. Van Damme R, Wilson RS, Vanhooydonck B, et al. Performance constraints in decathletes. Nature 2002;415:755.
22. Trappe S, Harber M, Creer A, et al. Single muscle fiber adaptations with marathon training. J Appl Phys 2006;101:721.
23. Fluck M, Hoppeler H. Molecular basis of skeletal muscle plasticity–from gene to form and function. Rev Physiol Biochem Pharmacol 2003;146:159.
24. Kubukeli ZN, Noakes TD, Dennis SC. Training techniques to improve endurance exercise performances. Sports Med 2002;32:489.
25. Coyle EF, Martin WH 3rd, Sinacore DR, et al. Time course of loss of adaptations after stopping prolonged intense endurance training. J Appl Phys 1857; 57:1984.
26. Meredith IT, Jennings GL, Esler MD, et al. Time-course of the antihypertensive and autonomic effects of regular endurance exercise in human subjects. J Hypertens 1990;8:859.
27. Wernbom M, Augustsson J, Thomee R. The influence of frequency, intensity, volume and mode of strength training on whole muscle cross-sectional area in humans. Sports Med 2007;37:225.

28. Schmutz S, Dapp C, Wittwer M, et al. Endurance training modulates the muscular transcriptome response to acute exercise. Pflugers Arch 2006;451:678.
29. Hickson RC, Rosenkoetter MA. Separate turnover of cytochrome c and myoglobin in the red types of skeletal muscle. Am J Phys 1981;241:C140.
30. Neufer PD. The effect of detraining and reduced training on the physiological adaptations to aerobic exercise training. Sports Med 1989;8:302.
31. Mujika I, Padilla S. Detraining: loss of training-induced physiological and performance adaptations. Part II: long term insufficient training stimulus. Sports Med 2000;30:145.
32. Wilkinson SB, Phillips SM, Atherton PJ, et al. Differential effects of resistance and endurance exercise in the fed state on signalling molecule phosphorylation and protein synthesis in human muscle. J Physiol 2008;586:3701.
33. Pilegaard H, Ordway GA, Saltin B, et al. Transcriptional regulation of gene expression in human skeletal muscle during recovery from exercise. Am J Physiol Endocrinol Metab 2000;279:E806.
34. Fluck M. Functional, structural and molecular plasticity of mammalian skeletal muscle in response to exercise stimuli. J Exp Biol 2006;209:2239.
35. Casaburi R. Principles of exercise training. Chest 1992;101:263S.
36. Suter E, Hoppeler H, Claassen H, et al. Ultrastructural modification of human skeletal muscle tissue with 6-month moderate-intensity exercise training. Int J Sports Med 1995;16:160.
37. McPhee JS, Williams AG, Stewart C, et al. The training stimulus experienced by the leg muscles during cycling in humans. Exp Physiol 2009;94:684.
38. Lindstedt SL, Wells DJ, Jones JH, et al. Limitations to aerobic performance in mammals: interaction of structure and demand. Int J Sports Med 1988;9:210.
39. Jensen L, Bangsbo J, Hellsten Y. Effect of high intensity training on capillarization and presence of angiogenic factors in human skeletal muscle. J Physiol 2004;557:12.
40. Laughlin MH, Roseguini B. Mechanisms for exercise training-induced increases in skeletal muscle blood flow capacity: differences with interval sprint training versus aerobic endurance training. J Physiol Pharmacol 2008;59(Suppl 7):71.
41. Dufour SP, Ponsot E, Zoll J, et al. Exercise training in normobaric hypoxia in endurance runners. I. Improvement in aerobic performance capacity. J Appl Phys 2006;100:1238.
42. Zoll J, Ponsot E, Dufour S, et al. Exercise training in normobaric hypoxia in endurance runners. III. Muscular adjustments of selected gene transcripts. J Appl Phys 2006;100:1258.
43. Esteve-Lanao J, Foster C, Seiler S, et al. Impact of training intensity distribution on performance in endurance athletes. J Strength Cond Res 2007;21:943.
44. Laursen PB, Jenkins DG. The scientific basis for high-intensity interval training: optimising training programmes and maximising performance in highly trained endurance athletes. Sports Med 2002;32:21.
45. Laursen PB, Shing CM, Peake JM, et al. Influence of high-intensity interval training on adaptations in well-trained cyclists. J Strength Cond Res 2005;19:7.
46. Hoppeler H, Klossner S, Vogt M. Training in hypoxia and its effects on skeletal muscle tissue. Scand J Med Sci Sports 2008;18(Suppl 1):38.
47. Stray-Gundersen J, Chapman RF, Levine BD. "Living high-training low" altitude training improves sea level performance in male and female elite runners. J Appl Phys 2001;91:8.
48. Paavolainen L, Hakkinen K, Hamalainen I, et al. Explosive-strength training improves 5-km running time by improving running economy and muscle power. J Appl Phys 1999;86:1527.

49. LaStayo PC, Pierotti DJ, Pifer J, et al. Eccentric ergometry: increases in locomotor muscle size and strength at low training intensities. Am J Physiol Regul Integr Comp Physiol 2000;278:R1282.
50. Saunders PU, Telford RD, Pyne DB, et al. Short-term plyometric training improves running economy in highly trained middle and long distance runners. J Strength Cond Res 2006;20:8.
51. Spriet LL, Tunstall RJ, Watt MJ, et al. Pyruvate dehydrogenase activation and kinase expression in human skeletal muscle during fasting. J Appl Phys 2004; 96:2082.
52. Billat LV. Interval training for performance: a scientific and empirical practice. Special recommendations for middle-and long-distance running. Part II: anaerobic interval training. Sports Med 2001;31:75.
53. Iaia FM, Hellsten Y, Nielsen JJ, et al. Four weeks of speed endurance training reduces energy expenditure during exercise and maintains muscle oxidative capacity despite a reduction in training volume. J Appl Phys 2009;106:73.
54. Tanaka H, Costill DL, Thomas R, et al. Dry-land resistance training for competitive swimming. Med Sci Sports Exerc 1993;25:952.
55. Mujika I, Padilla S, Pyne D, et al. Physiological changes associated with the pre-event taper in athletes. Sports Med 2004;34:891.
56. Saunders PU, Pyne D, Gore CJ. Endurance training at altitude. High Alt Med Biol 2009;10:14.
57. Ponsot E, Dufour SP, Zoll J, et al. Exercise training in normobaric hypoxia in endurance runners. II. Improvement of mitochondrial properties in skeletal muscle. J Appl Phys 2006;100:1249.
58. Mizuno M, Juel C, Bro-Rasmussen T, et al. Limb skeletal muscle adaptation in athletes after training at altitude. J Appl Phys 1990;68:496.
59. Ventura N, Hoppeler H, Seiler R, et al. The response of trained athletes to six weeks of endurance training in hypoxia or normoxia. Int J Sports Med 2003; 24:166.
60. Bergstrom J, Hermansen L, Hultman E, et al. Diet, muscle glycogen and physical performance. Acta Physiol Scand 1967;71:140.
61. Knechtle B, Boutellier U. [Nutrition in long physical endurance events]. Praxis (Bern 1994) 2000;89:2051 [in German].
62. Helge JW. Adaptation to a fat-rich diet: effects on endurance performance in humans. Sports Med 2000;30:347.
63. Berthelot G, Thibault V, Tafflet M, et al. The citius end: world records progression announces the completion of a brief ultra-physiological quest. PLoS One 2008;3: e1552.
64. Baker JS, Graham MR, Davies B. Steroid and prescription medicine abuse in the health and fitness community: a regional study. Eur J Intern Med 2006; 17:479.
65. Wagner EN. Wahnsinnige kriminelle Energie. Neue Zuercher Zeitung am Sonntag:1, 2006 [in German].
66. Lundby C, Thomsen JJ, Boushel R, et al. Erythropoietin treatment elevates haemoglobin concentration by increasing red cell volume and depressing plasma volume. J Physiol 2007;578:309.
67. Trepp R, Fluck M, Stettler C, et al. Effect of GH on human skeletal muscle lipid metabolism in GH deficiency. Am J Physiol Endocrinol Metab 2008; 294:E1127.
68. Wagner JC. Enhancement of athletic performance with drugs. An overview. Sports Med 1991;12:250.

69. Schmitt B, Fluck M, Decombaz J, et al. Transcriptional adaptations of lipid metabolism in tibialis anterior muscle of endurance-trained athletes. Physiol Genomics 2003;15:148.

70. Timmons JA, Jansson E, Fischer H, et al. Modulation of extracellular matrix genes reflects the magnitude of physiological adaptation to aerobic exercise training in humans. BMC Biol 2005;3:19.

71. Puntschart A, Claassen H, Jostarndt K, et al. mRNAs of enzymes involved in energy metabolism and mtDNA are increased in endurance-trained athletes. Am J Phys 1995;269:C619.

72. Saltin B, Henriksson J, Nygaard E, et al. Fiber types and metabolic potentials of skeletal muscles in sedentary man and endurance runners. Ann N Y Acad Sci 1977;301:3.

73. Messonnier L, Kristensen M, Juel C, et al. Importance of pH regulation and lactate/H+ transport capacity for work production during supramaximal exercise in humans. J Appl Phys 2007;102:1936.

74. Gonzalez-Freire M, Santiago C, Verde Z, et al. Unique among unique. Is it genetically determined? Br J Sports Med 2009;43:307.

75. Ahmetov I, Williams AG, Popov DV, et al. The combined impact of metabolic gene polymorphisms on elite endurance athlete status and related phenotypes. Hum Genet 2009 [Epub ahead of print].

76. Bray MS, Hagberg JM, Perusse L, et al. The human gene map for performance and health-related fitness phenotypes: the 2006–2007 update. Med Sci Sports Exerc 2009;41:35.

77. Scott RA, Fuku N, Onywera VO, et al. Mitochondrial haplogroups associated with elite Kenyan athlete status. Med Sci Sports Exerc 2009;41:123.

78. Longmore GD. Erythropoietin receptor mutations and Olympic glory. Nat Genet 1993;4:108.

The Human Genome and Sport, Including Epigenetics, Gene Doping, and Athleticogenomics

N.C. Craig Sharp, BVMS, PhD, DSc, FIBiol, FBASES, MRCVS

KEYWORDS
- Athleticogenomics • Epigenetics • Gene doping
- Genome sport

THE GENOME

Humans have 23 chromosomes containing approximately 3×10^9 bases and approximately 25,000 genes. Chimpanzees have 24 pairs of chromosomes, 13 of them identical to humans'. Currently, humans are thought to share 96% of chimp genes, and they may share 97% of gorilla genes. The human genome "library" consists of 23 chromosome "books," with a total of 25,000 gene "chapters," consisting of exon "pages," comprising codon three-letter "words," made up from the four nucleotide base "letters" of DNA. The synthesis of mRNA on DNA is termed, *transcription*, and the synthesis of a protein on RNA is termed, *translation*. Each cell contains approximately 15 cm of DNA, and the body total could stretch to the moon and back 8000 times. However, 97% of human DNA is "junk" (ie, only 3% of it codes for functional proteins or instructions). The remainder is more or less kept silent. For example, on chromosome 6, gene IGF2R has 7473 "meaningful" bases over a 98,000-base stretch, interrupted 48 times by introns. Introns equate to advertisements or junk mail; exons equate to useful information, for transcription into proteins or instructions and modifiers.

The 97% of the entire genome littered with junk, or selfish DNA, is present as pseudogenes, retropseudogenes, satellites, minisatellites, microsatellites, transposons (jumping genes), and retrotransposons—including several thousand complete human endogenous viral genomes, which make up 14% of the genome. A human endogenous viral genome example is LINE-1 (of up to 6000 codons), which in turn is parasitized by Alu sequences, 180 to 220 codons long (forming approximately 10% of the

Centre for Sports Medicine and Human Performance, Brunel University, Uxbridge, West London UB8 3PH, UK.
E-mail address: c.sharp90@btinternet.com

Endocrinol Metab Clin N Am 39 (2010) 201–215
doi:10.1016/j.ecl.2009.10.010
0889-8529/10/$ – see front matter © 2010 Elsevier Inc. All rights reserved.

endo.theclinics.com

genome), in turn containing hypervariable minisatellites approximately 20 codons long (whose discovery led to forensic genetic fingerprinting). So, some junk has an un-looked-for benefit.

Some introns seem helpful. Endogenous retroviruses have been acquired by the genome during evolution, and Dunlap and colleagues[1] observed that one of them in sheep, enJSRV, is essential for placental function. The investigators blocked its mRNA with antisense oligonucleotides, and the sheep embryos were unable to implant, suggesting the necessity of enJSRV to sheep. Also, there is evidence that other endogenous retroviruses may protect the host from infection by exogenous pathogenic retroviruses. So not all of the 97% of selfish DNA is simply parasitic.

EPIGENETICS

Epigenetics ("upon the gene'") relates to changes in gene function that are not due to changes in DNA sequence. It involves self-perpetuating gene-regulatory systems that are independent of DNA sequence alterations.[2] The term was defined by Riggs[3] and is the mechanism whereby chemical controls switch genes on or off, or turn them up or down, as a form of instruction manual to modulate genome function. Genetics may be described as the inheritance of information on the basis of gene sequence and epige-netics as the inheritance of information on the basis of gene expression. Probably a major function of the epigenome is to silence junk DNA. Leading gene mapper, Dr Stephen Beck, noted that the epigenome is "the way that every single exposure to the environment can leave its mark on the genome." Such environmental exposure could be the altered internal milieu of the muscle cell under the physiologic extremes of training, in terms of chemical interactions at the gene/epigene level. Differing susceptibilities to such chemical interactions could explain the better trainability of some competitors or the greater effectiveness of some training regimens.

Epigenetics also covers the effects on gene regulation of chromatin marks (modifi-cations to the DNA or its associated proteins), RNA interference (discussed later), and the higher-order structure of chromosomes. These changes are modulated, at least in part, by the action of histone chromosomal proteins. The epigenetic slate seems not necessarily to be wiped clean between generations—thus, external influences may moderate histones, possibly even causing structural changes, which may then be re-produced in progeny (ie, changes in the epigenome may be inherited). An example of such epigenetic inheritance is shown by agouti mice, which are obese and yellow-coated. When female agouti mice are fed vitamin B_{12}, folic acid, and choline during pregnancy, they produce litters that are brown-furred and thin compared with the fat yellow progeny of control mice. The extra nutrients silence the agouti gene by inducing the epigene to methylate it and switch it off.[2,4,5] Mutations were originally thought to be responsible for some of what are now known to be epigenetic changes.

Organisms have evolved mechanisms to influence the timing or genomic location of heritable variability (known as phenotypic plasticity). Pando and Verstrepan[6] have shown that what they call epigenetic switches increase the variability of specific phenotypes. Also, error-prone DNA replicases produce bursts of variability in times of stress. It seems that these mechanisms tune the variability of a given phenotype to match the variability of the acting selective pressure (ie, an aspect of the environ-ment: local, cellular, or otherwise). The genome is an intensely dynamic informational service, issuing and accepting instructions. Among other things, epigenetic plasticity suggests the possibility, although no sports examples have yet been published, that some influences of elite training and competition might be passed on to competitors' children. Although these observations tend toward Lamarckism (and even

Lysenkoism), they do not undermine Darwin's theory, but they do suggest that selection and variability are less independent than once thought. In 12 months over the years 2006 and 2007, 2500 articles and a new journal were devoted to epigenetics, and Nature in 2007 devoted an entire "Insight" to the topic.[7] Professor Marcus Pembrey of University College London said, in a 2005 BBC "Horizon" program, "Epigenetics links past, present and future, involving a paradigm shift in the way scientists are thinking about genetics and heredity."

GENDER TESTING

DAX is the critical female gene on the X chromosome. The SRY gene on the Y is the crucial male equivalent. DAX and SRY are antagonistic, and an SRY always dominates a DAX. But two DAXs defeat a single SRY. Some individuals are born XY but have two DAXs on their X, which makes them appear absolutely normal women, but they fail the former buccal smear test, because they have no Barr bodies, as they have only one X, and the Barr body is formed from the second, inactivated, X. Clinically, these cases form the androgen insensitivity syndrome. X-chromosome inactivation is a good example of an epigenetic change.[8] Turner's syndrome (XO) women also failed the genetic test; conversely, Klinefelter's syndrome (XXY) men passed it. However, the Barr body buccal smear test is no longer used in sport. While on the topic of gender, male sperm seem to have a potential problem in that the Y chromosome has only approximately 50 genes and is losing approximately five genes every 10^6 years. Hence, in 10^7 years, there may be no functional human Y chromosome.

APO AND SPORT

A family of genes, APO-A, -B, -C, and -E, is spread over various chromosomes. Chromosome 19 has the APO-E gene, whose protein effects the transition between very low-density lipoproteins and the triglyceride-accepting receptors. APO-E is polymorphic (ie, its variants E2, E3, and E4 differ in their effectiveness at manipulating triglycerides). APO-E3 is the "most effective" and also the most common; 80% of Europeans have one copy and 39% have two, but 7% have two copies of E4—the "least effective" (ie, it is associated with the highest risk of early heart disease). The further north in Europe, the more common is E4. Sweden and Finland have three times the frequency of E4 compared with Italy. So, is it the Mediterranean diet or Mediterranean genes that are responsible for a lower incidence of coronary heart disease? There is, of course, much more to coronary heart disease than simply APO genes, and these may also be relevant to sport,[9,10] which is why APO-E4 is discussed. Professional boxers with two E4 genes would seem to be at higher risk of early Alzheimer's disease, as a higher frequency of them (in whom E4 is unusually common) seems to manifest Alzheimer's or Parkinson's disease by age 50. Loosemore and coworkers,[11] in a robust meta-analysis, found no strong evidence to associate chronic traumatic brain injury with amateur boxing (four rounds of 2 minutes each with the outclassed rule to stop a match). It has also been suggested that this E4/E4 susceptibility might apply to other sports with head strike, including heading soccer balls. At the least, E4/E4 homozygotes should be made aware of their possible risk. (Woodpeckers, through their skull design, anatomically avoid much of the percussive shock of their high-velocity 10g force.)

GENETIC BASIS FOR CHRONIC FATIGUE SYNDROME (AND POSSIBLY UNEXPLAINED UNDERPERFORMANCE SYNDROME)

Workers on chronic fatigue syndrome (CFS), at St George's Hospital and Hammersmith Hospital, in London,[12,13] have noted differences in gene expression in approximately 35 genes, including the mitochondrial gene EIF4G1, which may be hijacked by some viruses, possibly leading to fatigue. Similar changes may help explain the fatiguing and debilitating Unexplained Underperformance Syndrome (UPS) in sport, often wrongly called the overtraining syndrome,[14] with the possible invaluable outcome of a serologic test. CFS is postulated as having a genetic basis, which suggests that UPS might share a similar type of causation. Hooper[13] has noted differences in gene expression in immune cells of CFS sufferers, which "could lead to a blood test, and even to therapeutic drugs." Kaushik and colleagues[14] at St George's Hospital, University of London, compared levels of gene expression of the leukocytes of 25 healthy subjects with 25 CFS patients (diagnosed with strict criteria). Differences were found in 35 of 9522 genes, analyzed using DNA chip technology. Due to the conflicting results of the few similar studies, they double-checked their own results using a more accurate real-time PCR, which confirmed that 15 of the genes were up to four times as active in CFS patients as in controls. The study has been scaled up on 1000 CFS patients and healthy controls, surveying many more gene products. To date, the larger study is confirming the earlier one. It is hoped that this work indicates that some aspects of CFS may be understood in molecular terms. The group has already discovered differences in blood proteins, presumably resulting from changes in gene expression, and they believe that the work might even lead to treatment, stating that, "a significant part of the pathogenesis (of CFS) resides in the leukocytes and in their activity. It will open the door to develop pharmacologic intervention."

Kaushik and colleagues[14] noted that several of the CFS genes identified play important roles in mitochondria, stating that, "the involvement of such genes seems to fit in with the fact that patients lack energy and suffer from fatigue." One of these mitochondrial gene products, EIF4G1, may be hijacked by some viruses, and cells may compensate by ramping up gene expression. Basant Puri, a CFS authority at the Hammersmith, notes, "The group's finding of upregulation of EIF4G1 is consistent with a subclinical persistent viral infection."[15] This fits in with the belief that CFS is sometimes triggered by viruses, such as Epstein-Barr, Q fever, enteroviruses, and parvovirum B19. Kaushik and colleagues have further noted that, "CFS often begins with a flu-like illness which seems never to go away." Of the other genes whose expression varies in CFS patients, some are involved in regulating the activity of the immune system. Immune turning-down could also account in part for the tendency to immunosuppression in CFS, and possibly similarly in UPS, patients. Of course, UPS is not CFS; nevertheless, similar etiologic mechanisms may be involved, and the importance of such work is that it might lead to a revelation of cause and, hence, of rational treatment, of the not uncommon UPS of fatigue, illness, and underperformance in sports competitors, especially those in aerobic endurance sport.

GENE THERAPY

Artificially synthesized genes may be introduced to a cell by direct DNA injection (especially to muscle and liver), by injecting cells in vitro with synthetic DNA, or parenterally or locally via a virus carrier, such as a retrovirus, an adeno-associated virus (AAV), or a liposome. Also, Lavitrano[16] has developed a vector that does not integrate with the host genome yet replicates independently—and when she added this nonviral episomal vector to pig sperm, which then fertilized ova, 12 out of 18 of the resulting fetuses carried the vectors in all tissues tested.

Retroviruses make DNA copies from RNA and insert them into a cell's genome. A gene therapist can delete a harmful gene and add the requisite correct gene or simply add the correct gene if the malfunctioning one was intrinsically harmless. This was first tried on humans in 1991 in a case of severe combined immunodeficiency (SCID), which has a single altered base in the ADA gene on chromosome 20. In this case, Culver and colleagues[17] removed lymphocyte stem cells from young Ashanti DeSilva, infected them with a retrovirus containing the correct synthesized ADA gene, and injected them back into her. Her lymphocyte count trebled, her antibody levels rose, and she made 25% the normal level of ADA protein (this treatment, however, ran into problems in other SCID patients, highlighting the uncertainty of gene therapy). Gene therapy has also shown success in hemophilia, in the use of the human vascular endothelial growth factor gene in peripheral vascular disease, and even, promisingly, in coronary heart disease.

Along similar lines, could there be gene therapy for Marfan syndrome? This gives a liability to aortic rupture—a cause of sudden death in sports that favor tall players, such as basketball and volleyball. It has a genetic basis on chromosome 15, which contains genes coding for height, joint mobility, and the elasticity/friability of skin and, critically, of the aorta. A mutation in the fibrillin-1 gene, which recapitulates the dominant negative mutation, produces the syndrome, especially in its vascular aspects.[18] Furthermore, genes encoding suitable growth factors could be of regenerative use in those sports injuries involving slower healing tissues, such as tendon, ligament, cartilage, and bone.

It is relatively easy to switch off genes but harder to turn their expression up. Kodadek[19] has synthesized a molecule, however, that can penetrate living cells and perform this increase. It is a peptoid, bound to a protein that activates gene expression and to a compound, ImPy7, that binds DNA. It has increased, by 300%, the expression of approximately 45 animal genes. In contrast, 2006 Nobel laureates Fire and Mello[20,21] discovered the gene-silencing mode of RNA interference, through observing that a strip of double-stranded sense and antisense RNA could silence the matching mRNA. Also, they noted that this double strand could cause copies of itself to be made, to spread between cells, and even to be inherited in progeny of organisms. This is an important way of controlling, for example, transposons. This is leading to high hopes that RNA interference may reduce the activity of genes that cause disease, but possibly on the sports side it may turn down genes, such as that coding for myostatin, thus increasing muscle growth, or such as ACTN3 to possibly increase aerobic endurance at the muscle cellular level.

GENE DOPING IMPLICATIONS FOR SPORT

Drug doping has markedly increased as an unfair malpractice in sport over the past 40 years,[22] and its newest manifestation promises to be gene doping, defined by the World Anti-Doping Agency (WADA) in 2004 as "the non-therapeutic use of genes, genetic elements and/or cells, which have the capacity to enhance athletic performance." A few possibilities are of such fitness genes are discussed.

ACE II

In 1998, Montgomery and colleagues[23] were the first to publish evidence of such a gene, their ACE fitness-gene. This is a 287 base-pair insertion ACE II allele, which gives lower ACE enzyme activity and enhanced endurance performance (possibly by diverting some ATP away from wasted heat generation and into energy production for generating muscle force). Another example is ACTN3,[24] a gene for speed (see Bray and colleagues' 2009 comprehensive gene map for a description of no fewer than 239 "fitness genes for performance and health-related fitness phenotypes,"[25] a map they regularly update).

Adeno-Associated Virus–insulin-like Growth Factor 1

Sweeney[26] has used an AAV, which infects muscle harmlessly, as a vector for a synthetic gene coding for insulin-like growth factor 1 (ILGF-1), which triggers replication of muscle satellite cells, which stimulates muscle hypertrophy. His group injected AAV–ILGF-1 into the muscle of one hind leg in rats, then strength-trained both legs. After 8 weeks, the experimental muscle showed nearly twice the strength gains of the control legs. Even treated but sedentary rats showed a 15% increase.

Myostatin

Myostatin is an inhibitor of muscle growth; tissues may need to be inhibited as well as stimulated (eg, at the conclusion of the healing process). Myostatin possibly acts by turning down sarcolemmal satellite cell function. A mutant, less active (ie, less inhibiting) myostatin is responsible for the highly exaggerated physique in Belgian Blue and Blonde d'Aquitaine beef cattle breeds.[27] In the racing whippet, a mutation in the MSTN gene involving the deletion of only two base pairs results in premature termination of mRNA, which translates a truncated, and less effective, form of myostatin, giving greater muscle mass and faster running speed in the heterozygous condition.[28] But whippets homozygous for the gene carry too much muscle and are actually slower.[28,29] In the mouse mdx-model of muscular dystrophy, blockading the activity of the normal inhibitory myostatin, by means of a specific monoclonal antibody, has also been shown to increase muscle size and force and power, again possibly by disinhibiting satellite cells. Experiments on mice, genetically engineered as Schwarzenegger mice to produce less effective myostatin, have shown that diminishing this antigrowth factor induces hypertrophy and, unusually, muscle hyperplasia, again possibly through stimulating satellite cell function. Just as in the cases of the two excessively muscled cattle breeds and the whippet, so there are possible human mutations with regard to myostatin and its receptor. A 3-year-old Michigan boy gained wide media publicity in 2009 due to, among other things, a variety of simple strength tests (including sit up, pull up, and grip measures), which indicated that he was equivalent to the upper percentiles of 6-year-olds in some tests and the lower percentiles of 7-year-olds in one test. His grip strength was 300% greater than that of a peer group of larger children. Nevertheless, he had fairly normal myostatin levels and the assumption is that a mutation may lie in his myostatin receptors being less effective (the opposite of the more effective natural erythropoietin (EPO) receptor mutation of the Maentyranta family [discussed later]). An equivalent hyperstrength case was described in another young boy, but it was due to a defective gene for mysostatin rather than a receptor error.[30] Some bodybuilders obtain myostatin inhibitors over the Internet, but that is simple doping, not gene doping. In a different context, the syrinx vocal organ of the ringdove contains superfast muscles[31] and one wonders if its code and accessories might be adapted for use in some future human sprinters?

Erythropoietin Receptor Gene

The 1960 and 1964 Nordic-skiing triple-Olympic champion, Eero Maentyranta, and his family members were shown (more than 30 years after his wins and after technical advances) to possess a favorably mutated EPO receptor gene,[26,32,33] which increased their hemoglobin to a family mean of 204 g/L^{-1} (183–231 g/L^{-1}) compared with unaffected members' 154 g/L^{-1} (136–174 g/L^{-1})—a significant increase in oxygen transport in debatably the most aerobic of all sports.

Regarding the gene for EPO itself, in mice and primates, the hematocrit has been shown to rise, from 50% and 40%, respectively, to approximately 70%, for 4 and 6 months, after a single injection of an EPO gene. In 2006, *The Times* (London) correspondent, Owen Slot,[34] suggested that the first stage in the gene doping battle had started, with the emergence of Repoxygen EPO gene, manufactured in 2002 on a trial basis by the company, Oxford BioMedica (Oxford, United Kingdom). Slot quoted a variety of comments: Michelle Vertoken (UK Sport's director of ethics and antidoping) was quick to condemn it. Dick Pound (chair of WADA), stated, "You would have to be blind not to see that the next generation of doping will be genetic." Professor Werner Franke (the German cell biologist largely responsible for exposing those behind the drug regimens of the former German Democratic Republic) attested, "This is the crossing of the Rubicon, a real advance in criminality." In his extensive article, Slot went on to note that gene doping, "the apocalyptic future of illegal performance enhancement," had already started in Germany, as evidenced by a court case there in Magdeburg, which identified the distribution among coaches of Repoxygen. The trial was of Thomas Springstein, coach and partner of Grit Breuer, twice European 400-m champion, who was banned for doping. A police house raid removed Springstein's laptop, containing an e-mail exchange with a Dutch speed-skating club, including a discussion of Repoxygen. In originally announcing the breakthrough product in June 2002, an Oxford BioMedica spokesman explained that Repoxygen, which had been developed primarily to treat serious anemia, involved switching on a gene in response to hypoxemia and then, when that had been normalized, it acted to "switch the gene off; providing an exquisite control mechanism for the production of EPO in situ." After developing the Repoxygen prototype, Oxford BioMedica did not put it into production as they judged it to be commercially nonviable, due to the easy availability of EPO itself. Larry Bowers, managing director of the US Anti-Doping Agency, said, after a meeting about anti-doping strategy in Atlanta in October 2002, that they saw Repoxygen as a significant threat but added that they were attempting to pioneer a test for such gene doping. Professor Alan Kingsman, Oxford Biomedica's chief executive, said that they did not develop it beyond testing in mice, "so it simply remains in the frig. And we maintain very close controls, so I'd be extremely surprised if anything we made got onto the black market." But, other laboratories may have reproduced it from information gathered from Oxford BioMedica's launch. Slot ended his article by quoting Kingsman as saying, "to make it would be very irresponsible for a number of reasons. To use it in the human body would be playing with fire."

The new generation of EPO itself is continuous erythropoiesis activator (CEA), but this is current doping practice, in which genetic manipulation is not involved.

Vascular Endothelial Growth Factor

A virus-activated vascular endothelial growth factor gene has been used in elderly human patients and shown to improve their lower limb vascular supply, by stimulating angiogenesis.[35] As increased levels of muscle microcirculation are a vital response to appropriate aerobic fitness training, vascular endothelial growth factor could conceivably have a beneficial sports physiologic function.

Signal Transduction Pathways

Signal pathways are responsible for increasing or lowering gene function, for example, those controlling fast and slow muscle function,[36] and could be subject to extraneous modification. It seems likely that the expression of the muscle myosin heavy chain

(MHC) isoform genes is controlled by unusual regulatory mechanisms. It was discovered that the slow and intermediate/fast MHC isoforms occur as clusters in two locations on the genome.[36] The slow MHC-I cluster can be found on human chromosome 14, where the MHC-I and cardiac muscle genes lie close together. But the intermediate/fast MHC cluster is on chromosome 17, which also contains the MHC IIa, the MHC IIb, and the MHC IIx genes plus the very fast extraocular MHC and the developmental MHC isoforms (MHC embryonal and MHC perinatal). It seems likely that the organization of functionally related MHC genes in two clusters is linked to their regulation. In contrast, most coregulated genes, such as those for glycolytic or mitochondrial enzyme pathways, are found in locations all over the genome. Weiss notes, "These observations suggest that aerobic exercise activates many signal transduction pathways which up-regulate slow genes and down-regulate fast genes by several different mechanisms."[36] Observations such as these may eventually lead to future training being put onto a sounder theoretic basis, exactly as the growing discipline of sport and exercise molecular physiology predicts, and not just to gene doping.

RISKS IN GENE THERAPY AND GENE DOPING

There are major current risks in gene therapy and potential gene doping, and three brief but serious examples are

1. Cancers: 2 of 13 patients in the SCID work (discussed previously) developed neoplasms, possibly through uncovered oncogenes or by unknowingly transmitted oncoviruses.
2. Severe autoimmune reaction to the product: this has happened with some EPO gene insertions in primates who, ironically, subsequently developed severe anemia, as their own indigenous EPO was also compromised.
3. Reaction to the carrier virus: for example, an 18-year-old man died of a reaction to the carrier virus of a gene to repair an inborn error of metabolism involving ornithene transcarbamylase. Due to its apparent inactivity, the dose of the AAV vector was increased at log intervals, but the Kupffer's cells then seem to have been overwhelmed and to have unleashed an "overwhelming cytokine firestorm, precipitating disseminated vascular coagulation leading to multiple organ failure and the adult respiratory distress syndrome" (E.B. Wheeldon, BVMS, PhD, FRCPath, personal communication, 2008).

A major worry regarding gene doping is that unscrupulous medicoscientific sports personnel may likely bypass the normal stringent safety tests for such procedures and expose competitors to immense risks, especially regarding the possible formation of replication-competent new viruses or other contamination, the prevention of which generates many of the high costs of the controlled laboratories. There is also the worrying possibility of shed virus vectors as a risk of infecting others. In the SCID work (discussed previously), the ethics are equivocal regarding the administration of a basically experimental treatment to patients who otherwise are facing a high risk of death; to administer an unproved technique to an extremely fit and healthy sports competitor who has no medical need of it whatever, however, is utterly beyond any ethical pale, apart from it being an antidoping infringement.

GENE DOPING TIME SCALE

A "substance linked to gene doping" was detected at the 2006 Winter Olympic Games, but there seem to have been no similar reports from the 2008 Summer

Olympic Games. WADA head Dick Pound said in late 2007 that he could see gene doping occurring "in six or seven years"; Oxford BioMedica's breakthrough product, Repoxygen, has been discussed previously.

Nevertheless, apart from its risks, gene transcription (natural or artificial) is far more complicated than it might seem, which will add to the time scale. For example, in all eukaryotic cells, transcription of every protein-coding gene begins with the assembly of a RNA–polymerase II preinitiation complex on the promoters (which modulate the protein expression). Then the promoters, in conjunction with a battery of enhancers, silencers, and insulators, define the combinatorial codes that specify the gene expression patterns, and there is as yet a marked lack of information about the promoters for most human genes.[37] Thus, it is not simply a matter of seamlessly splicing in a new gene—because a veritable web of checks and balances, reacting between the DNA, the epigene, the RNA, and the cytosol environment, all have to be activated or inactivated, expressed, and coordinated. This apparent axiom is stated merely to counter any belief that inserting a functional gene into a cell, for therapeutic or doping purposes, is in any way a straightforward, simple, easy, or robust process to actually perform, quite apart from safety aspects.

THE NONLEGAL FUTURE—GENE DOPING POSSIBILITIES

In spite of the cautions discussed previously, gene doping and the possibilities of epigene doping, are major potential problems in sport.

1. Future work of great promise for therapy (and of great worry for sport) may lie in the manipulation of transcription factors. For example, one possibility might be to activate the already existing but silent human gene for a faster variant of human fast myosin.
2. Possibly loaded retroviruses or stem cell methodology may be used to target a wide variety of tissues, such as bone marrow for erythrocytes; liver and kidney for Cori-cycle lactate-removing kinetics; myocardium for increased cardiac output; and skeletal muscle to influence fiber-type quality and percentage, sarcomere structure, creatine-phosphate level, mitochondrial number, glycolytic enzyme and chemiosmotic pathway kinetics, levels of myoglobin and intracellular dipeptide buffers, and muscle capillary numbers. The energy-storing viscoelastic effects of tendon and ligament may be increased through new variants of collagen and elastin. Alexander has shown that approximately 35% of the energy of the human stride, at distance-running speeds, is stored and released in the Achilles tendon and approximately 17% in the ligaments of the arches of the foot[38]; improvements here could increase the vital factor of running economy.
3. Even appropriate neurologic areas may be targeted (eg, the naturally occurring SCN9A channelopathy causes a congenital inability to feel pain).[39] Artificially induced, this could be a useful factor in sport. The SCN9A gene is located on chromosome 2 and relates to a sodium channel subunit that is strongly expressed in nociceptive neurons. Some athletes may naturally have reduced function in such encoded channels, giving a higher pain tolerance. (Such channels would be excellent targets for analgesics.) In 2005, the BBC reported on a young boy, Ben Whittaker, with just such a markedly diminished pain perception.[40] There is also the possibility that genes encoding for the analgesic peptides, endorphins, and enkephalins could be administered, also to increase pain tolerance. Of course, in endurance sport, such pain diminishment could interfere with Noakes and coworkers' proposed "central fatigue governor"[41] with serious antihomeostatic

consequences, although the governor might self-adapt to cater for such contingencies.

4. There is a potential for improving muscle glycogen storage via glycogen synthase overexpression, possibly useful in endurance sport.

5. There are mice transgenic variants, PEPCK and PGC-1α, which improve type I fiber percentages and metabolism and which stimulate myocardial growth (PI3K mice) (Henning Wackerhage, BSc, PhD, personal communication, Aberdeen University, 2009). Along these lines, Martin Evans from Cardiff, together with Americans Mario Capecchi and Oliver Smithies, were awarded the 2007 Nobel Prize in Physiology or Medicine for their discoveries of "Principles for introducing specific gene modifications in mice by the use of embryonic stem cells."

6. Ideas from work (discussed previously) led Wackerhage to construct a list featuring a supposed genetic supermouse, having noted that many transgenic mice with an improved exercise-related phenotype have been generated. He has listed murine fitness gene examples (**Box 1**) (note that turn-up in this list indicates adding a more effective gene or increasing its function, whereas turn-down indicates the opposite).

Box 1
Dr Henning Wakerhage's vision of a preliminary aggregation of fitness genes for a possible transgenic athletic supermouse

Higher hematocrit

    EPO turn-up

Myocardial hypertrophy

    MEK1, P13K turn-up

Fiber type

    Calcineurin turn-up

    Ras and MAPK turn-up

    PGC-1α turn-up

    PPAR-γ turn-up

    ACTN3 turn-down

Mitochondrial biogenesis

    PGC-1α turn-up

    PPAR-γ turn-up

Raised muscle glycogen

    Glycogen synthase turn-up

Endurance running

    PEC-C^{mus} turn-up

    PPAR-γ turn-up

Muscle hypertrophy

    Myostatin turn-down

    Insulin-like growth factor 1 turn-up

    PKB turn-up

Longer legs

    Growth hormone turn-up

DETECTION

The International Olympic Committee (IOC) introduced the phrase, gene doping, into its list of prohibited substances and techniques in 2003, and WADA's list followed suit. As the dope gene is in situ, its product is natural to the individual and consequently poses particular challenges to detection. Peter Schjerling of the Copenhagen Muscle Research Center has indicated that gene doping could be nearly impossible to detect, noting that such cell signals or products would probably be indistinguishable from the indigenous equivalents and may not even enter the blood. At present, proteomics is the most promising detection method, permitting, as it does, the screening of hundreds of proteins simultaneously, but the tester has to know which protein markers to look for, which is a difficult challenge. In addition, this would require biopsy sampling, which could be a major barrier. Until then, the way forward is probably through competitors' passports, containing records of main physiologic protein parameters, to be viewed regularly for notable alterations. Such passports have already been proposed regarding hemoglobin parameters and EPO and continuous erythropoiesis activator. It might also be possible to map a gene signature for competitors, then to regularly to screen them for deviations. What could be one of the most telling factors is that DNA, especially in laboratory storage conditions, is stable for amply long enough to enable science to catch up for retrospective detection, and this should be publicized. WADA gave a grant of $325,000 (£171,000; €200,000) to help create a prototype test to differentiate between natural hormones and those created via gene doping. The IOC has increased its testing budget by £2.1 m ($4 m; €2.47 m), half of which is earmarked for those laboratories developing a gene doping test. For the 2012 Summer Olympic Games, a higher percentage than ever of competitors will be tested at doping controls, with blood tests probably mandatory in all sports.

In a possible paradox, or conflict of sports interest, the Genetic Information Non-Discrimination Act has been introduced recently in the United States to stop possible discrimination on the basis of DNA genomic analysis revelations of ill-health genes (in the areas of life assurance and of employment contracts, to give two examples). It would be highly ironic if the Act might be invoked to defend exposed gene doped athletes against sanction by WADA or other sports agencies.

THE LEGITIMATE FUTURE—ATHLETICOGENOMICS

Athleticogenomics is a neologism coined by the author[42–44] to describe a probable new, but presumably wholly legitimate, sports development of the future. Athleticogenomics is not gene doping, but it would involve the integration of selected physiologic performance parameters with genome dataset information, and it is not only the encoded protein itself but also its rate of transcription and translation that is important; hence, such aspects of gene expression profiling may come to be of legitimate use to sports competitors. Transcription and translation rates may be particularly important regarding trainability. Trainability relates to the fact that phenotypically similar competitors (eg, rowers in an eight) may react at different rates and intensities to the same training stimulus, thus some are said to be more trainable than others—a much prized quality. Just as the science of pharmacogenomics may usefully elicit the beneficial or adverse interaction of a patient's genome with selected drugs, so an equivalent science of athleticogenomics (and athleticoproteomics) could help coaches to optimize training specifically. In 2009, Collins and colleagues[45] demonstrated that exercise improved cognitive responses in mice through enhancement of epigenetic mechanisms in neurons in the dentate gyrus. They tracked these down to the histone modifications, histone-H3-phophoacetylation and c-Fos induction of the appropriate genes in the neurons (ie, they saw epigenetic changes related to gene transcription). The point is that one could match training regimens with specific epigenetic changes, presumably mainly in muscle (not brain) in terms of accessing tissue samples by biopsy. This is not, of course, gene doping—it is more gene profiling and data utilization, and it also has potentially wide applications in talent identification, which would certainly include trainability identification.

Polymorphism chips are utilized in targeted genome analysis. Such gene-array microchips may hold more than 25,000 DNA probes and can investigate the activity of large numbers of selected genes. The widest use of this technique is currently in pharmacogenomics. In sports competitors, after an appropriate genome analysis, a specific training schedule could be designed and monitored, which would form the ultimate in personalized coaching—a type of laboratory fitness testing of the genome, paralleling the physiologic fitness testing of the body.

"The computational analyses of the completely sequenced genomes of many organisms are driving research and guiding experiments. A new generation of tools such as micro-arrays, advanced imaging systems and single-molecule techniques are fundamentally changing experimental protocols."—so wrote Nobel laureates Sydney Brenner and Richard Roberts in a letter to *Nature* in 2007.[46] A new generation of DNA sequencing machines is massively broadening horizons. Various groups have recently performed epigenetic studies, which were impractical with the old technologies. A recent approach[47] "fishes out all the DNA associated with a given marker, such as one of the histone proteins used to package genes in chromosomes (and which control which regions of DNA can be read)." The key to this is the new technology. Already in Australia, Professor Deon Venter, via the company Genetic Technologies, is reported to be offering, for A\$110, DNA tests on children for fiber assessment, regarding the ACTN3 R577R gene for type 11[24] and the R577X variant for type 1 fibers.[48] Gene ACTN3 codes for alpha-actinin-3, which produces a stronger Z-disc in the sarcomere of type II (fast) fibers, enabling them to withstand their higher power generation. Type 1 (slow) fibers tend to be homozygous for a premature stop codon polymorphism in gene ACTN3, termed R577X.[49,50]

Athleticogenomics, as defined previously, may be anticipating too far ahead, although it could be seen as an extension of a physiologic performance-testing laboratory and of a molecular physiology laboratory. It would not seem to be risk associated, however, nor, crucially, is it illegal. Ethically, however, it is beyond the altitude tent or the superswimming costume. As yet, the discipline barely exists; however, it certainly will proliferate, unless it is specifically barred in some way.

SUMMARY

The possibilities for gene therapy are excitingly promising, but the possibilities for gene doping are worryingly impending. Both are fraught with risks and with difficulties, far more so doping than therapy, as the latter will tackle specifically defined genetic errors with highly controlled methodology, especially in terms of safety. At present, a major worry of WADA and the IOC is the suspected difficulty in detection, but unsuspected advances in this area may well occur. As in other forms of doping in sport, the motives behind banning gene doping are to prevent the genuinely serious health risks and to reduce unfair competitive advantage.

FURTHER READING

Still probably the best quick entry to the whole general area is Matt Ridley's excellent book, *The Genome*.[51] Many parts of this article (too diffuse to be referenced specifically) were inspired or informed by Ridley. For an account of epigenetics, *Nature* devoted an entire "Insight" feature to seven excellent reviews of the topic.[7] Spurway and Wackerhage[52] have provided a highly authoritative bridge between genetics and sport, whereas McArthur and North have written on specific genes and sport.[53]

The Dutch were quick to note the threat of gene doping, and in 2004 devoted an issue of the annual publication of the Netherlands Centre for Doping Affairs to gene doping, authored primarily by Hidde Haisma, Professor of Therapeutic Gene Modulation at the University of Groningen, which forms a highly recommended concise introduction to the field, as does an equally quick off-the-mark publication from Scotland, Miah's deeply thoughtful book of gene doping moral philosophy,[54] with a first-rate complementary volume by Tamburrini and Tannsjo.[55] The British Association of Sport and Exercise Sciences has a lucidly thoughtful position statement on gene doping in press.[56]

ACKNOWLEDGMENTS

The author's abiding interest in the genetic code and the genome was triggered by James Watson himself, who inspirationally lectured to him in a postgraduate, cell biology, small-group short-course in Glasgow, run by Dr John Paul, circa 1959, at a time when the disciplines of cell and molecular biology were just emerging. Nobel laureate Sir James W. Black and Professor William F.H. Jarrett, FRS, guided his departmental physiopathologic interests, and Professors Sir James Armour and John G.V.A. Durnin later helped him into sports science.

REFERENCES

1. Dunlap KA, Palmarini M, Vareia M, et al. Endogeneous retrovirus regulates peri-implantation, placental growth and differentiation. Proc Natl Acad Sci 2006; 103(39):14390–5.
2. Waterland RA, Jirtle RL. Transposable elements: targets for early nutritional effects on epigenetic gene regulation. Mol Cell Biol 2003;23(15):5293–300.
3. Riggs AD, Porter TN. In: Russo VEA, Martienssen RA, Riggs AD, editors. Epigenetics: mechanism of gene regulation. Woodbury (NY): Cold Spring Harbor Laboratory Press; 1996. p. 34–53.
4. Doliny DC, Weidman JR, Waterland RA, et al. Maternal genisten alters coat colour and protects Avy mouse offspring from obesity by modifying the fetal epigenome. Environ Health Perspect 2006;114(4):567–72.
5. Waterland RA, Travisano M, Tahiliani KG. Diet-induced hypermethylation at agouti viable yellow is not inherited transgenerationally through the female. FASEB J 2007;21:3380–5.
6. Pando OJ, Verstrepan KJ. Epigenetic switches. Cell 2007;128(4):655–68.
7. Ecclestone A, DeWitt N, Gunter C, et al. Epigenetics; nature insight. Nature 2007; 447:395–440.
8. Lyon M. How X-chromosome inactivation was discovered. Biologist 2007;54(2):94–7.
9. Jordan BD. Chronic traumatic brain injury associated with boxing. Semin Neurol 2000;20(2):179–85.
10. Jordan BD, Relkin NR, Ravdin LD. Apolipoprotein E4 associated with chronic traumatic brain injury in boxing. JAMA 1997;278(2):136–40.

11. Loosemore M, Knowles CH, Whyte GP. Amateur boxing and risk of chronic traumatic brain injury: systematic review of observational studies. BMJ 2007;335: 809–19.
12. Budgett R, Newsholme EA, Sharp NCC, et al. Redefining the overtraining syndrome as the unexplained underperformance syndrome. Br J Sports Med 2000;34:67–8.
13. Hooper R. Chronic fatigue syndrome. New Sci 2005;187(2509):9–11.
14. Kaushik N, Fear D, Richards SC, et al. Gene expression in peripheral blood mononuclear cells from patients with chronic fatigue syndrome. J Clin Pathol 2005;58:826–32.
15. Puri BK. Long chain fatty acids and the pathophysiology of myalgic encephalomyelitis (chronic fatigue syndrome). J Clin Pathol 2007;60:122–4.
16. Lavitrano M. Pig lets vector stay. Proc Natl Acad Sci 2006;103:17672–7.
17. Culver K, Anderson F, Blaese R. Lymphocyte gene therapy. Hum Gene Ther 1991;2:107–9.
18. Nakamura T. Marfan's syndrome: a mutation in the fibrillin-1 gene. Nature 2002; 415:168–71.
19. Kodadek T. Turning up genes. 'Research highlights'. Nature 2007;446:472.
20. Wagner R, Sun L. Functional genomics: double-stranded RNA poses puzzle. Nature 1990;391:744–5 (Fire and Gallo ref).
21. Abbott A. Youthful duo snag a swift Nobel for RNA control of genes. Nature 2006; 433:488.
22. Sharp NCC. Drugs wipe out a sporting chance. Nature 1999;398:675.
23. Montgomery HE, Marshall R, Rayson M, et al. Human gene for physical performance. Nature 1998;393:221–2.
24. Yang N, MacArthur DG, Hahn AG, et al. ACTN3 genotype is associated with human elite athletic performance. Am J Hum Genet 2003;73(3):627–31.
25. Bray MS, Hagberry JM, Rankinen T, et al. The human gene map for performance and health related fitness phenotypes: the 2006–2007 update. Med Sci Sports Exerc 2009;41(1):35–73.
26. Sweeney HL. Gene doping. Sci Am 2004;291:36–43.
27. Sharp NCC. Doping, a misuse of science. Phys Soc Physiology News 2004;57: 15–6.
28. Shadan S. Run, whippet, run. MSTN gene and racing performance. Nature 2007; 447:275.
29. Mosher D, Quignon P, Sutter NB, et al. A mutation in the myostatin gene increases muscle mass and enhances racing performance in heterozygote dogs. PLoS Genet 2007;3(5):e79. Available at: Genetics.plosjournals.org.
30. Shuelke M, Wagner KR, Stolz LE, et al. Myostatin mutation associated with gross muscle hypertrophy in a child. N Engl J Med 2004;350(26):2682–8.
31. Elemans CPH, Spiers ILY, Muller UK, et al. Superfast muscles control dove's trill. Nature 2004;431:146.
32. de la Chapelle A, Traskelin A-L, Juvonen E. Truncated erythropoietin receptor causes dominantly inherited benign human erythrocytosis. Proc Natl Acad Sci 1993;90:4495–9.
33. de la Chapelle A, Sistonen P, Lehvaslaiho H, et al. Familial erythrocytosis genetically linked to erythropoietin receptor gene. Lancet 1993;341:82–4.
34. Slot O. Raising the bar in the cheating stakes. London: The Times; 2006.
35. Baumgartner I, Pieczek A, Manor O. Constitutive expression of phVEGF165 after intramuscular gene transfer promotes collateral vessel development on patients with critical limb ischemia. Circulation 1998;97:1114–23.

36. Weiss A, McDonough D, Wertman B, et al. Organization of human and mouse skeletal myosin heavy chain gene clusters is highly conserved. Proc Natl Acad Sci 1999;96:2958–63.
37. Kim TH, Barerra LO, Zheng M. A high-resolution map of active promoters in the human genome. Nature 2005;436:876–8.
38. Alexander RMcNeill. The human machine. London: Natural History Museum; 1992. p. 74–9.
39. Cox JC, Reimann F, Nicholas AK, et al. An SCN9A channelopathy causes congenital inability to experience pain. Nature 2006;444:9–11.
40. BBC. Available at: http://news.bbc.co.uk/1/hi/health/4195437.stm. Accessed March 2009.
41. Noakes TD, St. Clair GA, Lambert EV. From catastrophe to complexity: a novel model of integrative central neural regulation of effort and fatigue during exercise in humans. Br J Sports Med 2004;38:511–4.
42. Sharp NCC. The human genome and sport including epigenetics and athletico-genomics. J Sports Sci 2008;26(11):1127–33.
43. Sharp NCC. Introduction. In: Pitsiladis Y, Bale J, Sharp NCC, et al, editors. East African running: towards a cross-disciplinary perspective. Abingdon (UK): Routledge; 2007. p. 1–7.
44. Sharp NCC. Athleticogenomics. Peak Performance 2006;230:8–11.
45. Collins A, Hill LE, Reul M, et al. Exercise improves cognitive responses to psychological stress through enhancement of epigenetic mechanisms and gene expression in the dentate gyrus. PLoS One 2009;4(1):e4330.
46. Brenner S, Roberts R. Genome sequencing. Nature 2007;446:275.
47. Check E. Sequencing revolution ushers in new era. Nature 2007;448:9–11.
48. Parisotto R. It's in the genes. Blood sports; the inside dope on drugs in sport. Victoria (Australia): Hardie Grant Books; 2006. p. 207–22.
49. MacArthur DG, North KN. A gene for speed? The evolution and function of alpha-actinin-3. Bioessays 2004;26(7):786–95.
50. Santiago C, Gonzalez-Freire M, Serratosa L, et al. ACTN3 genotype in professional soccer players. Br J Sports Med 2008;42:71–3.
51. Ridley M. The genome. London: 4th Estate; 2000.
52. Spurway N. Top-down studies of the genetic contribution to the differences in physical capacity. In: Spurway N, Wackerhage H, editors. Introduction to molecular exercise physiology; genetics and molecular biology of muscle adaptation. Edinburgh (UK): Churchill Livingstone; 2006. p. 61–120 and 121–64.
53. MacArthur DG, North KN. Genes and human elite performance. In: Pitsiladis Y, Bale J, Sharp NCC, et al, editors. East African running: towards a cross-disciplinary perspective. Abingdon (Oxon): Routledge; 2007. p. 217–33.
54. Miah A. Genetically modified athletes: biomedical ethics, gene doping and sport. Abingdon (Oxon), and New York: Routledge; 2004.
55. Tamburrine C, Tannsjo T. Genetic technology and sport: ethical questions. Abingdon (Oxon), and New York: Routledge; 2005.
56. Wackerhage H, Miah A, Montgomery HE, et al. Genetic research and testing in sport and exercise science: a review of the issues. J Sport Sci 2009;27(11):1109–16.

Index

Note: Page numbers of article titles are in **boldface** type.

A

Endocrinol Metab Clin N Am 39 (2010) 217–241
doi:10.1016/S0889-8529(09)00123-6
0889-8529/10/$ – see front matter © 2010 Elsevier Inc. All rights reserved.

endo.theclinics.com

Moving?

Make sure your subscription moves with you!

To notify us of your new address, find your **Clinics Account Number** (located on your mailing label above your name), and contact customer service at:

Email: journalscustomerservice-usa@elsevier.com

800-654-2452 (subscribers in the U.S. & Canada)
314-447-8871 (subscribers outside of the U.S. & Canada)

Fax number: 314-447-8029

Elsevier Health Sciences Division
Subscription Customer Service
3251 Riverport Lane
Maryland Heights, MO 63043

*To ensure uninterrupted delivery of your subscription, please notify us at least 4 weeks in advance of move.

Printed and bound by CPI Group (UK) Ltd, Croydon, CR0 4YY

03/10/2024

01040452-0009